Neuropsychiatry
An introductory approach

Advances in the basic and clinical neurosciences have dramatically changed our knowledge of the neurobiological basis of cognition, emotion and behavior, with corresponding changes in the understanding and treatment of mental illness. This practical introductory guide to neuropsychiatry provides a starting point for anyone interested in brain–behavior relationships and the treatment of neuropsychiatric problems.

In part I, the authors introduce a neuropsychiatric approach to understanding basic and complex cognition, emotion, personality and psychological adaptation. Part II describes the fundamental methods of neuropsychiatry, including an outline of the neuropsychiatric evaluation and the mental status examination. The contribution of electrophysiology and medical imaging is also discussed. Part III reviews a range of topics in clinical neuropsychiatry, illustrating the practical application of concepts and methods previously discussed. From here, readers will be able to extend the approach to the management of neuropsychiatric disorders seen in clinical settings.

For students, residents, allied health clinicians and psychiatrists this is an invaluable introduction to the neurobiology, neuroanatomy neurophysiology, evaluation and treatment methods of clinical neuropsychiatry.

David B. Arciniegas is Research Associate and Staff Physician, Denver Veterans Affairs Medical Center, Director of the Neuropsychiatry Service and Assistant Professor of Psychiatry and Neurology at University of Colorado School of Medicine.

Thomas P. Beresford is Director, Laboratory for Clinical Studies in Psychiatry and Director, Clinical research Training in Alcoholism and Substance Abuse, Denver Veterans Affairs Medical Center, and Professor of Psychiatry at University of Colorado School of Medicine.

Neuropsychiatry

An introductory approach

David B. Arciniegas

and

Thomas P. Beresford
University of Colorado School of Medicine

Foreword by

Thomas W. McAllister

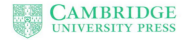

CAMBRIDGE
UNIVERSITY PRESS

PUBLISHED BY THE PRESS SYNDICATE OF THE UNIVERSITY OF CAMBRIDGE
The Pitt Building, Trumpington Street, Cambridge, United Kingdom

CAMBRIDGE UNIVERSITY PRESS
The Edinburgh Building, Cambridge CB2 2RU, UK
40 West 20th Street, New York, NY 10011-4211, USA
10 Stamford Road, Oakleigh, VIC 3166, Australia
Ruiz de Alarcón 13, 28014 Madrid, Spain
Dock House, The Waterfront, Cape Town 8001, South Africa

http://www.cambridge.org

First published 2001

Printed in the United Kingdom at the University Press, Cambridge

Typeface 11/14pt Minion   *System* QuarkXPress™   [SE]

A catalogue record for this book is available from the British Library

Library of Congress Cataloguing in Publication data

Arciniegas, David B. (David Brian), 1967–
Neuropsychiatry : an introductory approach / David B. Arciniegas and Thomas P. Beresford.
p. ; cm.
Includes bibliographical references and index.
ISBN 0 521 64311 2 – ISBN 0 521 64431 3 (pbk.)
1. Neuropsychiatry. I. Beresford, Thomas P. II. Title.
[DNLM: 1. Neuropsychology – methods. 2. Nervous System Diseases – therapy. WM
220 A674i 2001]
RC341 .A735 2001
616.8–dc21   00-066724

ISBN 0 521 64311 2 hardback
ISBN 0 521 64431 3 paperback

Every effort has been made in preparing this book to provide accurate and up-to-date information which is in
accord with accepted standards and practice at the time of publication. Nevertheless, the authors, editors and
publisher can make no warranties that the information contained herein is totally free from error, not least
because clinical standards are constantly changing through research and regulation. The authors, editors and
publisher therefore disclaim all liability for direct or consequential damages resulting from the use of material
contained in this book. Readers are strongly advised to pay careful attention to information provided by the
manufacturer of any drugs or equipment that they plan to use.

Everything should be made as simple as possible, but not simpler.

Albert Einstein, *Autobiographical notes*

Contents

Part I   Fundamental concepts in neuropsychiatry

Part II   A neuropsychiatric approach to evaluating the patient

Part III Applying the approach to neuropsychiatric disorders

Illustrations

Tables

Foreword

Having taught and practiced neuropsychiatry for 20 years, I am aware of the challenge to provide medical students, residents, allied health clinicians, and other colleagues with information about brain–behavior relationships that is interesting, easy to read, and relevant, yet not reductionistic, simplistic, and thus ultimately unhelpful. Like others, I have also struggled to keep up with the explosion of neuroscience knowledge, and to translate and apply this knowledge to clinical care. Neuropsychiatric reference materials presently available are often too big, too detailed, and digress into clinically irrelevant material, or are better classified as standard issue biological psychiatry, not neuropsychiatry. Reading them can be a daunting task, especially for the novice to the field.

Having attempted to fill this void myself with lectures and talks on various topics to psychiatric residents, medical students, and various groups of allied health clinicians in a piecemeal way over the years, I am aware of the daunting challenge that the authors faced in attempting their work. In fact, I confess to being just a little skeptical that they would succeed in following the goal of keeping it simple yet meaningful. Thus it was with great pleasure that I read each successive chapter. In my view the authors have consistently achieved their goal, whether outlining the historical context in which to place modern neuropsychiatry, distilling the critical elements of the neuropsychiatric evaluation, or defining the knowledge base needed to understand and treat the neuropsychiatric aspects of Parkinson's disease, traumatic brain injury and other disorders. In my view they have admirably struck the balance between supplying the basic and clinical science base needed to evaluate and treat patients competently, while not becoming bogged down in interesting but clinically irrelevant material.

I intend to use this text as the reference for our neuropsychiatry curriculum for medical students, residents, and others getting interested in the field. It is the ideal platform or foundation on which to grow a sophisticated knowledge of clinical neuroscience. I congratulate and applaud the authors for an outstanding contribution to both teachers and students of neuro-psychiatry.

Thomas W. McAllister, M.D.
Director, Neuropsychiatry Service
Professor of Psychiatry, Dartmouth Medical School

Preface

This book was developed with the hope of providing a starting point for anyone interested in brain–behavior relationships and the treatment of neuropsychiatric problems. The discoveries and advances of the basic and clinical neurosciences of the last 20 years have dramatically changed our understanding of the neurobiological bases of cognition, emotion, and behavior. While this progress is of great scientific and public interest, it also makes quite difficult the ostensibly simple task of determining how or where to begin one's studies, let alone attempting to assimilate this ever-growing body of information.

The first author, Dr. Arciniegas, has long been interested in the workings of mind and brain, and is a perpetual student of biology, psychology, and philosophy. His interests flourished during the latter stages of his specialty training, fed by the excitement of the recent advances in understanding brain–behavior relationships and by a desire to share this excitement with students and colleagues. The senior author, Dr. Beresford, approached these topics through his work with and study of patients whose medical illness presented with psychiatric symptoms. Dr. Beresford's interest in neuropsychiatry grew from an increasing sense of discomfort with commonly taught psychiatric diagnostic procedures, some of which mention the importance of the differential diagnosis but in practice do not always consider the relationship between psychiatric symptoms and brain disorders. The authors' two paths came together in the common interest of developing an accessible discussion of neuropsychiatry that might offer both a set of fundamental concepts and a practical approach to the understanding and treatment of neuropsychiatric problems.

Recalling de Maupassant's dictum that writing consists principally of putting ink on paper, Dr. Arciniegas began writing this work, first, as a series of lecture notes on the mental status examination, delirium, and dementia in his courses for psychiatric residents. Many of the students at these lectures commented that the accompanying handouts did not look like lecture notes but more like book chapters. These comments, along with Dr. Beresford's encouragement and the support of the Cambridge University Press, began the process of developing and expanding lecture notes into a useful guide to neuropsychiatry.

The goal was to make the material engaging but relatively simple, and therefore useful. The challenge in its writing was offering enough information to convey the richness of the material while not losing the notion of a practical, introductory guide to understanding neuropsychiatry among the seemingly endless details that might be included. The epigraph, *Everything should be made as simple as possible, but not simpler* (Albert Einstein), best captures the spirit of the effort to develop a substantive but readable text for relative newcomers, whether students, residents, or other clinical colleagues.

In producing the book over several years, Dr. Arciniegas wrote the basic text for all of the chapters but two – those on alcoholism and on coping mechanisms for which Dr. Beresford is responsible. Each author edited the other's chapters with an eye to practical use and writing style, and a skeptical eye towards content. Because of this process, both authors are very clearly responsible for the content of the work and own any errors that knowledgeable readers might find within its pages. These may appear, especially, in the necessary conflict between the complexity of the material and the intentional simplicity of its presentation. Where this conflict produces shortcomings, we ask the readers' indulgence.

Designed as a primer of concepts and methods, rather than an exhaustive survey of neuropsychiatric problems, the text divides into three parts. Part I, reviews the history and current state of neuropsychiatry, and then provides a neuropsychiatric approach to understanding basic and complex cognition, emotion, personality, and psychological adaptation. Part II, describes the fundamental methods of clinical neuropsychiatry, including an outline of the neuropsychiatric evaluation, and three detailed reviews of the mental status examination, clinical electrophysiology, and neuroimaging.

Part III, then examines several topics in neuropsychiatry with two purposes: a current review of information essential to the practice of neuropsychiatry; and an explicit application of the relevant concepts and methods of neuropsychiatry to these clinical problems. Topics included were selected to highlight the concepts included in Sections I and II. For example, delirium (Chapter 12) and dementia (Chapter 13) illustrate derangements of basic and complex cognition; obsessive–compulsive disorder (Chapter 14) and diminished motivation and apathy (Chapter 15) apply knowledge of frontal–subcortical circuitry to understanding a treatment of these problems; Parkinson's disease (Chapter

16) reviews all of these issues as well as the neurocircuitry of emotion; alcoholism and alcohol-related disorders (Chapter 17) offer a neuropsychiatric perspective on conditions where there are conflicting neurological, psychiatric, and public perspectives; and traumatic brain injury (Chapter 18) applies material from Parts I and II to a condition with many complex neuropsychiatric consequences. A host of other topics, such as multiple sclerosis, stroke, epilepsy, brain tumors, and so on, are not discussed in detail here in the interest of not distracting readers from purpose of this text, namely learning the neuropsychiatric approach itself. If this effort is successful, readers should be able to apply the concepts and methods of this approach to further learning about and to the care of patients with neuropsychiatric problems not discussed in detail here.

A worthwhile book affects not only its readers, but its writers as well. Dr. Beresford's enthusiasm for understanding and applying the basic science knowledge of brain functioning to clinical problems has grown, as has Dr. Arciniegas' patience for the delayed acceptance of neuropsychiatry by the larger, traditionally defined specialty fields of psychiatry and neurology. At the same time, Dr. Arciniegas' clinical work, research, and teaching in neuropsychiatry have led him to an even more strongly held unified view of brain and mind. Dr. Beresford remains the skeptic in this matter, and continues to find interest and usefulness in both unitary and dualist perspectives on the mind–brain problem. In this way, intellectual agreement and disagreement have stimulated productivity, and both authors have grown from the process of writing this book. Their ultimate hope is that readers of this work will find it also an occasion for growth.

David B. Arciniegas
Thomas P. Beresford

Acknowledgements

Many people offered support and encouragement during our work on this project, for which we are deeply grateful. Christopher Filley, M.D., C. Alan Anderson, M.D., Martin L. Reite, M.D., and Donald C. Rojas, Ph.D. were each engaged in innumerable discussions about the best method of approaching neuropsychiatry and the contents of this work, and all provided invaluable comments and suggestions. Dr. Rojas also contributed the cover figure for this publication. Brandon Martin, A.W. Emch, M.D., Benita Dieperink, M.D., R. Scott Babe, M.D., Heather Kennedy, M.D., Susie Harris, M.D., and Peter Wagner, M.D. made comments on the earliest versions of many chapters, often when still in the lecture note format, which proved very helpful while developing them into their final forms. Douglas Emch, M.D., Joseph (Will) VanDerveer, M.D., Yvonne Rollins, M.D., Robert Neumann, M.D., Lauren Frey, M.D., and Lindsey Sabec also graciously offered to review portions of the manuscript in its final stages of completion. Jeannie Topkoff provided many hours of assistance in the review, preparation, and assembly of the final manuscript, and her assistance deserves particularly grateful acknowledgement and thanks.

We are also deeply appreciative of the support, encouragement, and patience offered by Dr. Richard Barling, our editor at Cambridge University Press, during preparation of this book, and to Thomas W. McAllister, M.D. for his support and generosity in providing the Foreword. Keith A. Johnson, M.D. and J. Alex Becker, authors of *The Whole Brain Atlas* (http://www.med.harvard.edu/AANLIB/home.html), also deserve special thanks for their generous permission to use several of their brain images in Chapter 11. Finally and most importantly, we offer our deepest thanks to our families whose support, encouragement, and tolerance (even during the most irritable moments) of our efforts on this project was above and beyond the call of familial duty.

Part I

Fundamental concepts in neuropsychiatry

Neuropsychiatry – an introduction and brief history

Introduction

Neuropsychiatry may be defined as the study and treatment of cognitive, emotional, and behavioral problems caused by neurologic disorders. While this definition of neuropsychiatry accurately captures the clinical and research interests of many modern neuropsychiatrists, the field is more broadly and fully defined as the medical specialty dedicated to the study of brain–behavior relationships of all manner and to the treatment of patients suffering from disturbances in these relationships. The neuropsychiatrist subscribes to the philosophical position that mental states are brain states. As such, all disturbances of cognition, emotion, and/or behavior reflect brain disturbances. In this view, psychiatric illnesses are by definition neurologic illnesses. Additionally, it is further understood that many neurologic illnesses will entail disturbances of cognition, emotion, and behavior. Followed to its extreme, this definition suggests that any categorization of brain disorders as either exclusively neurologic or psychiatric is, at best, arbitrary. By extension, this definition suggests that psychiatry and neurology are themselves two somewhat arbitrarily defined divisions of the much broader medical specialty, neuropsychiatry.

This very broad and inclusive definition of neuropsychiatry, or other similar versions of it, is often met with skepticism and resistance among both psychiatrists and neurologists. Although modern psychiatrists are increasingly mindful of the biological bases of mental illness, most do not consider themselves neuropsychiatrists. Similarly, modern neurologists are aware of the neuropsychiatric sequelae of neurologic conditions (e.g., stroke, dementia, multiple sclerosis, etc.), but do not typically consider themselves experts in either the study or treatment of neuropsychiatric problems. Indeed, many clinicians in both specialties continue to make the distinction between disorders that are "organic" and those that are "functional," and regard the former as the province of neurology and the latter as the focus of general psychiatry. Certainly, this distinction facilitates referral to the physician whose training and experience are most likely to best serve patients – those with schizophrenia are best treated by psychiatrists, and those with strokes are best cared for by neurologists.

However, the last two decades of basic and clinical neuroscience research make clear that the distinction between psychiatric and neurologic conditions is not as unambiguous as has been presumed during most of the twentieth century. Further, it is becoming increasingly clear that neither specialty alone, at least insofar as they have been traditionally practiced, provides a framework in which the broad range of problems experienced by so many of our patients can be fully understood or optimally treated. For example, older patients with depressed mood may be in the early stages of a dementing illness – if the depression is the focus of treatment and the patient remains under the care of a general psychiatrist, will this result in optimal evaluation and treatment of the dementia as it progresses? If the patient is instead referred to a general neurologist, will the depression (including its impact on the patient's family) be optimally managed? What if electroconvulsive therapy for the dementing patient's treatment-resistant depression is indicated – who now is the best physician for the job? Similarly, if schizophrenia is indeed a disorder of impaired cognition (as has recently been suggested by many experts in the field), is it still a psychiatric disease, or is it now a neurologic disease? Who is best suited to care for these patients if the early (and fundamentally neurological) formulation of this problem, namely dementia praecox, turns out to be the most correct one?

If it is true that mental states are brain states, and therefore all disorders of cognition, emotion, and behavior are brain disorders, then dichotomizing brain disorders into those that are psychiatric and those that are neurological is indeed both arbitrary and artificial. History shows us that this dichotomization occurred relatively recently, as did the division of neuropsychiatry into the subdisciplines of psychiatry and neurology. It also may be suggested that these divisions are better explained as consequences of sociopolitical and medicopolitical forces than as the logical consequence of a valid and sound scientific thesis. A brief review of this history, beginning with the early origins of mind–body and mind–brain dualism and proceeding to the twentieth century, may permit a clearer understanding of how this schism between psychiatry and neurology developed. With this history understood we hope to encourage you to reconsider the traditional divisions between these specialties and the various disorders to which they lay claim. From the new perspective on neuropsychiatry that this review provides, we invite you to begin to engage in the study and treatment of your patients using the introductory approach to neuropsychiatry presented in this book.

A brief history

Although philosophers and physicians have long debated the nature of mind – whether it is spiritual–non-material or physical–material – resolution of this debate has been hampered by the lack of a technology of sophistication sufficient to permit scientific study of this problem. Many early philosophers believed that the body was infused with "vital spirits" which, when not present in the appropriate form or amount, produced mental and physical infirmity. Plato (fourth century BC) was an early advocate of this position, and in *Phaedrus* describes madness as "a divine release of the soul from the yoke of custom and convention . . . prophetic, initiatory, poetic, [and] erotic." Interestingly, although Plato is often referred to as an early mind–body dualist, it is not clear that his philosophy was entirely that of substance dualism. In the same passage from *Phaedrus* where he seemingly advocates a dualist position, he also describes another form of madness, one "produced by human infirmity," and ostensibly related to problems of the body–brain. Less ambivalent on this issue, Democritus (fourth century BC) offered a fundamentally materialist notion of the mind, claiming that since the world consists of nothing more than atoms and the void, the mind is simply a remarkably organized collection of atoms. Similarly, Hippocrates (fourth century BC) rejected entirely the notion of a divine origin of mental illness, stating his position quite clearly in *On the Sacred Disease*: "Men ought to know that from nothing else but the brain come joys, delights, laughter and sports, and sorrows, griefs, despondency, and lamentations . . . All these things we endure from the brain." However, without the scientific methods or tools needed to investigate these brain–behavior relationships, early philosophers and physicians were unable to make any definitive attributions of mental function to brain function.

Early western religions also subscribed to a version of Platonic mind–body dualism, making the mind indistinguishable from the soul. Since the soul was the province of the Church, it was therefore excluded from the realm of acceptable philosophical and scientific inquiry. In this context, such inquiries were potentially heretical and dangerous, and consequently there was little in the way of philosophical or medical dissent from the traditional dualist perspective for many centuries.

Restoring the study of brain–behavior relationships as an acceptable field of philosophical and scientific inquiry was accomplished almost single-handedly by Decartes (1596–1650). In *A Discourse on Method*, Decartes asserted that the brain is simply the material "machine" through which the non-physical mind–soul operated. In this light, the brain is simply another body part to be studied, and though the elements of the brain might be associated with certain functions of the mind, the operations of the brain are not equated with the mind itself. Instead, he suggested, mind consists of an entirely non-physical substance, removed entirely from the causality and physical laws of other material objects, and interfacing with the brain only through the pineal gland. In this fashion, Decartes offered a solution to the mind–body problem that simultaneously preserved religious notions of freewill, moral agency, and the soul and permitted investigation of the brain as the machine through which the mind operated in the physical world.

The historical importance of Decartes' work cannot be overstated, and must be recognized for its instrumental role in the genesis of neuropsychiatry. Indeed, in the remainder of the seventeenth century neuropsychiatry began to emerge as a distinct specialty, with the alienists as its practitioners, and began focusing on the humane treatment of the insane. However, while Decartes' dualist solution to the mind–body problem permitted humane treatment of those whose mind "machine" had malfunctioned, it nonetheless excluded from science any serious inquiry into the essential nature of the mind and mental processes, relegating such inquiries to philosophy and theology.

Despite Decartes' work and the societal/religious orthodoxy of the time, many Renaissance era neuropsychiatrists remained committed to the thesis that mental states are brain states, and that aberrations of mental functioning are the products of a disordered brain. Cullen (1710–1790) was the first among such physicians to include the mental disorders in his taxonomy of brain illnesses, and was the progenitor of the term "neuroses." In his classification of disease, the neuroses included the comata, adynamiae, spasmi, and vesaniae, with this latter group consisting of many of the classic "psychiatric" illnesses (e.g., mania, depression, psychosis, and dementia). His work influenced Coombe (1797–1847) in his classification of brain diseases into two major categories, "organic" and "functional." Coombe's intended use of these terms appears to have been to sort diseases of the brain into two categories based on the presence or absence of localizable abnormalities. It does not appear to have been his intention to establish a system in which some brain diseases are considered "real" brain problems and others are not considered brain problems at all, as is the more common usage of these terms today.

Griesinger (1817–1868) subsequently advanced the thesis that even normal mental processes are the direct result of brain activity alone, and echoed Hippocrates' view that the brain is itself the origin of all mental illness. According to Griesinger, psychiatry and neuropathology are the same field, with one language and one set of operative laws, and he suggested that we must "primarily and in every case of mental disease, recognize a morbid action of that organ [the brain]" (*Mental Pathology and Therapeutics*, 1857).

In the following 50 years, a host of German and French physicians began in earnest to examine the brain with respect to mental processes. Such efforts include those of Alzheimer (1864–1915) and Pick (1851–1924) in the study of the dementias, Kahlbaum's (1828–1899) description of catatonia, and Morel's (1809–1873) initial description of "demence precoce," and Kraeplin's (1856–1925) further characterization of dementia praecox. During this period of time, neurology began to develop as an independent field of study, most notably after the formation of the National Hospital for the "Relief of Paralysis, Epilepsy, and Allied Diseases" in Britain in 1860.

During that same time, Charcot (1825–1893) and his students began concentrating on the "neuroses," and pursuing a line of inquiry that turned the interest of psychiatry at the beginning of the twentieth century toward introspection, reflection, and consideration of the "person as a whole." Notably, as psychoanalysis became a more dominant force within psychiatry in the early twentieth century, this "person as a whole" became increasingly less whole with respect to a complete understanding of the neurology underlying neurotic conditions. Interestingly, this does not appear to have been the long-term objective of Freud (1856–1939), the progenitor of psychoanalysis. A neurologist by training, Freud was committed to a form of substance materialism.

"Research has afforded irrefutable proof that mental activity is bound up with the function of the brain as with no other organ. The discovery of the unequal importance of the different parts of the brain and their individual relations to particular parts of the body and to intellectual activities takes us a step further . . . " (The Unconscious, Section I, in *Collected Papers*, 1915.)

However, Freud believed that the science of his time was inadequate to the task of establishing clearly the relationship between the complex operations of mental processes, particularly in those patients afflicted with neuroses (which, at that time, were considered to be pathophysiologically distinct from the psychoses such as melancholia, schizophrenia, manic-depression, and the like). He subsequently evolved his theories of psychoanalysis to permit a departure from the current scientific methods of the day, and to facilitate an exploration of the neuroses within a purely psychological and self-contained framework. He was cautionary in his statement of his theories, however, and noted the limitations of this approach.

"Our mental topography has for the present nothing to do with anatomy; it is concerned not with anatomical locations, but with regions in the mental apparatus irrespective of their possible situation in the body. In this respect, then, our work is untrammeled and may proceed according to its own requirements. It will, moreover, be useful to remind ourselves that our hypotheses can in the first instance lay claim only to the value of illustrations." (The Unconscious, Section II, in *Collected Papers*, 1915.)

Freud believed that eventually science would become sufficiently sophisticated to permit a less metaphorical and more anatomical theory of mental processes. However, his theory is easily misinterpreted as supporting mind–body dualism, and appears to have further fostered a dualistic perspective on mind–body issues in both psychiatric practice and popular culture. As a result, the early part of the twentieth century witnessed the progressive movement of a significant part of psychiatry away from its neuropsychiatric foundations and the continued division of neurology and psychiatry into separate disciplines of study.

As the twentieth century progressed, neurology and psychiatry became increasingly polarized with respect to the focus and content of their studies. Neurology was interested in localizable pathology, the "organic" problems, and psychiatry was interested in the functioning of an individual's psyche, internally and interpersonally. These "functional" problems became the province of psychiatry, although again they are not the disorders to which Coombe had intended the term "functional" to refer. Further, as a result of being primarily interested in "nonanatomical" illnesses, psychiatry became increasingly less neurologic, and neurology as a field became increasingly less interested in "functional" disorders. Indeed, when previously "functional" disorders such as general paresis of the insane (neurosyphilis) were discovered to have an "organic" basis, neurology reclaimed them as under its purview with the ready agreement of most general psychiatrists. Because the vast majority of the "neuroses" eluded organic description using the science of that time, belief in the lack of a biological basis for the "functional" disorders became increasingly accepted in both fields, and the schism between psychiatry and neurology continued to widen.

As described in *The American Board of Psychiatry and Neurology: The First Fifty Years* (Hollender, 1991), the unification of these disciplines under the American Board of Psychiatry and Neurology (ABPN) in 1934 might have been expected to bring these fields closer together. However, it can be reasonably argued that the manner in which the ABPN was created contributed to the continued separation of psychiatry and neurology at least as much as did any fundamental philosophical differences between practitioners in each field. In the early 1930s, a group of neuropsychiatrists in the American Medical Association (AMA) suggested that psychiatry and neurology be united under a common board of examiners for the purpose of establishing criteria and examinations for certification to practice in these medical specialties. Their explicit purpose was not to make specific distinctions in training and clinical specialty between the fields, but instead to protect the public and the reputations of both fields by distinguishing qualified from unqualified practitioners.

In order to develop a board that would be widely accepted by the practicing clinicians of that time, the AMA solicited the participation of representatives from the American Psychiatric Association (APA) and the American Neurological Association (ANA) in discussions regarding the development of a unified examining board. In recommending a unified board, the AMA made clear its position that the content and practice of psychiatry and neurology overlapped substantially, and that both fields would be best served by an examining board that acknowledged their similarity.

However, ongoing tensions between the fields with respect to public legitimacy and scientific dominance limited the ability of the participating psychiatrists and neurologists to work together on this task, and influenced greatly the outcome of these discussions. Although the AMA representatives initiating these discussions were self-described neuropsychiatrists, in an almost paradoxical reaction to their AMA hosts' suggestion that the two fields be united administratively, the representatives from the APA and the ANA elected not only to disavow recognition of the field of neuropsychiatry but also to even more clearly divide the two specialties apart. First, Hollander notes, the APA and ANA representatives chose to demarcate sharply the lines for training and certification between psychiatry and neurology. Having done so, they then proceeded to heatedly debate the order in which the two fields should be represented in the Board's official title. Despite such academic posturing, however, the Board was nonetheless left to administer the same examination to candidates from both specialties for well over a decade. This outcome suggests that the AMA neuropsychiatrists may have been most correct in their assertion that the content and practices of these two specialties were indeed, at that time, fundamentally the same.

Over time, and as a consequence of training differences driven by the ABPN guidelines, the board examinations became increasingly focused on the candidate's field of training, either psychiatry or neurology. Nonetheless, even today 40% of the questions of each individual specialty's written examination remain based on the other specialty's material (i.e., 40% of the questions on the Part 1 examination in psychiatry are questions in neurology), explicitly acknowledging that much of the essential fund of knowledge necessary for competency in either specialty remains very similar. Interpreting this stance from a more philosophical perspective, one must at least consider the possibility that the AMA neuropsychiatrists' original position continues to be applicable today: that neurology and psychiatry remain scientifically inseparable and in practice require complementary knowledge bases and skills.

Nonetheless, the creation of ABPN left a legacy of an uneasy, if not occasionally hostile, alliance between psychiatrists and neurologists. Its creation also produced a cultural amnesia for the fact that the combined board was created in recognition of the similarity and overlapping areas of interest between psychiatry and neurology, and at the recommendation of a group of neuropsychiatrists. In the years since the Board's creation, a few leaders in both fields have made calls for a more substantial reunification of psychiatry and neurology. However, modern attempts to unite the fields in everyday practice have met with little acceptance outside of only a few academic and private institutions. Similarly, requests to the ABPN for the establishment of Added Qualifications in Neuropsychiatry (and its neurology-based counterpart, Behavioral Neurology) have not thus far been successful.

An introductory approach to neuropsychiatry

From the certitude arising out of our own training histories, neurologists and psychiatrists may each believe that their specialty offers the more interesting, more scientific, and more useful approach to understanding patients with disorders of cognition, emotion, and behavior. In fact, exclusive and narrowly focused training in either specialty alone cannot offer a comprehensive scientific approach to patients with such problems nor can it prepare clinicians fully to provide competent care for patients with complex neuropsychiatric disorders. This is not to suggest that all practitioners should undertake full training in both neurology and psychiatry, although such a suggestion would be the logical extension (albeit a rather extreme extension) of this view. Instead, and probably more realistically, this view suggests that, at a minimum, the fundamental methods of evaluation and treatment in both fields are equally valuable and complementary, and that training in either field should include sufficient experience in the other so as to permit the fullest possible understanding of the problems with which patients present and the varieties of therapies for them.

Therefore, we will abandon herein the medicopolitical arguments of the last 150 years regarding the areas of scientific inquiry and clinical practice "owned" by psychiatry and neurology, and instead focus on their complementary scientific and clinical perspectives in our consideration of these issues. When possessed of the variety of perspectives on cognition, emotion, and behavior offered by both specialties, our understanding and treatment of patients with neuropsychiatric problems may be improved to our own and our patients' benefit.

We believe it is this complementarity of method and practice that defines neuropsychiatry today. The neuropsychiatrist is a clinician conversant and facile in the language and techniques of both psychiatry and neurology, and one who approaches the problems and care of patients with that neuropsychiatric perspective. The neuropsychiatrist is often a consultant to patients and their families, to other general psychiatrists and neurologists, and a powerful advocate for and liaison in the development of optimal methods of caring for neuropsychiatrically complex patients.

The content and structure of this book is based on this conceptualization of neuropsychiatry. We believe that understanding disorders of cognition, emotion, and behavior requires knowledge of a broad range of issues in neurobiology, neuroanatomy, neurophysiology, and methods of clinical evaluation, as well as an appreciation of the neuropsychology, psychodynamics, family, and culture of individuals with these conditions. Of course, we cannot entirely divorce ourselves from the perspectives of our own specialty training and practice so there will at times be greater or lesser attention paid to each of these aspects as we progress through the following chapters. Nonetheless, even where we may not attempt to offer a comprehensive review of the topics presented, we hope that both the content and style of this book will reflect our desire to integrate the funds of information needed to practice clinical neuro-psychiatry. If we are successful in our efforts, we hope to provide you with an introductory approach to neuropsychiatry that will be useful in your clinical practice and form a good foundation from which to pursue a more detailed study of neuropsychiatry.

2

Essential behavioral neuroanatomy

Introduction

This chapter provides a brief review of the neuroanatomy most relevant to neuropsychiatry and clinical neuroscience. Because this is a review, the material presented is intentionally oversimplified. Our aim is to re-familiarize the reader with the major structural and functional areas of the brain, and to establish a common frame of reference for the material presented in subsequent chapters. For those interested in a more complete review of neurobehavioral anatomy, the relevant are chapters presented in Fogel et al. (1996), Yudofsky & Hales (1997), Feinberg & Farah (1997), and Mesulam (2000).

Form and function

Descriptions of behavioral neuroanatomy usually relate brain structure to function, and often contain lengthy lists of specific brain areas and their functional correlates. These descriptions follow from lesion studies of brain areas and their value cannot be understated. While informative, such lists can be difficult to remember for those beginning their studies of neuropsychiatry. Therefore, we suggest a more basic but also more practical method for remembering neuroanatomy that mixes structural and functional descriptions to build a brain, as it were, from the brainstem to the neocortex, following the brief outline in Figure 2.1. The rationale for this organization is similar to that outlined in Chapter 9, namely that normal function at each ascending level is to some degree predicated on normal function at the lower levels. For example, normal declarative memory, that memory for events in time and space which can be described using language, involves at least several medial and lateral temporal areas, heteromodal cortex of the parietal lobe, and some frontal structures. Normal functioning of declarative memory is logically predicated on relatively normal arousal and attention, functions that involve several lower

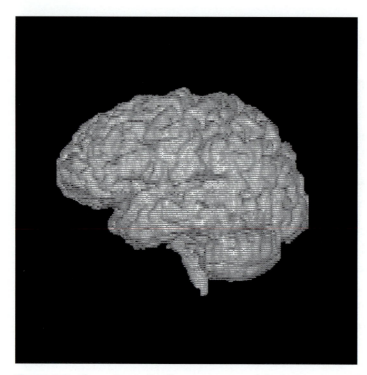

Telencephalon – neocortex, white matter, and subcortical nuclear complexes

Limbic System (functional) – collection of medial structures including the cingulate gyrus, hippocampus, amygdala, and other medial temporal gyri, thalamus (esp. dorsal and anteromedial), hypothalamus, and limbic midbrain area

Basal Ganglia (functional) – caudate, putamen, globus pallidus (interna and externa), and substantia nigra

Diencephalon – thalamus, hypothalamus, pituitary gland, pineal gland

Reticular Formation – collection of brainstem nuclei running from the rostral midbrain to the medulla, and with its functional components:

Brainstem:
Mesencephalon – midbrain
Metencephalon – pons and cerebellum
Myelencephalon – medulla

Figure 2.1   Three-dimensional reconstruction of the brain, view of the left hemisphere.

brain areas such as the elements of the reticular formation and diencephalon, as well as higher areas such as medial temporal, parietal, and frontal structures. If the lower levels are markedly dysfunctional, functioning of higher areas will also be compromised. In clinical (and somewhat crude) terms, it is difficult to learn, and report on, new information when one is comatose.

Given this notion of relative hierarchical functioning of the brain, we will begin at the level of the myelencephalon, and progress through those elements listed in the above outline toward the telencephalon. Selected images from an MRI (magnetic resonance imaging) scan of a normal brain are included to place these descriptions in the context of the neuroanatomy as we might encounter it clinically.

Myelencephalon

The myelencephalon is the medulla oblongata (Figure 2.2). It is the lowest level of the brain and is the junction between the brain and the spinal cord. Its

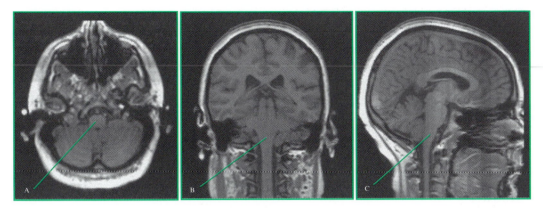

Figure 2.2 T1-weighted magnetic resonance image of the brain showing the myelencephalon in axial (A), coronal (B), and sagittal (C) views.

ventral (anterior) surface lies against the basilar portion of the occipital bone, and its dorsal (posterior) surface is wedged in a groove along the ventral surface of the cerebellum. At the medulla, both the descending motor (pyramidal) tracts and the ascending sensory dorsal columns (vibration, proprioception) decussate. The ascending spinothalamic tracts (pain, temperature) run through the medulla on their way to the thalamus.

The medulla also contains the most caudal portions of the serotonergic nuclei, as well as medullary opiocortin (adrenocorticotropin, β-endorphin, and melanocyte stimulating hormone) neurons, and adrenergic neurons. These systems are involved in modulation of ascending and descending signals, and also have modulatory effects on the reticular formation.

The medulla contains cranial nerve nuclei X (vagus), XI (accessory), and XII (hypoglossal) and the lowest portions of the nuclei for cranial nerves V (trigeminal) and VIII (vestibular).

Metencephalon

The pons ("bridge") and the cerebellum comprise the metencephalon (Figure 2.3). The ventral surface of the pons lies against the occipital bone, and its dorsal surface lies along the ventral surface of the cerebellum. It contains bundles of transversely oriented fibers originating in the pontine nuclei and entering the cerebellum via the cerebellar peduncles. As its name suggests, the pons represents a bridge between the motor, sensory, and other

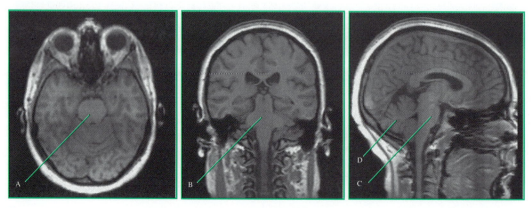

Figure 2.3 T1-weighted magnetic resonance image of the brain showing the metencephalon. The pons is indicated in the axial (A), coronal (B), and sagittal (C) views. The cerebellum (D) is also shown in the sagittal view.

information processing pathways between the cerebrum and the cerebellum, conveying, for example, the corticopontine, corticobulbar, and corticospinal tracts.

One of the important diffusely projecting pontine nuclei is the locus ceruleus, a noradrenergic nucleus that is the principle source of most cerebral norepinephrine. The locus ceruleus is an important component of the reticular formation, and is particularly important in its ascending activating projections. The pons also contains lower portions of the serotonergic nuclei (pontine raphe nucleus), the projections of which enter the reticular formation. The cranial nerve nuclei VI (abducens), VII (facial), and portions of the nuclei for cranial nerves V and VIII are also contained in the pons.

Although the cerebellum is in many texts not explicitly described as a part of the brainstem, it is part of the metencephalon and hence is included at this point in our review. The cerebellum is a bihemispheric organ subserving coordination and integration of primary motor and sensory function. In particular, the timing, sequence, and coordination of muscle activation initiated by cerebral neurons are further organized by the cerebellum. Additionally, the cerebellum appears to play a role in cognition and memory, including at least motor learning and reflex modification. Although the role of the cerebellum in more complex aspects of cognition is not entirely known at the present time, it may be that its role in cognition parallels those aspects of motor function that it also facilitates, for example refinement of the timing, sequence, and coordination of certain aspects of cognition.

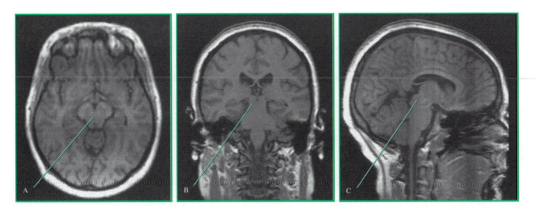

Figure 2.4 T1-weighted magnetic resonance image of the brain showing the mesencephalon in axial (A), coronal (B), and sagittal (C) views.

Mesencephalon

The mesencephalon is the midbrain (Figure 2.4). Its ventral surface lies along the basilar portion of the occipital bone, and its dorsal surface forms an isthmus between the cerebrum and the cerebellum. The midbrain is connected to the cerebrum by the cerebral peduncles, which contain the ascending and descending tracts between the brainstem and the neocortex.

The midbrain contains two important reflex centers: the visual reflex center (superior colliculus) and the auditory reflex center (inferior colliculus). The centers are connected to one another by the medial longitudinal fasciculus, a fibre bundle involved in head and neck reflex movements in response to visual and vestibular stimuli. Accordingly, the midbrain also contains cranial nerves III (occulomotor), IV (trochlear), and the most superior portions of cranial nerves V and VIII.

The midbrain also contains several functionally important nuclei. The major dopaminergic nuclei, the substantia nigra and the ventral tegmental area, are located in the midbrain. The substantia nigra is the principal source of dopaminergic input to the basal ganglia (the nigrostriatal or mesostriatal pathway) and is critically important in the regulation of "extrapyramidal" motor function. The ventral tegmental is the principal source of dopaminergic neurons projecting to limbic structures (mesolimbic pathway) and to the neocortex (mesocortical pathway).

At least two major sources of cerebral serotonin are also located in the midbrain, although the serotonergic nuclei extend into the medulla and pons as well. The mesencephalic serotonergic include the dorsal raphe nucleus and the central superior nucleus. These nuclei project diffusely to the neocortex and are substantially involved in the functioning of the reticular formation and in the regulation of multiple frontal-subcortical and limbic-subcortical circuits.

The area surrounding the cerebral aqueduct in the midbrain is the periaqueductal gray matter, also known as the limbic midbrain area. The periaqueductal gray matter (abbreviated as PAG in some texts) is part of the functional limbic system. It receives input from a variety of cortical, limbic, diencephalic, and brainstem areas and is extensively interconnected to the major nuclei of the reticular formation. The limbic midbrain area contributes significantly to modulation of pain sensation, defensive reactions to immediate threat, emotional expression, sexual behavior, feeding, and metabolism. Given its interconnections with limbic structures, prefrontal cortical areas, and the reticular formation, the periaqueductal gray may also play a role in modulating attention to internal and external stimuli involved in survival, emotion, and memory.

Reticular formation

The reticular formation is a collection of brainstem nuclei and their projections, and derives its name (Latin, *reticulum*, little net) from its net-like organization. The reticular formation extends rostrally from the medulla toward the midbrain and into the diencephalon, and includes the intralaminar nuclei of the thalamus and certain aggregations of subthalamic cells (zona incerta). In essence, the reticular formation is that part of the brainstem located in the space not otherwise occupied by the cranial nerve nuclei, supplementary sensory and motor nuclei, and other ascending/descending white matter tracts.

The nuclei that form the reticular formation are many, but may be most easily grouped into three anatomic and functional areas: a median and paramedian zone, comprised of the serotonergic raphe nuclei; a medial zone, which appears to serve an integrative function for both motor and sensory pathways; and a lateral zone, which includes dopaminergic, noradrenergic, adrenergic, and cholinergic cell groups. The functioning of this lattice of cell groups is complex, and a detailed description of their functions and interactions is well beyond the scope of this work. Put most simply, the rostral nuclei from all three zones are essential for arousal, consciousness, and the waking state, while the caudal nuclei are essential for automatic breathing and a series of reflexes including those involving the vestibular, cardiopulmonary, gastrointestinal, and genitourinary systems.

It may also be helpful to conceptualize the function of the reticular formation as dividing into an ascending reticular activating system (ARAS) and an ascending reticular inhibiting system (ARIS).

- ARAS: this collection of nuclei is located in a narrow isthmus between the cerebrum and cerebellum, and includes the locus ceruleus (pontine), the ventral tegmental area (midbrain), and cholinergic nuclei (Ch5 and 6). These nuclei project to a number of areas, including the thalamus, subthalamic nucleus, limbic areas, and neocortex. The principal function of the ARAS is to maintain a state of wakefulness, and to participate in modulating attention to both ascending sensory input and internal stimuli (e.g., percepts, emotions, and thoughts). The degree to which it is able to maintain arousal and attention depends on both intrinsic neuronal firing activity and the effects of external (including both environmental and visceral) stimulation or exogenous substances.
- ARIS: this "system," comprised by the raphe nuclei, is used here as a theoretical construct, as it is not to our knowledge specifically described as such elsewhere. Nonetheless, we find this concept useful for remembering the importance of those portions of the reticular formation that modulate or attenuate (e.g., provide inhibitory tone to) the activity of the ARAS. In other words, attenuating wakefulness (or promoting sleep) is not simply a function of decreasing activation but also of increasing inhibition, and in particular via increased activity of the serotonergic nuclei. A relatively clear example is sleep, which appears to be driven by medullary portions of the reticular formation (Coenen, 1998). The effect of the serotonergic portions of the reticular formation is to promote neuronal hyperpolarization, and therefore decreased firing, in areas involved in wakefulness, including the thalamocortical circuits. These ascending serotonergic projections of the reticular formation therefore oppose the activation from adrenergic, noradrenergic, dopaminergic, and cholinergic systems. Similarly, the mesencephalic raphe nuclei (dorsal raphe and central superior nuclei) modulate the activity of the ARAS and may be involved in promoting behavioral inhibition (Robbins, 1997), perhaps via their role in the frontal-subcortical circuits (see Chapter 4). While the effect of the raphe nuclei and their diffuse projections is far more complex than this simplification suggests, the concept of an "inhibitory" system will be a useful one in the many chapters that follow.

Diencephalon

The thalamus and hypothalamus, the pituitary gland, and the pineal body (Figure 2.5) comprise the diencephalon. The thalamus is a central brain

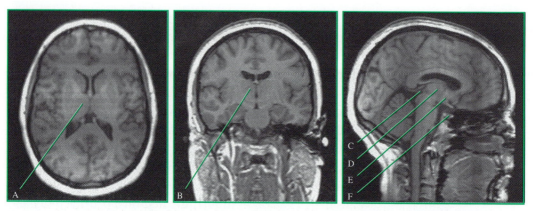

Figure 2.5 T1-weighted magnetic resonance image of the brain at the level of the diencephalon. The thalamus is shown in axial (A), coronal (B), and sagittal (D) views. The other diencephalic structures, including the pineal body (C), hypothalamus (E), and pituitary (F) are also shown in the sagittal view.

structure that serves as a relay center for information ascending from spinothalamic tracts to the cortex, descending from cortical areas to the reticular formation and the spinal cord, and traversing between cortical and subcortical structures. The thalamus is comprised of multiple smaller nuclei, a detailed discussion of which is again beyond the scope of this presentation. However, it is useful to think of the thalamus as a central relay station and to note that its various nuclei are topographically related to the cortical areas to which they are connected. Hence, the anterior thalamus is reciprocally connected to frontal areas, the superior and posterior areas of the thalamus are connected to parietal and occipital lobes, the inferior portion of the thalamus connects the orbitofrontal, insular, and temporal areas, and the ventral thalamus receives input from limbic areas. The thalamus also receives extensive afferent input from ascending sensory tracts, participates in the activity of reticular formation, and is a major component of the multiple frontal-subcortical circuits discussed in later chapters. The various thalamic nuclei also are extensively connected to one another.

The hypothalamus is important for integrating the functioning of the autonomic nervous system and for expressing the effects of the higher cerebral functions (especially limbic activity) via the autonomic nervous system and the pituitary. The hypothalamus is also comprised of several smaller nuclei. Simplistically, the hypothalamic nuclei control: sexual drive (anterior), satiety (ventromedial), appetitive behavior (lateral), and arousal for "fight /flight" reactions (posterior).

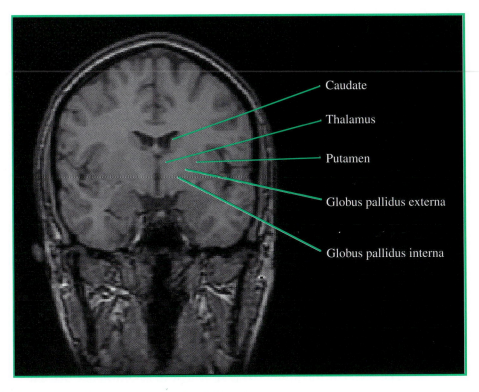

Figure 2.6 The basal ganglia. Also shown is the thalamus.

As mentioned in the previous section, it has been suggested that the reticular formation may have a diencephalic extension. The diencephalic component of the reticular formation not only includes the reticular nucleus of the thalamus, but also may include the major cholinergic nuclei (Ch1–4), including the nucleus basalis of Meynert (Ch4). Selden et al. (1998) have described the major cortical cholinergic pathways, and note that limbic (Ch1 and 2, hippocampus; Ch3, olfactory tubercle) and neocortical (Ch4) cholinergic pathways are involved in modulating cortical activity.

Basal ganglia

The term basal ganglia refers to several subcortical gray matter nuclei or "ganglia." The basal ganglia (Figure 2.6) include the caudate ("tail-shaped"), the putamen ("shell"), and the internal and external portions of the globus pallidus ("pale body"). The caudate and the putamen together are often referred to as the striatum, and may be simplistically viewed as the major input site to the basal ganglia, receiving input from the entire neocortex and from the substantia nigra.

Although the basal ganglia have traditionally been discussed in the context of motor function, it has become increasingly clear over the last decade that these nuclei also comprise essential components of the pathways serving executive functioning, social behavior, and motivation. To that end, Nieuwenhuys et al. (1988) have also suggested that the concept of these structures as "extrapyramidal motor nuclei," functionally driven by but external to the descending motor pathways, requires serious reconsideration. The basal ganglia both receive input from, and direct output to, multiple frontal-subcortical circuits involved in not only motor function but also in the most complex aspects of cognition (see Chapter 4).

Functionally, the various loops between the cortex and the basal ganglia all follow a similar pattern: neocortex to striatum, striatum to globus pallidus (direct and indirect pathways), globus pallidus to thalamus, and thalamus to neocortex. The subthalamic nucleus, amygdala, and inputs from the reticular formation also play important roles in these circuits, and may be thought of as components of the functional basal ganglia, as we shall see in subsequent chapters. For the present, it is sufficient to acknowledge that the basal ganglia are responsible for fine motor, postural, and facial coordination, and figure importantly in motivation, executive function, and the modulation of social behavior.

Limbic system

The limbic system is a collection of structures on the medial aspects of the cerebral hemispheres, forming a ring (from Latin *limbus*) of connections to one another. The limbic system is the anatomic substrate for emotions, survival functions (eating, fighting, fear, sexual desire/mating, grooming, nurturing), and is also important in episodic memory (memory for events, or memory that has spatial and temporal contexts). Of note, the circuit of Papez (1937; Figure 2.7) was the first pathway hypothesized as a possible substrate for the appreciation and expression of emotion in humans. This early view of the neural substrates of emotion suggested that information from the brainstem/ARAS is received in the hippocampus, and from there is transmitted to the mammillary bodies. The mammillary bodies are a processing station for both emotional and memory information. Information from the mammillary

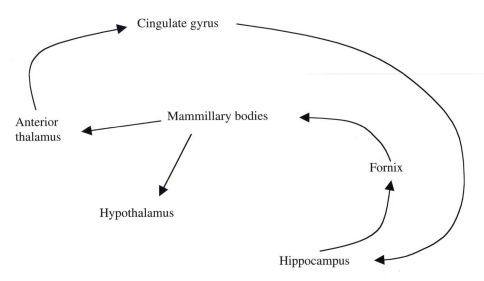

Figure 2.7 The Circuit of Papez, an early (1937) model for the neural substrates of emotion.

bodies is sent to the anterior thalamus, and relayed to the cingulate gyrus. The cingulate gyrus plays a role in the conscious appreciation/internal experience of emotion. The cingulate gyrus returns information to the hippocampus where the circuit begins again. Simultaneously, the mammillary bodies relay information to the hypothalamus, where autonomic centers (acting in concert with additional limbic connections to the ARAS and basal ganglia) initiate outward expression of emotion. As discussed further in Chapter 5 dealing with emotion, although this circuit is no longer regarded an adequate model for the neural substrates of emotion, more modern derivations and elaborations of the Papez circuit remain a source of study in a number of neuropsychiatric disorders (e.g., obsessive–compulsive disorder).

The limbic system is a complex collection of reticular, diencephalic, medial temporal and paralimbic frontal areas. For our purposes, the basic limbic system anatomy includes the cingulate and orbitofrontal gyri, hippocampus, hypothalamus, thalamus (dorsal and anteromedial), amygdala, medial temporal cortex, and the limbic midbrain (periaqueductal gray) area (Figure 2.8). These structures are organized into and connected by several major pathways, including the stria terminalis, the medial forebrain bundle, the fornix, and multiple frontal-subcortical circuits. These areas are reciprocally connected to one another and to other areas of the brain, particularly the reticular nuclei and frontal-subcortical circuits. The limbic system receives input from and

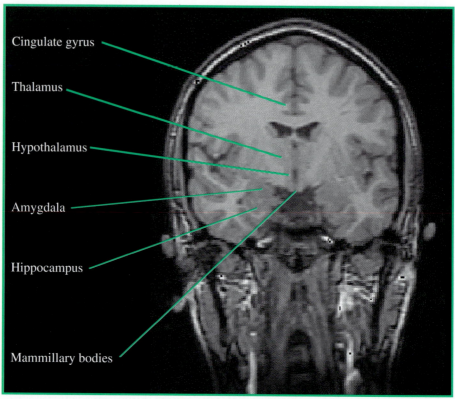

Figure 2.8 Several important limbic structures. T1-weighted coronal magnetic resonance image of the brain at the level of the hippocampal formation.

directs output to these areas in a continuous fashion, and plays a major role in directing both cognition and behavior toward content with high emotional/survival value.

The Papez circuit (Figure 2.7) is an inadequate model for the neurocircuitry of emotion, since our present understanding suggests that the neurocircuitry involved is much more complex. However, for our present purposes the Papez circuit can be usefully applied as an introduction to a few fundamental concepts in the neurobiology of emotion. First, the Papez circuit suggests the presence of a continuous circuit that regulates internal emotional states and drives the outward (including somatic) expressions of emotion. Experience of positive emotion may involve the cingulate gyrus (as above) and multiple additional connections with the septal nuclei and other frontotemporal areas, while experience of negative emotion most likely involves the amygdala and other frontotemporal areas. The external expression of emotion involves both hypothalamic modulation of autonomic (e.g., visceral) function via sympathetic and parasympathetic pathways and also basal ganglia-mediated automatic motor responses to limbic activity. Limbic input to the ARAS is also important in the development of affective responding since such input modifies level of arousal. The combination of limbic and ARAS inputs to frontal-subcortical circuits thereby affects motivational state and influences behavioral responses.

It may be argued that some limbic responses, particularly those to emotionally charged stimuli, are "hard-wired," either innately (genetically conserved) or in response to earlier experiences (memory of the particular organism). Those responses that have facilitated survival become increasingly automatic, blending innate and learned responding to affect (and sometimes limit or at least constrain) future behavior. If true, then it makes some sense that the limbic system should have developed evolutionarily to subserve both emotion and new learning (episodic memory) – those emotional reactions with high survival value are best remembered so that they may be repeated. In this light, it also makes sense that the type of memory mediated by limbic structures should be episodic memory, memory that involves spatial and temporal contextual cues, which may provoke memories of similar situations in response to elements of current stimuli.

Indeed, the limbic system is heavily involved in episodic memory. Simplistically, the principal limbic structures that mediate this type of memory include the amygdala, hippocampus and mammillary bodies, which participate in affective responding and begin the process of encoding events into memory. Further, the involvement by the more "emotional" elements of the circuit (e.g., extended amygdala and cingulate areas) most likely affects significantly the types of things to which attention is paid and memories are created. Strong emotion (either positive or negative) associated with input for memory serves as strong internal reinforcement (i.e., has high survival value) for learning and the development of permanent memories; conversely, input without significant emotional impact (i.e., low survival value) results in less strength for memory input and learning.

Neocortex (telencephalon)

The telencephalon, or neocortex, includes the cerebral hemispheres and their lobar divisions (frontal, parietal, temporal, and occipital) and is involved in the

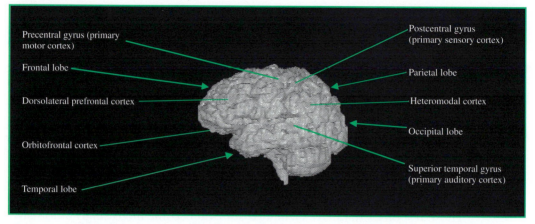

Precentral gyrus (primary motor cortex)

Frontal lobe

Dorsolateral prefrontal cortex

Orbitofrontal cortex

Temporal lobe

Postcentral gyrus (primary sensory cortex)

Parietal lobe

Heteromodal cortex

Occipital lobe

Superior temporal gyrus (primary auditory cortex)

Figure 2.9 The neocortex (telencephalon). Lateral view of the left hemisphere using a three-dimensional reconstructed magnetic resonance imaging of the brain. The major lobar divisions are illustrated, as are several specific gyri discussed in the accompanying text. Arrows indicate the major neocortical lobes while the markers indicate the location of specific gyri.

perception, association, interpretation, and response to information received from both external and internal sources (Figure 2.9). Although discussed earlier in the context of structure, the subcortical structures (e.g., anatomic basal ganglia) and also the white matter projections from below and between neocortical structures (e.g., internal capsule) are parts of the functional telencephalon.

Localization of function in the neocortex has historically depended on lesion or cortical stimulation studies. General concepts correlating cortical regions with specific behavioral characteristics have been established, although the structural boundaries by which the cortical lobes and gyri are anatomically defined do not always necessarily indicate strict functional boundaries. Indeed, the functional boundaries of the telencephalon include subcortical and white matter structures: it is possible to find impairments in complex cognition (e.g., executive function, social intelligence, motivation) caused by damage to these areas. For brevity, in this chapter we will consider neocortical function in terms of the cortex alone, and defer detailed discussion of the frontal-subcortical circuits to Chapter 4. Table 2.1 summarizes the major functions of each cortical lobe.

We find it helpful to think of the neocortex as dividing into two general functional types: primary and association (secondary, tertiary, or quaternary) cortices. Primary motor cortex is responsible for generating descending signals for voluntary movement and the primary sensory cortex is responsible for receiving input from the ascending sensory pathways. Added to these primary cortical areas are the association cortices. The association cortex in closest proximity to the primary cortex is referred to as secondary association cortex. Secondary motor association cortex is responsible for elaborating and generating the impulses that are then developed into motor output by the primary motor cortex. Secondary sensory association cortices organize input from the primary sensory areas (e.g., visual, auditory, tactile, olfactory, gustatory) and compare that input with previously experienced (encoded) sensory inputs. Information from the sensory association cortex is then further communicated to tertiary and quaternary association areas for further elaboration, comparison, and integration into the individual's cognition, emotion, and behavior.

Motor function is subserved by the primary motor cortex located in the precentral gyrus. This motor area has an adjacent association cortex, where motor patterns are organized and transmitted to the primary motor cortex. Sensory function is subserved by the postcentral gyrus (tactile and proprioceptive), the medial and superior temporal lobe (olfactory/gustatory and auditory, respectively), and the occipital lobe (visual). Each primary sensory area is unimodal (serving only one sensory type), and has a unimodal secondary association area associated with and adjacent to it. These unimodal secondary association areas serve elaborative and comparative functions to the primary sensory area.

Two additional association areas are critical to normal and complete function of the human brain, and therefore warrant additional description. First, the inferior parietal lobule (comprised of the supramarginal and angular gyri) receives input from all of the secondary association areas, and is therefore referred to as cross-modal (heteromodal) or tertiary association cortex. This area facilitates integration of the various sensory cortices, giving humans the ability to associate sights with sounds, sight with touch, smell with sight, and so on. This tertiary association cortex also receives input from the reticular formation, the limbic system, and the frontal lobes (see below), which both modulate and integrate emotional and sensory experiences, most likely based on their relative emotional valence or survival value.

Second, the frontal lobes serve as quaternary association areas for the synthesis, elaboration, and regulation of emotional, cognitive, and behavioral/motor processes. The frontal lobes are the most phylogenetically recent

Table 2.1. The major divisions of the neocortex, and some of the major functions subserved by each neocortical area

Frontal	Temporal	Parietal	Occipital
Motor planning	Primary auditory cortex (lateral)	Tactile sensation	Vision
Voluntary movement	Language recognition (left lateral)	Heteromodal sensory association	Visual perception and association
Social behavior and judgment			
Motivation	Auditory prosody (right lateral)	Visuospatial function (right)	
Complex cognition	Memory (medial)	Some elements of praxis (right)	
Language production (left)	Fight/flight reactions (medial)	Reading (left)	
Language/motor prosody (right)	Taste (medial and lateral)	Calculation (left)	
	Smell (medial)	Stereognosis (left)	

addition to the brain, and the last to mature in the child. Their connections to the rest of the brain are richly reciprocal.

Input to the frontal lobes largely originates from four areas: the tertiary sensory association cortices (heteromodal cortex); the secondary association cortices; and limbic-subcortical and reticular areas. Sensory information largely projects to the lateral convexities of the prefrontal cortices, and limbic information projects to the basilar (orbitomedial) surface of the frontal lobes. Subcortical structures (striatum, globus pallidus, subthalamic nucleus, and thalamus) form five major circuits with various frontal gyri, including primary motor cortex, frontal eye fields, dorsolateral prefrontal cortex (made up of the middle and superior frontal gyri), orbitofrontal cortices (gyrus rectus and medial orbital gyrus, medially, and lateral orbital gyrus and medial inferior frontal gyrus, laterally), and the anterior cingulate gyrus. Reticular formation afferents project diffusely throughout the frontal lobes, modulating arousal and attention related to the various sensory and limbic inputs. Output from the frontal lobes is essentially reciprocal to these same structures, as well as to frontal motor areas bilaterally.

The functions of the frontal lobes may be most simply related to the activity of the five major frontal-subcortical circuits described above: motor (voluntary motor function); frontal eye fields (eye movements); dorsolateral prefrontal (executive function); lateral orbitofrontal ("social intelligence"); and anterior cingulate (motivation and emotional experience). The latter three of these circuits are discussed in detail in Chapter 4, but all five circuits share a common neural organization involving the connections between the frontal lobes, the striatum (caudate and putamen), the globus pallidus interna and externa, the subthalamic nucleus, and the thalamus.

The prefrontal-subcortical circuits (in particular those involving dorsolateral, orbitofrontal, and anterior cingulate areas) integrate cognitive, emotional, and motivational information with somatosensory information received from the secondary sensory association and heteromodal cortices. Frontal-subcortical circuits (especially those involving the dorsolateral prefrontal cortex) likely have efferents to the tertiary and secondary association cortices that facilitate directed attention to sensory and emotional information with high survival value, meaning information that is recognized as important by virtue of activating "hard-wired" or innate neural networks involved in the recognition of dangerous or valuable stimuli or by activating networks that have been reinforced by experience. These reciprocal cortico-cortical circuits are postulated to serve as an active guidance process to control

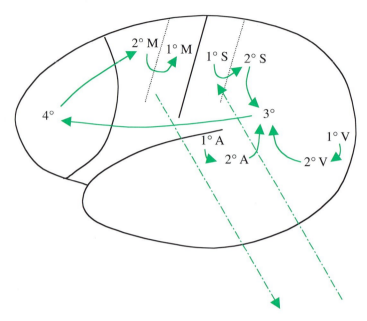

Figure 2.10 Schematic diagram of the pathways between the primary, secondary, tertiary, and quaternary cortical areas. The flow of information from ascending input to motor output illustrates a simple view of the processing of stimuli as it leads to the generation of a behavioral response. M, motor; S, somatosensory; A, auditory; V, visual. 1°, primary cortical area; 2°, secondary association cortex; 3°, heteromodal cortex; and 4°, prefrontal cortex.

and determine to which internal or environmental stimuli attention is directed, which mental processes that will be continued, and when and how any change in mental direction occurs. Both the prefrontal cortices and pre-motor cortex participate in the generation of motor behaviors. Figure 2.10 provides a very simple view of how motor responses may be generated. Primary sensory areas receive ascending information, and transmit this area to their respective secondary association areas where the information is com-pared to previous experienced stimuli. Secondary association areas send afferents to the tertiary association cortex, where ongoing limbic and frontal afferents modulate attention and processing of information. The tertiary asso-ciation area then sends information to the quaternary (prefrontal) areas, where the information is elaborated and responses are generated. The prefron-tal cortices project afferents to the premotor (motor association) cortices, which organize these inputs into necessary motor patterns that are finally transmitted to the primary motor cortex for production of voluntary motor behavior.

Summary

The structural and functional neuroanatomy presented in this chapter conceptualizes brain function as building sequentially on the structure and function of lower and more fundamental areas of the brain. An intact brainstem allows normal function of the reticular system, which allows normal function of the diencephalon, limbic system, and basal ganglia, that facilitate activity in the neocortex. All of these areas are necessary for the higher cortical functions that characterize the cognition, emotion, and behavior upon which normal functioning and neuropsychiatric health are built. In the chapters that follow, we will examine several fundamental neuropsychiatric functions and problems, using the basic framework presented here to relate clinical phenomena to the underlying anatomy.

3

Basic cognition

Introduction

Broadly defined, cognition includes all those mental processes associated with thinking. More specifically, cognition refers to the essential processes by which things are known, such as perception, attention, memory, recognition, language, imagination, reasoning, planning, and judgment. Cognition is the process of making sense of sensory inputs, of remembering events and procedures, of making generalizations, analogies, and explanations, and of developing means of communication. The cognitive mental status examination (detailed in Chapter 9) is designed in such a way that these functions may be divided into their simplest elements (attention, language, memory, praxis, recognition (or gnosis), and the "higher cortical functions" or complex cognition) both for the purposes of scientific inquiry and clinical evaluation. When functioning in any of these major domains is impaired, a cognitive disorder must be considered in the differential diagnosis.

Many neuropsychiatric disorders (e.g., schizophrenia, major depression, traumatic brain injury, Parkinson's disease, etc.) produce cognitive disturbances, and in some of these illnesses impaired cognition is an essential feature of the presentation. For example, patients with schizophrenia typically demonstrate disturbances in perception (hallucinations), concentration and early working memory, some aspects of language, and may have serious problems in reasoning, judgment, and other aspects of complex cognition. Interestingly, despite having clear impairments in cognition, such patients have not been regarded as suffering from a cognitive disorder per se; at least not since Kraeplin's description of this problem as dementia praecox. Nonetheless, cognitive impairments are common among patients with schizophrenia, often significantly affecting their functional abilities and clinical outcome, particularly as reflected in their ability to live independently, to participate meaningfully in planning, and to adhere to treatment.

An understanding of the basic elements of cognition, the terms used to describe them, and the presentation of impairments in each major cognitive domain is prerequisite to any discussion of neuropsychiatric syndromes. Hence, in this chapter we will focus on the basic elements of cognition and the language used to describe disorders of impaired cognition. In Chapter 4, we will define complex cognition and its disorders. Although a select set of neuropsychiatric disorders that involve impaired cognition (e.g., delirium, dementia, apathy) are presented in detail in later chapters, we will conclude our discussion of basic and complex cognition with a brief overview of the clinical implications and management issues relevant to the care of patients with cognitive disorders. This discussion will be, by design, rather brief since many of the same issues are reiterated in later chapters on delirium, dementia, motivation and apathy, and traumatic brain injury. As in Chapter 2, we have organized the material according to a relative hierarchy of function, beginning with the more basic functions and then proceeding through those of increasing complexity.

Arousal

Arousal, or level of consciousness, is a function of the activity of the reticular formation, including brainstem and thalamic components and their projections throughout the brain. Clinically, levels of arousal are usually described using terms such as alertness, somnolence, lethargy, obtundation, stupor, semi-coma, and coma. Although definitions have been offered for each of these terms, clinical use of each term does not always follow its formal definition and can be quite confusing. Additionally, such language is not particularly useful to describe patients who are not only alert but also hyperaroused, as in some deliria and in mania. Consequently, we echo the suggestion of Strub & Black (1985) that use of any qualitative term should be accompanied by a brief description of: (1) the level of stimulus (verbal, physical, and/or noxious physical) necessary to arouse the patient; and (2) the patient's behavioral response (becomes alert, meaningfully engages, responds unintelligibly, withdraws, and/or does not respond) to the stimulus. For example, a patient would be most helpfully described as "somnolent: aroused easily to verbal stimulation, meaningfully engaged with the interviewer during the examination, and gradually returned to sleep upon conclusion of the examination." This type of statement provides a clear picture of the patient's ability to respond to and engage with the environment.

Attention

Attention is the ability to focus the brain's conscious activity on a stimulus or a task. Attention is needed for functions such as conversations, reading, watching a television program, or creating a train of thought. Impairments in attention include a loss of selective (or "phasic") attention, sustained attention (or concentration), or both. The ability to shift attention, sometimes referred to as multitasking, is also considered by some researchers to be a function of attention.

Selective attention appears to be a more basic function than sustained attention. Selective attention is the process by which one selects a target stimulus upon which to focus. Clinically, this function is demonstrated by the ability to focus attention on a meaningful and relevant stimulus in the environment and to exclude from attention those stimuli that are irrelevant (see Chapter 9). Selective attention is most dependent on the brain's level of arousal, which is mediated by ascending activating input from the reticular formation, but also requires thalamic, hippocampal, and prefrontal functions that filter irrelevant sensory and cognitive stimuli information and direct attention to those that are relevant based on their emotional, motivational, or "survival" valence (see Chapter 5). Additionally, normal selective attention further involves a complex network of structures comprised by the reticular formation, hippocampal formation, thalamus, frontal lobes, and also the right parietal lobe to filter and direct attention, and then to begin holding (sustaining) that information so that it may be considered and acted upon.

Sustained attention (or concentration) is predicated on selective attention, in that once the initial focus on a stimulus occurs, the focus on that stimulus is maintained over a period of time and even in the face of additional competing stimuli. This function provides not only concentration, but also freedom from distraction. Clinically, sustained attention is evidenced by the ability to maintain attention on a simple task such as counting (Trail Making Test part A), and is believed to be a prerequisite for new learning (or memory). Although sustained attention is a basic cognitive function, it is also highly dependent on the interaction between the reticular formation, subcortical structures, medial temporal structures, frontal lobes, and right parietal lobe. Damage to any part of this network can disrupt sustained attention and produce functional impairment, either decreasing the duration of concentration or increasing susceptibility to distraction.

Though the type and degree of impaired attention varies based on the location and severity of the disturbance causing it, such impairments are commonly produced by neurological and medical problems (see Chapter 12). However, it is important to recognize that most patients do not typically suffer a complete failure in selective and sustained attention, but instead demonstrate some degree of incomplete or variable impairment. Consequently, the deficits with which attentionally impaired patients present may be subtle, and may require detailed testing of selective and sustained attention to demonstrate both their presence and severity.

Impairment of the basic function of attention predictably results in deficits in more complex cognition. Often, the apparent memory problems reported by patients are simply the direct consequence of impaired selective and sustained attention. Since attention is necessary for registration of information, it is crucial to the development of working memory. By failing to attend to stimuli adequately, such patients do not sufficiently register the information and encode it for later recall. The evaluation, if not also the actual functions, of language, praxis, recognition, and more complex cognition all similarly depend on relatively normal attention.

Language

Language is the means by which symbolic communication (verbal or written) occurs. Its constituent elements include: (1) fluency, the ability to produce spontaneous grammatically normal language without undue word-finding pauses; (2) comprehension, the ability to recognize auditory or written symbols as language and to understand and interpret them; (3) repetition, the ability to repeat verbal or written language without error; and (4) naming, the ability to attach a symbolic label to an object in the environment regardless of the sensory mode through which it is presented (which distinguishes this function from recognition, which is discussed later). A basic schematic diagram relating these areas to their underlying neuroanatomy is illustrated in Figure 3.1; each of these language functions is further described in Chapter 9.

Aphasia

Aphasia is the loss or impairment of language due to brain damage of any etiology. Essential to this definition is an understanding of language as the ability to handle (encode, decode, and interpret) the symbols used within a cultural group for the communication of feelings, thoughts, and information. The

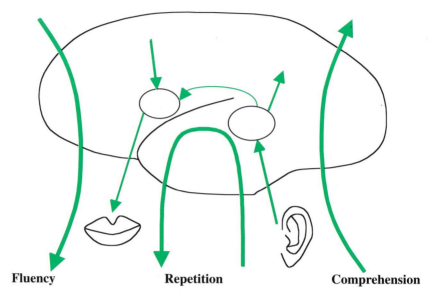

Fluency   **Repetition**   **Comprehension**

Figure 3.1 A schematic representation of language areas and their connections. Three discrete language pathways are defined: a motor/fluency pathway – motor association cortex to Broca's area to output via speech or writing; a sensory/comprehension pathway – sensory input to Wernicke's area to secondary and tertiary association areas; and a repetition pathway – input to Wernicke's area, then to Broca's area via the arcuate fasciculus, then output. Importantly, the repetition pathway can operate even when higher comprehension or motor planning areas are impaired, sometimes producing a parrot-like repetition (or echolalia) of information by patients so affected.

types of communication at issue are spoken or written, and the person with aphasia is understood to have lost the neural circuitry coding for language in motor areas, sensory areas, or both.

The concept of aphasia was first introduced in 1861 by Broca when he described a patient who had lost the ability to speak following damage to the left frontal lobe. This description was the first of its kind, and set the stage for correlating clinical behavior with anatomy, especially with regard to lateralization of hemisphere function and language. Wernicke followed in 1874 with a description of a different form of language disruption resulting from posterior injury, thereby illustrating an anterior/posterior dichotomy in language function. However, this concept of aphasia lost favor from the early 1900s through the 1960s and was replaced by a "holistic" concept. The "holistic" theory vaguely localized language to the thalamus, with variation in individual presentations produced by damage to associated areas. It also regarded language as a single, unitary, nondivisible function.

A return to our current localizationist approach followed from the work of Geschwind during the 1960s, when he clearly demonstrated that disconnnection of dominant hemisphere cortical areas produces distinctive language impairments. This approach has since been expanded in the fields of cognitive science, linguistics, artificial intelligence, neuropsychology and medicine, and has most recently incorporated neuroimaging to increase the power of structural/functional correlates of language.

Aphasia syndromes

The aphasias represent a collection of distinct language impairments with specific neuroanatomic correlates. Though rarely seen in their pure form in clinical practice, they are described so herein (see Figure 3.2). Additional discussion of the neurobiology and evaluation of the aphasias is included in Chapter 9. Current terminology and classification of aphasias is based on the work of the Boston Aphasia Group (Benson, 1981), although a few additional language disturbances are also presented in the following list.

- *Broca's* – non-fluent, non-repeating, intact comprehension (though relational words may be poorly understood), +/− naming, impaired writing, +/− impaired reading.

    Pathology: dominant frontal opercular area; usually associated with right-sided weakness.

    When Broca's aphasia occurs after strokes involving only the cortex, prognosis for some recovery of fluency is better than when there is also deep involvement (e.g., basal ganglia or internal capsule injury).

- *Wernicke's* – fluent (with paraphasias), non-repeating, non-comprehending, +/− naming, impaired reading and writing.

    Pathology: posterior superior temporal lobe/superior temporal gyrus; may therefore also be associated with superior quandrantanopia.

- *Conduction* – fluent, non-repeating, comprehending, +/− naming (often due to paraphasic intrusions), fair reading comprehension (though reading aloud presents a problem), impaired writing.

    Pathology: anterior inferior parietal lobe or supramarginal gyrus or arcuate fasciculus; may be associated with cortical sensory loss, and paresis or visual field defects.

Type of aphasia	Fluency	Repetition	Comprehension	Naming
1. Broca's	Impaired	Impaired	Normal	Impaired
2. Wernicke's	Normal	Impaired	Impaired	Impaired
3. Conduction	Normal	Impaired	Normal	Impaired
4. Transcortical Motor	Impaired	Normal	Normal	Impaired (mildly)
5. Transcortical Sensory	Normal	Normal	Impaired	Impaired (mildly)
6. Mixed Transcortical	Impaired	Normal	Impaired	Impaired
7. Global	Impaired	Impaired	Impaired	Impaired
8. Anomic	Normal	Normal	Normal	Impaired

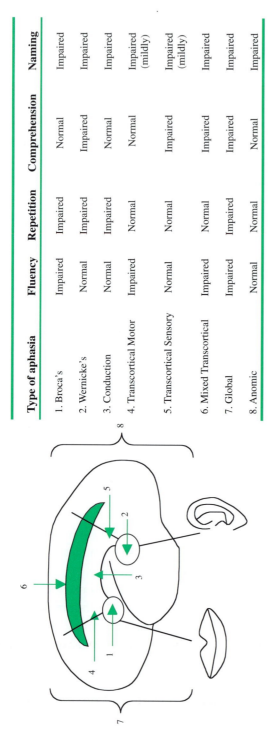

Figure 3.2 Lesions of the language areas and their connections, with accompanying table outlining the classic aphasia syndromes associated with damage to these areas.

- *Global* – all modalities impaired.

  Pathology: dominant hemisphere damage, most often middle cerebral artery infarct; usually associated with contralateral hemiplegia and hemiparesis.
- *Transcortical Aphasias* – the primary distinguishing factor of these aphasias is the ability to repeat spoken language in the face of distinct language impairment. These aphasias illustrate repetition as a linguistically distinct function.
    (i) *Transcortical motor*, like Broca's, but with intact repetition.

      Pathology: supplementary motor area or in tissue connecting it to the frontal opercular area.
   (ii) *Transcortical sensory*, like Wernicke's, but with intact repetition.

      Pathology: angular gyrus.
  (iii) *Mixed transcortical*, global, but with intact repetition.

      Pathology: vascular border zone in frontal and parietal areas.
- *Anomic* – primary problem is word-finding difficulties.

  Pathology: not consistent, though seen with injury to the dominant hemisphere angular gyrus; may be associated with alexia or agraphia.
- *Subcortical* – usually initiated with a period of mutism, then abnormal speech (hypophonia and articulation problems); finally, variable picture of aphasia, with impairment in several modalities while relatively sparing repetition.

  Pathology: variable, but subcortical; prognosis for recovery better if lesion is entirely subcortical, worse if more extensive (i.e., additional cortical involvement).
- *Amelodia* – "motor aprosodia" or flat, monotonous speech, with no ability to produce melody when singing, sparse use of gestures, and decreased facial grimacing; whether aprosodias such as this constitute a separate class of disorders or instead simply reflect damage to the prosodic elements of language predicated on non-dominant hemisphere function is a matter of some debate; for simplicity, we include this problem in our discussion of language disorders.

  Pathology: non-dominant frontal opercular area; may be associated with depression; an apparently "depressed" patient with this finding deserves neuroimaging of the brain as otherwise "silent" infarctions of this area are possible.
- *Verbal dysdecorum* – decreased ability to monitor and control contents of verbal output; often confabulates; consequently, seems socially inappropriate.

Pathology: non-dominant frontal lateral convexity; may present to psychiatrist with primary complaint of inability to keep/make friends; often difficult to treat, but underlying cause should be addressed to prevent further injury, if possible.

Memory

Memory is a general term for the mental processes that allow individuals to store experiences and perceptions for recall at a later time. While memory may be described in a number of ways (verbal vs. visual, declarative vs. procedural, etc.), we will offer only a general overview of memory function and its major categorizations in this section, and defer a more detailed discussion to the chapter on mental status examination. We will first describe memory in terms of three useful temporal distinctions: immediate; recent; and remote. We will then briefly present a categorization of memory with respect to its underlying neurobiology.

Immediate (or "working") memory is predicated on attention and language. While, sustained attention is characterized by the ability to maintain one's focus on a stimulus, immediate memory is characterized by the ability to briefly maintain focus on the content of that stimulus after it has been withdrawn from the environment (e.g., keeping the stimulus "in mind"). For example, on the Folstein Mini-Mental State Examination (Folstein et al., 1975), the task of registering and immediately repeating three items is a task of immediate memory. This function may also be assessed using other registration tasks such as digit span.

Recent memory is a complex function, and is dependent on attention, language, memory, emotion, and on some aspects of complex cognition. Recent memory may be most easily assessed by determining the patient's orientation to person, place, time, and situation. In other words, remembering who, where, when, and why are all elements of recent (and, in particular, declarative) memory. This function may also be assessed by the patient's ability to recall the short list of items used to assess immediate memory after a delay of several minutes.

It is important to note that orientation alone should not be used as an index of memory or as the sole measure of a patient's mental status, as is too often the case in many evaluations in hospital or clinic settings. Among delirious patients, impaired orientation to year, month, and place is not universal, thus if only these items are used to assess recent memory a large number of delirious patients will go unrecognized.

Assessment of memory using tasks that require new learning during an examination may produce results that are more clearly referable to recent memory than are those regarding orientation. Although these tasks are described in Chapter 9 ('Mental status examination'), the method of clinically assessing recent memory that we use combines orientation to person, place, time, and situation with registration and recall of three items (two complex items and one abstract item, such as "apple pie, red Cadillac, honesty"). With regard to the three items, we prefer to use complex objects that may be recalled in parts (e.g., "apple") or misrecalled ("red car"), and to use an abstract object for which encoding and recall cannot be obviously facilitated by visualization. We find this method is relatively more sensitive to subtle memory impairments than the use of three simple and concrete objects. In addition to recent verbal memory, recent visual memory and procedural memory should also be assessed, as deficits in these areas may have implications for the differential diagnosis of the cause of memory impairment. Methods for assessment of these functions are included in Chapter 9.

Remote memory is the most complex form of memory, and is dependent on normal functioning of attention, language, and the other memory functions. Without question, it is the aspect of memory that is most difficult to separate not only from the more basic functions upon which its development is predicated, but especially from other aspects of complex cognition required for retrieval, manipulation, and application of remote memories. At the bedside, remote memory is most commonly assessed by asking the patient to recall events of both a personal and historical nature. Personal events must be verifiable by a reliable source other than the patient; performance of recall on historical information must be interpreted in the context of the patient's intelligence, education, and social experience.

As has been repeated several times in the preceding sections, the proper function of memory depends on a large number of brain structures, and is predicated on attention and language (hence the discussion of memory at this point in this chapter). Structures identified as critical to memory are the amygdala, hippocampus, mammillary bodies, thalamus, sensory cortices, secondary and tertiary (parietal) association areas, and prefrontal cortices, at least as regards episodic memory (that of events with temporal and spatial characteristics, often heavily dependent on language). The mechanisms by which memories are encoded and retrieved are complex, but may be simplistically viewed as requiring the activity and integration of several sub-systems.

First, an intact medial temporal system capable of assigning affective valence to incoming stimuli in order to prioritize stimuli for attention and encoding is required. This function is most likely dependent on the activity of the extended amygdala, without which there may be impairments in learning of emotionally important information (that which is relatively important for future survival) – not surprisingly, this function is sometimes referred to as "emotional learning" and may be deficient in disorders in which there is significant amygdala injury (e.g., Klüver–Bucy syndrome).

Second, the hippocampal formation (including the amygdala) is needed to hold, integrate, and begin encoding complex multimodal sensory and cognitive information via a process referred to as long-term potentiation. Although the exact mechanisms by which this process operates in humans is not yet fully understood, the general idea of this process is that the hippocampus first stores incoming information by facilitating the establishment of a temporary neural network to represent the stimulus being encoded. This almost certainly involves the dorsolateral prefrontal and anterior cingulate-subcortical circuits and projections to and from all of the areas of association cortex relevant to the stimulus. In so doing, temporally and contextually associated stimuli from multiple sensory, emotional, and cognitive domains are simultaneously represented within the network. In response to: (1) repeated presentation of these stimuli; (2) strong affective loading of stimuli; (3) similarity of new stimuli to previously encoded material (permitting association within already established networks); or (4) a combination of these and other factors, relatively stable associative neural networks are developed via strengthening of the synaptic connections between groups of neurons within the network. Although multiple neurotransmitters are possibly involved in this process, N-methyl-D-aspartate (NMDA) receptors within, and connected to efferents from, the hippocampus have received much attention for their role in long-term potentiation. Importantly, these distributed memory networks are not themselves hippocampal, but instead appear to involve distributed networks linking sensory, heteromodal association, motor, limbic and paralimbic areas, and prefrontal cortices.

Third, frontal-subcortical circuits (discussed further in chapter 4) are required for the organization and retrieval of memories via activation of these representational neural networks. Although the frontal-subcortical circuits are needed for free recall of encoded material, it appears that their processing of recalled information may be facilitated by responses to either ongoing internal processes or via activation of these networks by new external stimuli, particularly those with high emotional (or survival) value. External stimuli that are similar to ones previously experienced and encoded appear to activate these networks relatively automatically, which may be the basis for a variety of experiential phenomena ranging from simple learning to the pathological intrusive memories of posttraumatic stress disorder.

Disorders of memory

Identifying the various roles for the elements of memory systems and the clinical phenomena that they underlie becomes important when one wishes to create a differential diagnosis for the various memory disorders seen in clinical practice. For example, bilateral amygdala damage will decrease the ability to learn emotionally important material and to respond appropriately to stimuli with significant survival value; however, it may have a much more attenuated effect on declarative memory if the damage does not also affect the hippocampi. For example, a patient with bilateral amygdala damage (i.e., Klüver–Bucy syndrome) cannot associate newly presented and previously known dangerous stimuli. This may result in a condition referred to as *psychic blindness*, in which the patient repeatedly places himself in danger despite being able to articulate the risk of so doing. The failure to avoid danger appears to be due to a failure to learn or appropriately recall the emotional or survival importance of stimuli and not one of simple amnesia for the stimuli.

By contrast, a patient with pure bilateral hippocampal injury may retain the capacity for affective responding and learning, but lose the ability to develop declarative (language based) memories. Clinically these patients will demonstrate impairments in encoding of new material, and consequently also in recent recall (one cannot recall that which was never learned). By contrast to the hippocampally-injured patient, those with frontal-subcortical dysfunction may be able to encode new material, but often exhibit difficulty with spontaneous recall (suggesting mild impairment) and/or recognition (suggesting more severe impairment). Such differences are relatively important when trying to distinguish between an Alzheimer's type dementia (impaired encoding) and the memory impairment more typical of Parkinson's disease or other disorders involving frontal-subcortical dysfunction (impaired spontaneous retrieval which improves with semantic or recognition cues, suggesting relatively preserved encoding).

Many other neuropsychiatric disorders produce impairment in memory, either transiently or permanently and often in a relatively classic pattern. For example, alcohol amnestic disorder (Korsakoff's psychosis) is the result of microinfarctions of the outflow tracts from the hippocampi (see Chapter 17). In this condition, although the hippocampus itself may be able to participate in the direction of attention and initiate its own internal processes related to the encoding of memories (long-term potentiation), the outflow tract from the hippocampus is interrupted and consequently new information cannot be encoded in the appropriate association areas or network. As a result, these patients are profoundly amnestic with respect to new learning, although immediate memory (registration) remains relatively intact.

In the *Diagnostic and Statistical Manual of Mental Disorders*, 4th edition, referred to as DSM-IV (American Psychiatric Association, 1994), amnestic disorders are characterized by impairment in memory in the absence of other significant cognitive impairments. Individuals with an amnestic disorder are most often impaired in their ability to learn new information (anterograde amnesia). Less often, they are unable to recall previously learned information or past events (retrograde amnesia). This rule – that anterograde memory deficits are typically more severe than retrograde memory deficits – is known as Ribot's law. The feature that distinguishes this problem from dementia is the absence of other impairments such as inattention, aphasia, apraxia, agnosia, dysexecutive functioning and the like.

As noted above, the ability to recall new information is almost always impaired in an amnestic disorder. Problems in recall of previously learned information are much more variable, and dependent on the locus and extent of neuronal injury. Although there are a few reported cases of selective retrograde amnesia due to anterior temporal damage, in general the loss of remote memory without concurrent loss of new learning (recent memory) should be regarded with caution, as it may possibly be a conversion symptom (i.e., conversion disorder). This phenomena violates Ribot's law, and is sometimes described as "soap opera amnesia" – although we certainly do not advocate the use of this fairly judgmental term clinically, it is a helpful phrase by which to remember the difference between a memory disorder and more "hysterical" amnestic symptoms.

Amnestic disorders are often preceded by an evolving clinical picture that includes confusion and disorientation, occasionally with attention problems that suggest a delirium. Confabulation, often evidenced by the recitation of imaginary or partially true events, may be noted and is easily misinterpreted as delusional thinking. Rather than volitional or delusional attempts at deception, confabulation probably represents the patient's best effort to offer a meaningful response given severe memory deficits and, at best, fragmentary recollection of information. Profound amnesia may result in disorientation to time and place, but rarely to self. Frequently, patients have little insight into their amnesia despite fairly severe impairments, and confrontation of the patient may lead to paranoid accusations by the patient against their confronter or others.

Quantitative neuropsychological testing is often helpful in characterizing the specific nature and extent of the memory impairment, and may be quite helpful in treatment planning. Some individuals will have greater difficulty with either visual or auditory memory, and when preservation of function exists in a specific domain, compensatory strategies may be devised to capitalize on that strength.

Treatment of amnestic disorders follows the rule "treat the underlying cause." Cerebrovascular events, traumatic brain injury, neurotoxic exposure, tumor, infection (e.g., herpes encephalitis), substance abuse, sustained nutritional deficiency, and surgery are all in the differential diagnosis for etiologies of amnestic disorders. Clearly, the treatment will vary greatly depending on the cause, and consultation with the appropriate specialty (neurology, medicine, neurosurgery, etc.) may be required to institute definitive therapy; additional issues in treatment are discussed at the end of Chapter 4.

Praxis

Praxis is the ability to integrate comprehension and execution of a task. Consequently, the apraxias (or, when mild, dyspraxias) are acquired impairments of skilled purposeful movement despite intact motor function, sensory function, and comprehension of the purposeful movement at issue. Clinically, apraxia represents a failure to integrate comprehension and execution of a specific task on command, although in its severest form such failures may also occur spontaneously (for example, a dressing apraxia in a severely demented patient might leave the individual unable to independently dress each morning).

Praxis appears to be a dominant hemisphere function – skilled purposeful movements are neurally represented in a fashion and location relatively similar to language. Movement "memories," "engrams," or "maps" are principally coded in the dominant hemisphere circuitry. Injury to this circuitry seems to result in loss of the integrated representations of purposeful movements, and therefore an inability to "retrieve" the necessary motor (procedural) memories for these movements. Viewed in this fashion, apraxia can be thought of, in a very rudimentary way, as a motoric form of memory dysfunction – patients lose memory for "how" a task is performed. Conversely, apraxias may be likened to executive functions (discussed in Chapter 4) in that patients appear to suffer impairment in the planning, sequencing, organization, and initiation of purposeful movements Not surprisingly, the apraxias are commonly encountered with both aphasia, especially non-fluent aphasia, and dysexecutive function given the overlap of praxis maps with the frontal opercular area and dorsolateral prefrontal cortex.

Apraxia syndromes

- *Limb-kinetic* – loss of the usual agility, efficiency, and precision of the affected side, frequently manifest in tasks involving fine coordination or demanding motor skills (e.g., picking up objects, dressing, pantomiming).

  Pathology: contralateral premotor area, specifically interrupting the corticospinal tracts at the level of the cortex.
- *Ideomotor* – failure to carry out motor acts on verbal command despite intact comprehension, normal strength, and easy spontaneous performance of the same act; the best example of disconnection between understanding an act and its performance; the term specifically refers to difficulty performing a single task (for example, "take this piece of paper in your right hand") rather than a sequence of acts (as on the Mini-Mental State Examination, "take this piece of paper in your right hand, fold it in half, and place it on the table").

  This is the most common form of apraxia, and may be evident in limbs, axial, or facial musculature; it is usually bilateral; since neural coding for these movements is in the dominant hemisphere, an insult to that hemisphere will result in loss of coded information for execution on both sides of the body.

  This form of apraxia is most clinically obvious when asking the patient to pantomime tasks; typically, patients are better able to imitate or spontaneously perform the commanded action, although with more severe apraxia this is less true.

Several forms of *ideomotor apraxia* exist, and warrant individual discussion:
- *Buccofacial* – difficulty in voluntary oral/facial movements, such as blowing out a match.

    Pathology: left frontal operculum; frequently seen with aphasia.
- *Limb* – disconnection of cortical areas, resulting in difficulty with hand/arm or leg movements.

    Pathology: left perisylvian area, or anterior corpus callosum.

    Callosal (sympathetic) apraxia (special case of limb apraxia), in which apraxia is seen in the nonparetic left hand. This is thought to reflect left hemisphere damage to either "memory" circuitry for the movements, or damage to tracts communicating these patterns from left hemisphere to right hemisphere (i.e., the corpus callosum). Interestingly, in patients where the damage is in the left portion of the anterior corpus callosum, this apraxia may only be evident in the left hand, with intact function of the right hand.
- *Axial* – disconnection of relevant cortical areas needed for integration and execution of axial movements.

    Pathology: lesion of the arcuate fasciculus, or left temporal lobe; frequently presents with comorbid conduction aphasia.
- *Ideational* – failure to perform voluntary sequential motor acts even when each constituent act can be performed in isolation; example of such a sequence might include folding a letter, putting it in the envelope, sealing it, and putting a stamp on it, although the patient is capable of any one of these tasks alone; represents a defect in overall planning, and among the apraxias it is the most comparable to executive impairment.

    Pathology: not well-defined, as it may occur in frontal, bifrontal, and parietal damage, though again left hemisphere injury to distributed praxis "memories" or "maps" may be implicated as well.

Agnosia

From gnosis, meaning knowledge, the term agnosia (absence of knowledge) was coined by Freud in 1891 in his early monograph on aphasia. Fundamentally, an agnosia is an acquired impairment of recognition in which a normal percept (an item being perceived) appears to have been stripped of its meaning. It is usually seen in a given patient in only one sensory modality at a time, and is manifest by the patient's inability to recognize (or name) an object presented in only that modality. Unlike aphasia, however, when the object is presented in a different sensory modality, it can be correctly recognized and named (i.e., its language representation is not lost, only its neural representation in a single modality).

The agnosias can be grossly divided into apperceptive and associative types. Apperception refers to the synthesis of sensory elements into a unified mental "image," where association refers to the matching of a mental "image" with previously encoded images. Agnosias are generally classified by affected sensory modality.

Agnosia syndromes

- *Visual* – a failure to recognize visually presented objects.
  - (i) *apperceptive*, parts of objects are seen, but a unified image cannot be synthesized, and therefore the object is not recognized.

    Pathology: usually seen with bilateral occipital lesions with partial cortical sparing.
  - (ii) *associative*, can recognize, draw, copy, and match multiple presented objects, but cannot accurately identify these objects; may appear clinically like a sort of "memory failure" (often Mr. Magoo-like) for visual items.

    Pathology: best thought of as verbal–visual disconnection; may be seen with occipitotemporal damage.

  Special examples of visual agnosia:
  - (i) *prosopagnosia*, failure to recognize familiar faces despite knowing that the percept is a face and can point out its features; it is usually associated with other visual agnosias, including simultagnosia (see below); it has been suggested that prosopagnosia may be a special case of simultagnosia for faces;

    Pathology: appears to be bilateral ventromesial occipitotemporal lesions, although it may be seen in patients with only right hemisphere lesions.
  - (ii) *central achromatopsia*, inability to identify colors despite otherwise intact visual recognition; may occur only in affected hemi-field.

    Pathology: classically, central achromatopsia results from injury to the inferior occipitotemporal region either of the right hemisphere (causing a fairly pure left hemiachromatopsia) or the left hemisphere (in which case it may be associated with *alexia*, or difficulty reading).

(iii) *simultagnosia*, failure to synthesize elements of an object into a whole image even though the constituent elements can be properly identified.

Pathology: may be seen following injury to the inferolateral portion of the dominant hemisphere or bilateral injury to the superior visual association cortices.

(iv) *alexia (without agraphia)*, a visual agnosia for written words, despite otherwise intact language functions, in which the patient loses the ability to read; while the patient may retain the ability to write but still not be able to read that which they have just written.

Pathology: injury to the left visual cortex and the pathways from the right visual cortex to language areas of the dominant hemisphere.

- *Auditory* – a failure to identify items when presented in the auditory domain only, but not if presented using other sensory (tactile, visual, olfactory) modalities. This is distinct from aphasia, in which the item cannot be identified regardless of the modality of its presentation because the language representation for the item is lost. For example, a patient (who has been a longstanding cat owner) with one kind of this agnosia (see below) might identify a cat by sight, but be entirely unable to identify a cat by its characteristic "meow."

(i) *apperceptive*, recognizing "what kind" of sound (i.e., sound discrimination).

Pathology: largely a right (nondominant) hemisphere function.

(ii) *associative*, recognizing "what it means" (semantic content).

Pathology: largely a left (dominant) hemisphere function.

Special examples of auditory agnosia:

(i) *pure word deafness*, superficially looks like Wernicke's aphasia with respect to comprehension and fluency, but reading and writing are perfectly intact; hears, but doesn't understand.

Pathology: dominant hemisphere primary auditory cortex is intact but disconnected from its association areas.

(ii) *auditory sound agnosia*, inability to recognize nonverbal sounds (i.e., bells, music, ambient noises).

Pathology: non-dominant primary auditory cortex is disconnected from its association areas.

- *Tactile* – a failure to identify objects by touch despite being able to identify them through other modalities.
    - (i) *apperceptive*, inability to recognize an object by its size, shape, texture, and/or weight.

        Pathology: dysfunction of the postcentral gyrus of the hemisphere contralateral to the side of the body to which the stimulus is presented, although disruption of either ipsilateral and/or contralateral fibers connecting primary somatosensory (tactile) cortex to its secondary association areas in the dominant hemisphere alone can produce an apperceptive tactile agnosia.

    - (ii) *associative*, inability to recognize the type of object presented despite the ability to identify its size, shape, texture, and/or weight.

        Pathology: dysfunction of the posterior parietal cortex of the hemisphere contralateral to the side of the body to which the stimulus is presented, although disruption of either ipsilateral and/or contralateral fibers connecting tactile tertiary association areas and/or to language areas in the dominant hemisphere alone can produce an associative tactile agnosia.

Special examples of tactile agnosia:
- (i) *astereognosis*, probably the most familiar agnosia, it is a form of tactile associative agnosia in which the patient is unable to identify an object placed in one hand using only tactile sensation. For example, when testing for this agnosia clinically, a patient (with eyes closed) asked to identify a paper clip placed in the hand might note its small size, its cool temperature, its smooth surface and curves, its light weight, but be entirely unable to associate these qualities with the object "paperclip." However, with eyes open and visualizing the object, the patient immediately identifies it as a paperclip.

    Pathology: may involve either dominant or nondominant sensory association cortices and their connections to the language areas of the dominant hemisphere; in the case of dominant hemisphere lesions, astereognosis may be seen in both hands.

- (ii) *graphesthesia* is sometimes used to test posterior column function (localization of tactile stimuli), but it also serves as an indicator of possible loss of recognition in the tactile domain when other tests of posterior column function are normal (e.g., proprioception, vibration).

Pathology: if not due to posterior column disease, it is most likely due to the disruption of fibers connecting the secondary tactile association areas to language areas in the dominant hemisphere.

Summary

The basic elements of cognition include arousal, attention, language, memory, praxis, and recognition. Disturbances of the most basic functions of arousal and attention are generally seen in delirious states, and also involve disturbances in more complex cognition. Disorders of language (aphasias), memory (amnesias), praxis (apraxias), and recognition (agnosias) may occur independently, although the homology of their representations in the brain frequently results in their co-occurrence.

These basic functions are not in and of themselves sufficient to permit normal complex cognition. Complex cognition appears to depend on the ability of the prefrontal cortex to integrate, select, and manipulate the information provided by each of the more basic functions. Examples of complex cognition include a fund of information, calculation, problem solving, abstraction, judgment, and insight. Detailed discussion of complex cognition is presented in the next chapter, along with some general treatment strategies for patients with impaired basic or complex cognition.

4

Complex cognition

Introduction

In the preceding chapter we reviewed the "basic" elements of cognition, namely arousal, attention, language, memory, praxis, and recognition. In the model that we have been following, cognition is relatively hierarchically organized in a parallel fashion to the neuroanatomy upon which it is predicated. As stated earlier, the most basic element of our functional neuroanatomy is reticular formation and its diencephalic extensions, which mediate arousal and play an inexorable role in attention. As we move "up" the brain, both the functional neuroanatomy and related cognitive functions become increasingly complex. Eventually, we arrive at the functional neuroanatomy and aspects of cognition that are the focus of this chapter, namely the frontal lobes and complex cognition.

The frontal lobes are the most recently evolved area of the primate brain, and among primates they appear to be most developed in human beings. Even as early as the sixteenth century the size of the frontal areas fostered their recognition as one of the three major "prominences" of the brain. They were subsequently described as discrete "lobes" of the brain by Willis in the seventeenth century. However, clarifying the function of the frontal lobes has been a difficult task that has occupied the work of many basic and clinical researchers over the last 150 years.

By many accounts, the modern task of understanding the function of the frontal lobes in human beings has its clearest beginnings in the case of Phineas Gage reported by Harlow in 1848. Gage, a 25 year-old foreman for the Rutland and Burlington Railroad, Vermont (USA), suffered a serious penetrating brain injury involving (at least) the orbitofrontal lobes when an iron tamping rod was projected through his skull by an explosion. Amazingly, Gage survived his injury – however, he subsequently experienced a remarkable change in his personality. Prior to his injury he had been regarded as a man of "temperate habits, and possessed of considerable energy of character." After his accident,

Gage became "childish, capricious and obstinate," and showed remarkably poor judgment in his interactions with others. Interestingly, despite this change in personality, he appeared to largely retain his previous level of intelligence and motivation, and although he was not consistently employed due to his behavior he was reasonably self-sufficient until his death 13 years later. Similar case studies and a wealth of clinical experience in the century since suggest that his personality change was a direct result of damage to the orbitofrontal lobes.

The case of Phineas Gage is remarkable in many ways, but it is particularly interesting as an illustration of the role of the frontal lobes, particularly with respect to a function that we will refer to herein as "social intelligence." After destruction of the orbitofrontal areas, particularly on the left but probably bilaterally, Gage appears to have developed serious problems with social judgment: he used profanity (a more serious problem in his era), was rude and inconsiderate of others, and had a penchant for acting impulsively at inappropriate times.

Returning to our model for understanding cognition, complex functions such as executive function, social intelligence, and motivation are the products of relatively discrete but complex neuroanatomic circuits involving the prefrontal cortices and several subcortical structures. In general, the neurocircuitry we will describe herein is a useful model for introducing the functional neuroanatomy of complex cognition, but it must be regarded only as a helpful simplification. It is perhaps more accurate to think of the neural substrates of complex cognition as parallel, distributed, and reciprocally interconnected networks built upon the neurocircuitry of more basic aspects of cognition. The relationship between basic and complex cognition is therefore relatively hierarchical. Certainly, disorders of arousal and attention (see Chapter 12) sufficiently disrupt basic cognition such that impairment in these functions almost invariably entails some impairment in one or more aspects of complex cognition. However, the reverse also may occur: disruption of complex cognition often entails disturbances in some aspects of basic cognition. For example, orbitofrontal injuries like that of Phineas Gage frequently result in impairments in sustained attention (distractibility) and in emotional regulation. In other words, affecting the top of the hierarchy does not necessarily leave entirely intact those cognitive functions at the bottom.

In this chapter, we will review "complex" cognitive functions, including executive function, personality/comportment/empathy (which we will refer to as social intelligence), and motivation. During this review, we will echo the suggestion made by many other authors that while the "complex" cognitive functions synthesize and elaborate the activities of the "basic" cognitive functions, they are ultimately inseparable from them. As a detailed discussion of these functions and their putative neurobiological bases is well beyond the scope of this work, our discussion here will be, by necessity, relatively brief. Interested readers are referred to Mega & Cummings (1994) and Mega et al. (1997) for a more detailed review, as much of the model presented here is derived from their cogent synthesis of the scientific literature on the neurocircuitry of complex cognition. We hope that this chapter will summarize some of the important features of complex cognition, the relevant structural and functional neuroanatomy, and the clinical problems that may arise from disturbances in complex cognition.

Defining complex cognition

Complex cognition may be divided into three major areas, executive function, "social intelligence," and motivation. Executive function refers to a collection of abilities including categorization and abstraction, systematic memory searching and information retrieval, information, problem solving, self-direction, independence from external environmental contingencies, maintenance of and fluent shifting between information or behavior sets, use of language to guide behavior, and generation of motor behavior. These functions, and their relation to more basic cognitive functions like new learning, language, and visuospatial skills, constitute the functions that are most immediately regarded as "intelligence." Problems in executive functioning feature prominently and most obviously in the dementias (e.g., frontotemporal dementias and advanced Alzheimer's disease), stroke, traumatic brain injury, and schizophrenia, among others. The serious functional consequences of impaired executive functioning are intuitively evident based on the set of abilities that comprise executive function. However, it should not go unstated that even milder impairments in executive function may seriously interfere with the ability to meet the everyday demands of modern life, particularly as regards, for example, the ability to maintain housing, responsibly manage finances, and provide adequate self-care.

As Gardner (1983) and Goleman (1995) have pointed out, however, intelligence is probably better defined more broadly, including not only the complex information processing provided by executive function, but also social intelligence and the motivation to make use of all of these skills. Accordingly, the second area of complex cognition of interest here is social intelligence, which we define as a collection of abilities that mediate social knowledge and behavior, including social appropriateness, exercising restraint over aggressive, sexual, and appetitive impulses, organizing appropriate grooming behaviors, and developing appropriate empathy for and nurturance of others. These abilities constitute a large portion of what is frequently referred to as comportment, or the way in which one behaves interpersonally or socially.

The third area of complex cognition we will consider is motivation and the conscious experience of emotion. This domain of cognition consists of the ability to integrate executive function and social intelligence with emotion, and to use the products of this process to develop and guide behavior. In this chapter we will describe this cognitive domain only briefly, since we discuss disturbances of motivation (apathy) and also emotion and emotional dysregulation in later chapters.

Neurocircuitry of complex cognition

These three major domains of complex cognition are subserved by three of the five parallel and reciprocally connected frontal-subcortical circuits (the other two subserve "extrapyramidal" motor and eye movements, as noted in Chapter 2). Executive function is mediated by the dorsolateral prefrontal circuit (Figure 4.1), social intelligence is mediated by the lateral orbitofrontal circuit (Figure 4.1), and motivation and the conscious experience of emotion are mediated by the anterior cingulate circuit (Figure 4.2).

Each circuit involves the same basic anatomic elements (Figure 4.3), including the relevant portion of the frontal lobe, the striatum (caudate/putamen), globus pallidus, the substantia nigra, and the thalamus. As a result of this organization, impairments of complex cognition, sometimes also referred to as "frontal lobe syndromes," may result from injuries at locations other than the frontal lobes. Interruption anywhere in these circuits may produce phenomenologically similar "frontal lobe syndromes" independent of a lesion specific to the frontal lobes themselves. Each circuit uses the same basic pattern of excitatory and inhibitory neurotransmitters at each stage of the circuit.

Although the neurocircuitry is substantially more complex than this very simple representation suggests (see Figure 4.4) and is, at the present time, incompletely understood, the basic neurocircuitry involves:

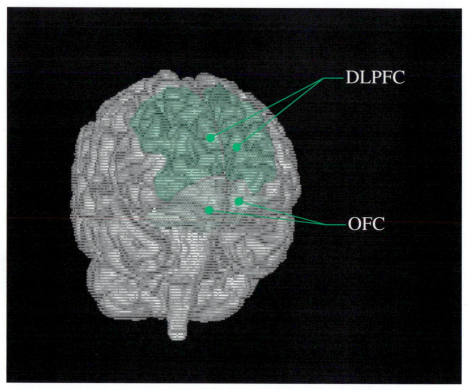

Figure 4.1 Three-dimensional reconstruction of the brain, anterior view. Shaded areas roughly indicate the dorsolateral prefrontal cortices (DLPFC) and orbitofrontal cortices (OFC).

(1) dopaminergic (excitatory) inputs from the ventral tegmental area to the frontal lobes;

(2) glutamatergic (excitatory) projections from the frontal lobes to the striatum and serotonergic (functionally inhibitory) projections from the dorsal raphe nucleus to the striatum;

(3) GABA-ergic (inhibitory) projections from the striatum to the globus pallidus (interna and externa) and substantia nigra;

(4) GABA-ergic (inhibitory) projections from the globus pallidus externa to the subthalamic nucleus;

(5) glutamatergic (excitatory) projections from the subthalamic nucleus to the globus pallidus interna;

(6) GABA-ergic (inhibitory) projections from the globus pallidus interna to the thalamus;

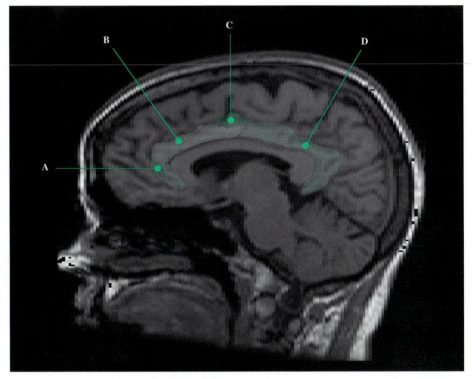

Figure 4.2 Sagittal view of the cingulate gyrus and its major divisions: the infracallosal cingulate or visceral effector region (A), the anterior cingulate or cognitive effector region (B), the skeletomotor effector region (C), and the posterior cingulate or sensory processing region (D).

(7) glutamatergic (excitatory) projections from the thalamus back to the frontal lobes.

The relative anatomic positions of the frontal cortices are preserved in the topography of each circuit, including the topography within the subcortical nuclei. As a result, small injuries to the subcortical and white matter tracts within the circuits may produce relatively discrete dysfunction in one, but not all, of the frontal-subcortical circuits.

These frontal-subcortical circuits operate in parallel, and all make use of the same basic set of neurotransmitters at parallel sites in the circuit. As a result, augmenting the function of a neurotransmitter in one circuit with a medication (e.g., a selective serotonin reuptake inhibitor, or SSRI) may have unwanted effects on the function of a parallel loop. For example, decreasing

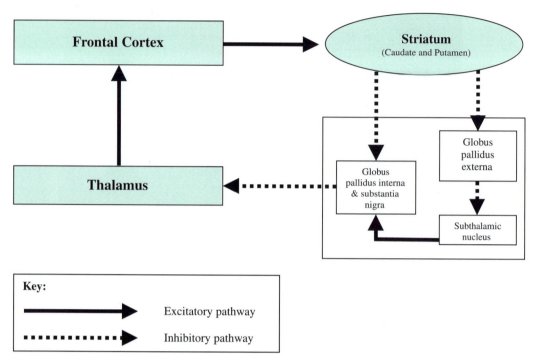

Figure 4.3 General outline of frontal-subcortical circuitry.

the over activity of the orbitofrontal cortex (as in obsessive–compulsive disorder) with an SSRI may have the intended effect of decreasing cognitive activity related to social intelligence (e.g., obsessing about sex or aggression). However, this same treatment may have the unintended consequence of simultaneously diminishing activity in the anterior cingulate circuit, thereby decreasing motivation and the conscious experience of emotion.

Dorsolateral prefrontal circuit

This circuit originates from the dorsolateral prefrontal cortex (DLPFC, Brodmann areas 9 and 10). Figure 4.5 offers a rough illustration of this circuit in the context of an axial magnetic resonance image (MRI) of the brain. Connections from the DLPFC project to the dorsolateral head of the caudate. From the caudate, there are two principal projections that form the direct and

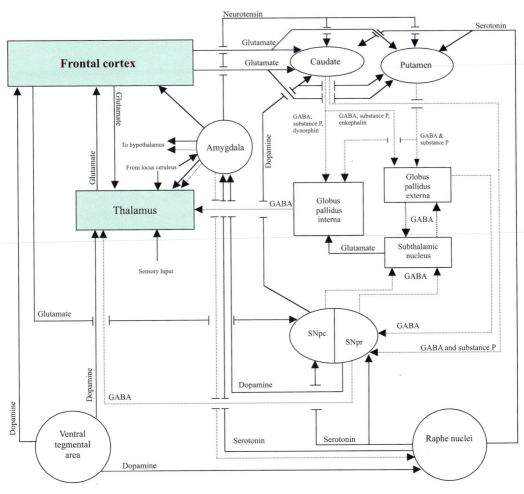

Figure 4.4 A more complex schematic diagram of the neurocircuitry of complex cognition. Complex though it may appear, even this diagram is, at best, a tremendous over simplification of networks involved in complex cognition. Solid lines indicate excitatory connections, dashed lines indicate inhibitory connections. Of note, the serotonergic afferents to the striatum (caudate and putamen) appear, in this model, to effect behavioral inhibition. Abbreviations: GABA, gamma-aminobutyric acid; SNpc, substantia nigra pars compacta; SNpr, substantia nigra pars reticulata.

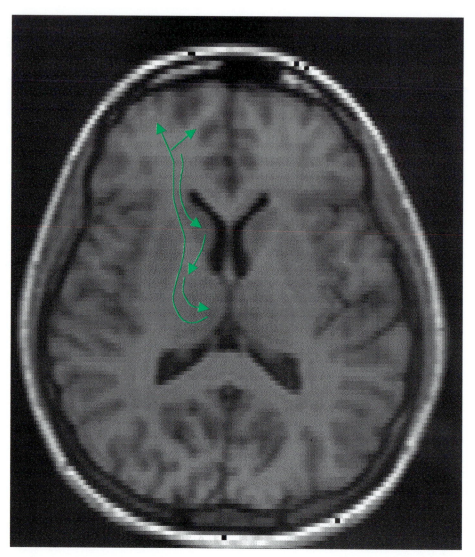

Figure 4.5 A schematic depiction of the dorsolateral prefrontal-subcortical circuit. This axial magnetic resonance image depicts the approximate pathway of this circuit, from right dorsolateral prefrontal cortex (DLPFC, superior and middle frontal gyri) to striatum (caudate), to globus pallidus (not shown), to thalamus, and back to the DLPFC.

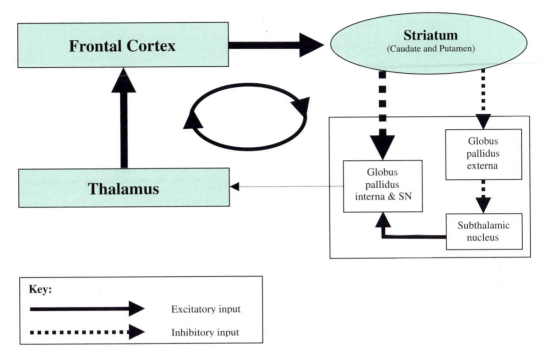

Figure 4.6 An illustration of the functional effects of activity in the direct basal ganglia pathway. Frontal input increases striatal inhibitory output to the globus pallidus interna and substantia nigra (SN). Inhibitory output from these structures to the thalamus is therefore reduced, and the thalamus is disinhibited. Excitatory thalamic output drives the frontal cortex to continue firing, and the circuit is perpetuated (as depicted by the circle in the center of the diagram).

indirect basal ganglia pathways, the different effects of which are illustrated in Figures 4.6 and 4.7, respectively.

The direct pathway consists of the globus pallidus interna (mediodorsal portion) and the substantia nigra pars reticulata (rostrolateral portion). When the caudate receives excitatory input from the DLPFC, it sends inhibitory input into the direct pathway, the effect of which is reciprocal disinhibition of the thalamus, and therefore perpetuation of this activity is this circuit (Figure 4.6).

Activity of the direct pathway is balanced by activity of the indirect pathway. The indirect pathway consists of the globus pallidus externa (dorsal portion), the subthalamic nucleus (lateral portion), and their return to the globus

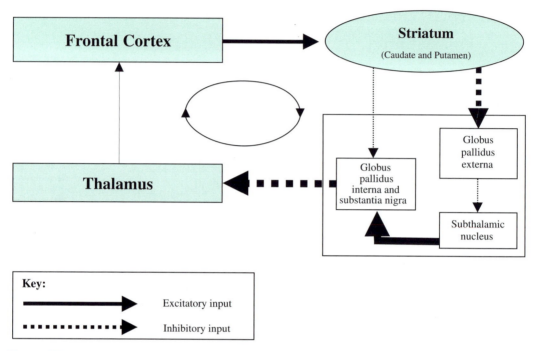

Figure 4.7 An illustration of the functional effects of activity in the indirect basal ganglia pathway. Frontal input increases striatal inhibitory output to the globus pallidus externa. This results in reduced inhibition of the subthalamic nucleus. The relatively disinhibited subthalamic nucleus is then able to send excitatory output to the direct basal ganglia structures, and facilitates inhibition of the thalamus. Excitatory thalamic output is reduced, decreasing drive to the frontal cortex and reducing reverberant activity in this circuit (as depicted by the circle in the center of the diagram).

pallidus interna. The globus pallidus externa inhibits activity of the subthalamic nucleus, which would otherwise send excitatory afferents to the globus pallidus interna, thereby producing inhibition of thalamic activity. When the caudate receives excitatory input from the DLPFC, it sends an inhibitory signal to the globus pallidus externa. Inhibition of the globus pallidus externa reciprocally disinhibits the subthalamic nucleus, which consequently sends 'an excitatory signal to the globus pallidus interna. Once activated, the globus pallidus interna sends an inhibitory signal to the thalamus. Being inhibited, the thalamus no longer continues to send excitatory signals back to the DLPFC, and therefore activity in this circuit decreases (Figure 4.7).

Within the DLPFC circuit, the balance between the indirect and direct pathway subcircuits appears to be very important to the kind of cognitive flexibility that we associate with normal executive function. As discussed before, this circuit is required for organizing information, developing strategies for this organization, searching memory, facile shifting between and integration of information, and developing sequences of motor responses to information. Injury to the DLPFC produces impairments of these functions, although the degree of impairment may not be uniform across them all.

We offer this possible explanation for such discrepancy in the severity of specific impairments in patients with dysexecutive syndromes – it may be that differences in the extent to which there is injury to or dysfunction of the direct pathway, indirect pathway, or both as they project from the various portions of the DLPFC and into this circuit predicts differences in clinical presentation. As indicated in Figure 4.1, the DLPFC represents a fairly large area of each frontal lobe. Injury to only one portion of the DLPFC or only one hemisphere (as might occur with a stroke) would not be expected to affect all aspects of executive functioning. By contrast, injury to the subcortical structures might be expected to have a broader impact on executive function (as in Parkinson's disease, Huntington's disease, or subcortical stroke). Hence, differences in the location and extent of injury to the circuit would be expected to offer some predictive value with regard to clinical presentation. We offer here a simplified but clinically useful way of making sense of such phenomena, although the validity of this approach requires further research.

The apparent consequence of activity in the direct pathway is increased activity in the circuit as a whole. In other words, this pathway "turns on" the information processing circuitry. Therefore, injury to the direct pathway (or the cortex driving it) should result in difficulty generating and synthesizing information. Clinically, impairment in this pathway should manifest as poor word list generation, reduced design fluency, poor recall of both recent and remote memories, concrete interpretation of categories and proverbs, and impaired performance on neuropsychological tasks like the Wisconsin Card Sorting Test (a neuropsychological task that tests set shifting and maintenance, strategy generation, and organization of information). In essence, the clinical presentation of impaired direct pathway activity should be one of too little information processing. This is indeed a common clinical finding among patients with DLPFC dysfunction, for example patients with left dorsolateral frontal stroke or schizophrenic patients with prominent "hypofrontality."

By contrast, injury to the indirect pathway should have a somewhat opposite, though also functionally impairing, effect. Since the apparent result of activity in the indirect pathway is to "turn down" activity of the circuit, injury to the indirect pathway should result in difficulty terminating information processing. In other words, once the circuitry for processing information is "turned on," the patient may have difficulty turning it off. Clinically, impairment in this pathway would manifest as perseveration, poor set shifting, a tendency toward "stimulus-bound" behavior (inappropriately placing the hands of the clock on "11" and "10" when asked to indicate ten minutes after eleven; see Chapter 9), poor go/no-go performance, and impaired performance on serial tasks. Again, these are common findings among patients with dysexecutive syndromes.

Importantly, these two types of clinical presentation are not at all exclusive, and both are often seen concurrently among patients with DLPFC circuit dysfunction. Assuming normal motivation, the relative prominence of either impaired generation and manipulation of information or impaired termination of activity may depend to some degree on the extent of dysfunction in either the direct or the indirect DLPFC circuit.

Additionally, some authors have suggested that there may be hemispheric differences in executive function, akin to those seen in emotion (see Chapter 5). The left hemisphere may be more involved in "turning on" functions, including initiation, generation, sequencing, and so on, whereas the right hemisphere may be more important in "turning off" functions. If correct, one might predict more difficulty with initiation and planning in patients with left hemispheric dysfunction and more perseveration and stimulus bound behavior in patients with right hemisphere dysfunction. While such observations may be made clinically and neuropsychologically, certainly exceptions to this sort of lateralization of executive function are commonly observed. Nonetheless, this may be a useful concept to entertain in this introductory approach to neuropsychiatry.

Lateral orbitofrontal circuit

This circuit originates from the lateral orbitofrontal cortex (Brodmann areas 10, 11 and 47; Figure 4.8), after which it follows essentially the same sort of course as outlined for the DLPFC circuit. The specific elements of this circuit include the ventromedial caudate, a direct pathway course through the most medial portion of the globus pallidus interna and the rostromedial portion of the substantia nigra pars reticulata, and an indirect pathway course through the dorsal globus pallidus externa, the lateral portion of the subthalamic

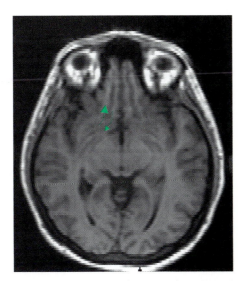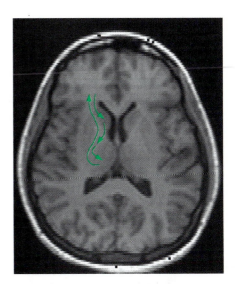

Figure 4.8 The lateral orbitofrontal-subcortical circuit. These axial magnetic resonance image slices depict the approximate pathway of this circuit. The image on the left is about mid-level through the orbits, between which are the orbitofrontal cortices. The dashed arrows in the left image indicate the input and output from the right orbitofrontal cortex, which ascends to the circuit depicted in the right image. As with the dorsolateral prefrontal-subcortical circuit, the circuit follows the same basic pathways, proceeding from cortex to striatum (caudate), to globus pallidus (not shown), to thalamus, and back to cortex.

nucleus, and a final output through the ventral anterior thalamus and medio-dorsal thalamus back to the orbitofrontal cortices. As with the DLPFC circuit, the apparent result of activity in the direct pathway is increased activity of the orbitofrontal circuit, and the result of activity in the indirect pathway is an overall decrease in the activity of the orbitofrontal circuit.

As with the DLPFC circuit, the lateral orbitofrontal-subcortical circuit is critically important to the manner in which one interacts with the world. As noted earlier, the specific aspects of complex cognition related to the orbito-frontal circuit are those we have called "social intelligence," and include social appropriateness, the ability to exercise restraint over aggressive, sexual, and appetitive ("limbic") impulses, organizing appropriate grooming behaviors, and developing empathy for and nurturance of others. In discussing the func-tion of this circuit with our students, we sometimes use the metaphor of the "limbic police" – this circuit polices the improper expression of limbically-driven behaviors, and may either be ineffective (with a resulting "limbic riot" of inappropriate behavior) or overly restraining (with a resulting "limbic martial law" and excessive focus on restraining these behaviors, as in obsessive–compulsive disorder). Metaphors aside, proper functioning of the circuit as a whole, intrinsically and with respect to the input it receives from the other frontal-subcortical circuits and from other parts of the brain (particularly the limbic system), is required for normal "social intelligence."

When there is injury to this circuit, and to either of the pathways within it, social intelligence may be severely disrupted. As with the DLPFC circuit, we find it useful to conceptualize the disturbances arising from the orbitofrontal-subcortical circuit in terms of dysfunction of the direct versus the indirect pathway; however, the validity of this conceptualization requires further research for validation. For example, the result of direct pathway activity should be to increase focus on restraint of limbic behaviors (to send the limbic police into action). Consequently, impaired functioning of the direct pathway should result in a lack of appropriate behavioral restraint: patients may be tactless and say things without exercise of good social awareness; they may be impulsively aggressive, sexually inappropriate, or have unrestrained appetitive behaviors; they may lack empathy for others, and experience little or no remorse, guilt, or other feelings related to their inappropriate behaviors. Phineas Gage seems to fit this picture well. Similar presentations are common among patients with traumatic brain injuries, tumors of the orbital floor, mania, Huntington's disease, and patients with either primary or acquired sociopathy.

By contrast, the indirect pathway facilitates inhibition of the thalamus, or a decrease in the behavioral restraint afforded by orbitofrontal circuit activity – some degree of sexual, aggressive, appetitive, and other such behaviors are necessary for survival. Dysfunction of the indirect pathway should therefore result in an overactivity of "social intelligence:" excessive concern and contemplation of cognitions and affects related to aggression ("did I hurt someone?"), sex ("I've been having dirty thoughts I can't stop"), appetitive behavior (over- or under- eating and possibly hoarding), over concern for others, and excessive grooming (cleanliness). In other words, overactivity of the direct pathway in the orbitofrontal circuit, in the absence of adequate balancing activity from the indirect pathway, would predictably result in the classic symptoms of obsessive–compulsive disorder. This notion is discussed in more detail in Chapter 14.

Interestingly, some patients, for example those with Huntington's disease and traumatic brain injury, may concurrently demonstrate dysfunction referable to both direct and indirect pathway subcircuits. These patients may have obsessive–compulsive symptoms and also be unpredictably aggressive and socially inappropriate. Certainly, the actual processes underlying such mixed presentations are highly complex, and tax the usefulness of the framework presented here. Nonetheless, it is useful to conceptualize such behaviors as arising out of a relative imbalance in activity or pathological activity in these pathways, and we find this conceptual framework useful when considering one or another pharmacological intervention for disturbances in these symptoms (discussed further below).

Anterior cingulate circuit

Motivation and the conscious experience of emotion are believed to arise from the activity of the anterior cingulate circuit. This circuit has received more attention and scientific investigation than the DLPFC or orbitofrontal circuits, and the literature in this area is proportionately more complicated. While we acknowledge this state of affairs, we present here the anterior cingulate-subcortical circuit in the same manner as the others in this chapter, in the hope that this simplified explanation will make easier the pursuit of a richer understanding of the constitution and function of this circuit for interested readers. With this in mind, we return to this circuit in more detail in Chapter 15.

The anterior cingulate-subcortical originates from the anterior cingulate gyrus (Brodmann area 24; Figure 4.9), and projects first to the ventral striatum (ventromedial caudate and ventral putamen). This circuit more obviously involves two structures not mentioned in our earlier discussions, namely the nucleus accumbens and the olfactory tubercle. Similar to the general pathways outlined for the other frontal-subcortical circuits, the anterior cingulate circuit also contains two basal ganglia pathways. The direct pathway passes through the globus pallidus interna (rostromedial and ventral pallidum) and the substantia nigra pars reticulata (rostrodorsal) to the thalamus (mediodorsal). The indirect pathway first passes through the globus pallidus externa (rostral pole) and the subthalamic nucleus (medial), and then projects to the globus pallidus interna and subsequently to the thalamus. From the thalamus, afferent projections return to the anterior cingulate gyrus.

The anterior cingulate circuit appears to be critical for the development of motivation, and may play a role in the conscious experience of emotion. Motivation is best described as the direction, intensity, and persistence an individual has toward achieving specific goals, and is the process by which the behavior and emotional reaction associated with achieving those goals is started, directed, and sustained. The primary clinical phenomenon associated

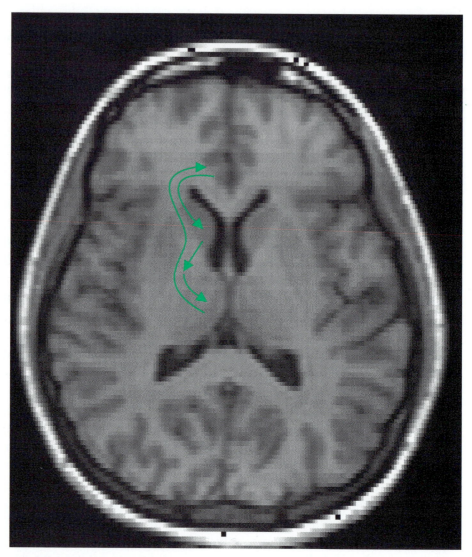

Figure 4.9 The anterior cingulate-subcortical circuit. This axial magnetic resonance image depicts the approximate pathway of this circuit. The starting and ending arrows in this figure arise out of the right anterior cingulate gyrus. The pathway follows the same general course as that described for the dorsolateral prefrontal- and lateral orbitofrontal-subcortical circuits (see Figure 4.5).

with dysfunction of this circuitry is diminished motivation (or, in increasingly extreme forms, apathy and abulia) – a reduction in goal-directed motor, emotional, and cognitive activity due to diminished motivation. Even in the context of normal executive function and "social intelligence," impairment of the anterior cingulate circuit can produce profound disability simply by virtue of eliminating the drive to process or respond to the information in the other frontal-subcortical circuits. This is a common clinical finding among patients who have suffered cingulate injuries due to traumatic brain injury, stroke, or tumor, and among those with neurological illness that affects the circuit's subcortical relays (Huntington's and Parkinson's disease) or white matter tracts (multiple sclerosis).

It has also been suggested that the anterior cingulate circuit may be involved in the conscious experience of emotion, an idea that appears to originate with Papez' original description of the circuit that bears his name (see Chapter 2). If this circuit does subserve the conscious appreciation of emotion, then the clinical phenomenon that would arise from its dysfunction would be anhedonia, the inability to experience pleasure or, more generally, feeling. Whether conscious experience of emotion is truly related to the anterior cingulate circuit alone or to the interaction of this and other frontal-subcortical circuits is unclear, although it is addressed in more detail in Chapter 5. As a preliminary statement, it seems most likely that dysfunction of this circuit reduces the drive to act on emotional (limbic) and other complex cognitive inputs, giving the appearance of a lack of emotion but not necessarily supporting the conclusion that the emotion is entirely absent.

As an example that may, however, combine both aspects of this circuit (motivation and experience of emotion), consider the patient with "negative" symptoms or the "deficit syndrome" of schizophrenia. Abnormalities in the structure and function of the cingulate gyrus have been described in schizophrenia, and the "negative symptoms" (in particular apathy and anhedonia) may be a reflection of the degree to which activity in this circuit is impaired. Since at least a portion of activity of the anterior cingulate gyrus is driven by dopaminergic projections from the ventral tegmental area, medications with antidopaminergic properties would reduce the activity in the cingulate gyrus, and hence also in the circuit as a whole, clinically worsening motivation and anhedonia. Given this view of the anterior cingulate-subcortical circuit, it is easy to understand why the administration of typical antipsychotic medications worsens the negative symptoms of schizophrenia and why many patients are reluctant to remain compliant with such therapies.

As noted earlier in this chapter, understanding the parallel neuroanatomic nature of these frontal-subcortical circuits may make clearer the association of untoward medication side effects. Not only do typical antipsychotics reduce dopaminergic activity in the anterior cingulate-subcortical circuit, they simultaneously reduce activity in the DLPFC circuit and in the lateral orbitofrontal circuit. While such an effect on this latter circuit might reduce aggression and inappropriate behavior, this effect predictably entails exacerbation of problems with executive function, motivation, and emotional experience. Understanding the mechanics of these circuits as they relate to clinical presentation is essential for selecting treatment rationally. In our example of the patient with schizophrenia and negative symptoms, it would appear to be better to choose an agent with less robust dopaminergic blockade (e.g., an atypical antipsychotic) so as not to predictably worsen apathy and anhedonia.

Since we have been speculating about the clinical phenomena arising from either inactivity within the basal ganglia pathways, a few tentative comments within that framework may also be made here. As with the other frontal-subcortical circuits, activity in the direct pathway has the effect of "turning on" the circuit and producing the clinical behavior with which the circuit is associated. In the case of injury to the anterior cingulate-subcortical circuit direct pathway, diminished motivation appears to be the primary clinical consequence. This is the most common clinical presentation of dysfunction in this circuit, and is that most frequently discussed in reference to this circuit.

Although dysfunction of the indirect pathway is not often discussed, the possible behavioral effects of disruption of this subcircuit are potentially interesting. If the function of the indirect pathway is to "turn down" activity in the circuit, then dysfunction of the indirect pathway would have the effect of leaving the motivation circuit "turned on." For example, the relationship between dysfunction of the indirect pathway in the lateral orbitofrontal circuit and simultaneous (parallel) dysfunction of the indirect pathway in the anterior cingulate circuit might usefully inform the association between obsessions and compulsions (a driven motor behavior related to the obsessions). It is also tempting to speculate that there may be a spectrum of clinical phenomena that might be associated with "hyperfunction" of the anterior cingulate-subcortical circuit, ranging from excessive drive to act (e.g., compulsions) to moderately excessive motivation (e.g., the "workaholic") and perhaps even to relatively adaptive forms of increased motivation seen in some very successful and productive persons.

Complex cognition and personality

Personality is defined in the DSM-IV (American Psychiatric Association, 1994) as "enduring patterns of perceiving, relating to, and thinking about the environment and oneself," and personality traits are aspects of the personality that are exhibited in social and personal contexts. When personality is discussed in the context of complex cognition, it is most often related to lateral orbitofrontal activity. While it is certainly true that lesions in the lateral orbitofrontal circuit may produce dramatic changes in a person's relationship to the outside world, the concept of personality entails more than one's social behavior, or comportment alone. The definition of personality used in psychiatry (e.g., that given in the DSM-IV) echoes this belief, stating that personality is the collection of processes related to perceiving, thinking about, and relating to both the environment and oneself. In other words, personality is derived from the interaction and integration of basic cognition (perception, attention, memory, language, performance abilities), all aspects of complex cognition, including executive function, social intelligence, motivation, and also emotion. Given this understanding, we believe that attribution of personality to orbitofrontal function alone is inadequate – we will return to this discussion in greater detail in Chapter 6.

Treatment of cognitive disorders

While cognitive impairments are attributable to focal neurological damage or dysfunction of distributed neural networks, such damage is invariably the result of an underlying process (neurodegeneration, stroke, tumor, trauma, infection, alcoholism, etc.) and therefore treatment must be considered in the context of treatment for the underlying problem. Often, these underlying problems will also disrupt areas subserving emotion and behavior. In other words, impairments in basic or complex cognition are often accompanied by secondary psychiatric symptoms or syndromes (depression, mania, anxiety, psychosis, etc.).

Even if only present as an isolated cognitive impairment, most of the problems presented in this and the preceding chapter produce serious personal and social problems for the patient, and may require a substantial change in lifestyle for both the patient and his or her family. This is particularly true for patients with aphasia. The problem of sudden language dysfunction is regarded by rehabilitation specialists as being of the same magnitude of stress as hemiplegia, sudden blindness, or initial diagnosis of a terminal illness. The change in physical status is acutely disabling, particularly if the impairment is accompanied by further neurological or medical problems.

Cognitive disorders also frequently result in change in social and family position. Such patients often need intensive caretaking in the early stages of rehabilitation, and often may only recover incompletely. These disabilities also carry a perceived (and often real) threat to the patient's economic status. Additionally, recreational options may become limited. Such disabilities frequently limit the flexibility of (or sometimes precipitously make entirely unavailable) the patient's usual repertoire of coping skills, often resulting in significant stress, grief, and possibly depression.

Not surprisingly, grief and depression are common reactions to the onset of many cognitive disorders. The usual "grief models" applied in psychotherapy surrounding other major life events or losses may not apply to many of these patients, however, and a not uncommon perspective in the rehabilitation community is that the patient never really "accepts" major neurological disability. Instead, they accommodate to and compensate for it, but the process of coping with disability never ends. In counseling around such adjustment issues, education, competence building, problem solving, realistic goal setting, and family interventions should be a major focus of treatment.

With the acute onset of cognitive impairment, depression may develop and often requires alteration in rehabilitation treatment strategies. In some cases, location of the lesion may facilitate the development of such depressions (discussed more in the next chapter). Treatment of these acute depressions with antidepressant medications is not always necessary, as some depressive reactions may resolve before these medications could exert an antidepressant effect. However, if the depressive reaction persists beyond the first week, or is clearly impeding participation in rehabilitation, treatment with antidepressants should be initiated. Agents with significant anticholinergic (e.g., tricyclics) or sedating (e.g., benzodiazepines) properties should be avoided as brain injured patients tend to be more susceptible to medication side effects. Selective serotonin reuptake inhibitors are often a good choice, and those with short half-lives may be preferable because they can be more quickly eliminated should intolerable side effects develop.

Treatment of agitation may also be necessary. In general, benzodiazepines should be avoided, as they will predictably further impair memory and may increase the risk of falls. BuSpar (buspirone) and Inderal (propranolol) may be helpful in decreasing impulsive aggressive behavior. Low-dose valproate has also been suggested to be helpful in decreasing agitation in cognitively impaired patients. Unless the patient's agitation is fueled by psychosis (hallucinations, delusions), typical antipsychotic medications should be regarded as agents of last choice as there is otherwise no clear psychopharmacological rationale for their use, their side effects and risks of their use may outweigh potential benefits, and some authors have suggested that they may actually impair neuronal recovery in the acute injury phase.

Working with the family of a patient with a cognitive disorder is also extremely important. Family involvement has been shown to be a significant predictor of the patient's discharge either to home or to an institution after acute rehabilitation. Additionally, lack of family interaction with the patient is a more significant predictor of subsequent rehospitalizations than lesion location, patient age, length of initial hospitalization, dysphasia, mental status exam, or socioeconomic status (Evans et al., 1987). Consequently, psychiatric intervention with patient and family may be invaluable for both functional outcome and cost of treatment. Family members should also be encouraged to make use of community or organized support resources concerning the type of cognitive disorder faced by their family member.

Rehabilitation for the patient and family should focus on reinforcing remaining strengths and developing useful compensatory strategies for the disability. Neuropsychological testing may be useful in designing such cognitive training programs.

Finally, competency issues are often raised during rehabilitation. The evaluation is often complicated by the presence of language dysfunction, but the patient should not be summarily dismissed as incompetent due to the presence of aphasia. A careful evaluation, informed by the observations of family, caregivers, neuropsychological testing, and patient interview is needed to make a competency determination. The patients' ability to understand and participate in decisions that affect them may often rely more on functional measures including their social interactions, their behavior (including treatment compliance), their degree of self-concern (versus neglect), and whether they are able to demonstrate their wishes through non-verbal means.

Competency evaluations of this sort will often take several sessions. It is frequently the case that patients with cognitive disorders such as Broca's aphasia understand more than they are able to make known easily, and therefore should be given the benefit of the doubt with respect to legal decisions while the competency evaluation is ongoing. Additionally, the psychiatrist may be needed to help assess the competence and reliability of the caregivers – patients with cognitive disorders are at great risk of exploitation by unscrupulous caregivers or "interested" third parties.

Summary

As we have considered complex cognition here, it is clear that each of three major domains (executive function, social intelligence, motivation) is essential to normal functioning in everyday life. Executive functioning is referable to activity in circuits involving the dorsolateral prefrontal cortex, social intelligence is mediated by the lateral orbitofrontal circuit, and motivation and the conscious experience of emotion involve (at least) the anterior cingulate circuit. Each of these circuits includes a direct and an indirect pathway, and the balance of activity between these pathways may determine the contribution of the overall circuit to cognitive, emotional, and behavioral responses.

The function of each domain of complex cognition influences, and is influenced by, the activity in each of the other domains, since the circuits operate in a parallel and reciprocal fashion. Additionally, each domain has a similar functional relationship to more basic aspects of cognition. The frontal-subcortical circuits described in this chapter are similar in their organization, both anatomically and with respect to their pharmacologic makeup. Understanding the basic organization of these circuits makes clearer both the relationship between clinical phenomena and their underlying neural bases and also the effect of pharmacological and behavioral interventions on complex cognition.

5

Emotion

Introduction

Recognizing the importance of emotions and emotional regulation to all manner of brain-behavior relationships is essential to the practice of neuropsychiatry. However, emotion and emotional dysregulation have not yet undergone the extent and intensity of neuroscientific study as have cognition and cognitive disturbances. Consequently, there is at present no clear consensus on the proper description of either emotions or their disturbances, and we must be circumspect about the validity of the perspective that we will offer in this chapter – as more research on the neuroscience of emotion accumulates, it is likely that we will need to revise substantially our current understanding of the neuropsychiatry of emotion. The comments of William James, a pioneer in psychology during the late nineteenth century, in his work *Principles of Psychology* (1890, republished, 1950) continue to serve as an appropriate caution:

"We should, moreover, find that our descriptions [of emotions] had no absolute truth; that they only applied to the average man; that every one of us, almost, has some personal idiosyncrasy of expression, laughing or sobbing differently from his neighbor, or reddening or growing pale where others do not. We should find a like variation in the objects which excite emotion . . . [and] the internal shadings of emotional feeling, moreover, merge endlessly into each other . . . The result of all this flux is that the merely descriptive literature of the emotions is one of the most tedious parts of psychology. And not only is it tedious, but you feel that its subdivisions are to a great extent either fictitious or unimportant, and that its pretences to accuracy are a sham."

Given this cautionary note, a number of reasonable clinical descriptions of emotion and emotional dysregulation (including James' own) have been offered. Such descriptions are generally concerned with the more stereotyped disorders of emotional regulation (e.g., depression, mania, pathological laughing and crying), and in many regards the classification of these problems and their treatments is remarkably more consistent and useful than James might have predicted. The most recent edition of American Psychiatric Association's *Diagnostic and Statistical Manual of Mental Disorders* (DSM-IV), while limited in its usefulness in cases that do not conform to stereotypic disorders, nonetheless offers a phenomenologic approach to the prototypical disorders of emotion that has been demonstrated repeatedly to be both valid and reliable (American Psychiatric Association, 1994).

There are, however, far fewer satisfying neurobiological accounts of emotions and emotional disturbances, and deciphering the scientific literature in this area presents a substantial challenge to clinicians interested in better understanding and providing care to patients with such problems. In an attempt to make this challenge more manageable, this chapter describes first a framework for the description and evaluation of emotion and emotional dysregulation. We then offer an overview of the neurobiology of emotion, and finally we offer a neuropsychiatric approach to treatment of patients with emotional problems.

Emotion and emotional dysregulation

From a neuropsychiatric perspective, emotions may be thought of as brain-behavior states established by the interaction between somatic sensations and responses and limbic, paralimbic, and neocortical processes, the product of which is the generation, maintenance, and regulation of both subjectively experienced emotional feelings (e.g., joy, sadness, anger, fear) and objectively observed emotional responses (e.g., laughing, crying, rage, panic). As James noted, there is considerable variability both between and within individuals in the experience and expression of ostensibly similar emotions, even given identical environmental triggers for those emotions. Some of this variability is possibly a function of the complexity of the neurobiological systems upon which emotions are predicated, a complexity that occurs at both macroscopic network levels and at microscopic cellular (perhaps even genetic) levels. Consequently, there are few necessarily true statements that can be made about the phenomenology or neurobiology of emotions in either normal or pathological states.

For example, sadness refers to an emotional state consisting of either decreased or increased muscle tension, decreased heart and respiratory rates, fatigue, tearing and nasal congestion, attention to the cause of the experience, and to associated cognitions and physical sensations, all of which are brought into awareness and are experienced as a feeling of sadness. If any one of these elements is absent from the set, the remainder might still be considered to constitute a state of sadness by the individual experiencing it, a keen observer, or both. Not every one of these elements is sufficient or even clearly necessary to establish a state of sadness. This is reflected in the DSM-IV criteria for a major depressive episode, in which not even the subjective experience of sadness is necessarily needed to make the diagnosis provided that the neurovegetative and cognitive (anhedonic) components of this emotional state are present in sufficient number and severity.

Therein lies the difficulty in describing emotions: there is tremendous variation in the way they are experienced and expressed. Given this difficulty, singular descriptions of emotional states like depression are untenable. Most authors therefore approach the study of pathological emotional states by delineating their constituent elements, from which the phenomenology and neurobiology of emotions may be more systematically pursued and easily understood.

Some authors suggest a simple division of emotional experience and expression into two major categories – mood and affect. In this framework, mood describes an individual's internal experience of a subjective emotional state, and affect describes the observable external and somatic expression of that emotional state. The advantage of this approach is that it creates an easily understood division between the experience and expression of emotion, and is particularly useful when describing conditions in which there is a relatively clean dissociation of emotional experience and expression, as in pathological laughing and crying.

However, the simplicity of this approach is offset by its limited clinical utility and potential for generating confusion when describing patients whose symptoms do not conform to prototypical forms. For example, some patients do experience alterations in their subjective emotional state (which are usually emotionally congruent) during an episode of pathological crying. If mood is the patient's subjective emotional state, then this change is described as a "depressed mood." Indeed, some patients describe their episodes as "mood swings" or "depression." However, many patients intuitively reject this description of their problem, noting that they are not "depressed" *per se*, but are instead suffering from uncontrollable episodes of short-lived but intense sadness. However, having learned to describe all subjective emotional states as "mood," clinicians unfamiliar with disorders of pathological affect hear the patient's complaints of "mood swings" as suggestive of a mood disorder, and may therefore not pursue the type of evaluation and treatment needed by patients with pathological affect. This is the principal liability of the "mood = subjective state and affect = expression" method of describing emotion – the unintended consequence of suggesting the presence of a DSM-IV-type mood disorder (e.g., major depression or bipolar disorder) where there is only a subjective emotional disturbance of much shorter duration and narrower scope.

An alternative, and in our view, a more clinically useful method of describing emotion, is an extension of those suggested by Adams et al. (1997b), the American Psychiatric Association (1994), and Woyshville et al. (1999), in which mood is used to refer to a relatively pervasive and sustained emotional baseline over time (the emotional "climate") and affect refers to the present emotional state (the emotional "weather"). In this framework, mood describes the predominant emotional state over a relatively long period of time (i.e., days to weeks) while affect describes the more transient (minutes to hours) emotional variation that occurs in the context of that mood. As a consequence of this definition, both mood and affect may be described according to their objective (expressed and observable) and subjective (experienced) components. The subjective and objective components of mood and affect may be further described according to their variability, duration, and intensity, contextual appropriateness, and the extent to which they are subject to voluntary control (Figure 5.1).

Regardless of which of these two frameworks one chooses to use to describe emotion, we suggest that the approach to describing emotions should be similar to the one for describing alterations of consciousness (see Chapter 3), namely that any qualitative term should be accompanied by a brief description of the clinical phenomena to which it refers. For example, a patient with a "depressed mood and relatively flat affect" might be more precisely described by briefly stating:

"The patient stated that his mood had been persistently, intensely, and unwaveringly sad over the last two weeks. He reported that he had no obvious reason for these feelings, and in fact the circumstances of his life were the best they had been in many years. Despite this, he felt unable to overcome his sad feelings. The patient's wife corroborated his report, stating that his mood had been observably sad over the last two weeks, as evidenced by his continuously sad facial expression, frequent tearfulness, heavy sighs, and markedly decreased speed of speech and movement. Throughout the interview, the patient demonstrated little change in his facial expression, looking entirely and invariably sad. He also reported no change in his subjective affective state in response to a joke that he and his wife stated he would ordinarily find amusing."

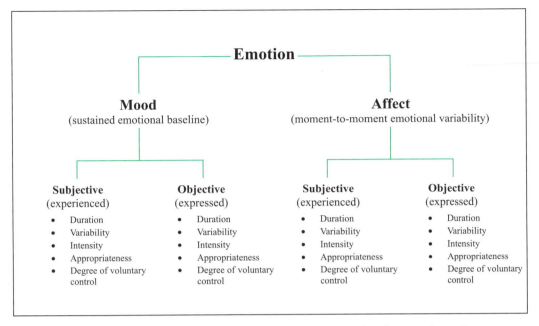

Figure 5.1 Outline of the suggested approach to the description and evaluation of emotion.

In light of this example, we prefer use of the second framework noted above, as it offers a more detailed and clinically meaningful description of mood and affect, their respective objective and subjective components, and the duration, variability, intensity, contextual appropriateness, and degree of voluntary control of each component.

Neurobiology of emotion

The neurobiology of emotion has a long, complex, and at times contentious history. The view that emotions and emotional disorders are the products of the brain is not a recent one, although at various points in history the view that emotions are the products of the brain has been extremely unpopular, if not frankly heretical (see Chapter 1). During the twentieth century, however, this view that emotions are based in the brain has re-emerged as the dominant one in neuropsychiatry. From this understanding of emotion, a number of theories regarding the relevant neuroanatomy and neurochemistry have been offered. A complete review of this literature is well beyond the scope of the present work, so we will provide here only a brief overview of those areas needed for an introduction to the neuropsychiatry of emotion. Readers interested in more detailed reviews of this subject should consider the works by Mega et al. (1997), Heilman (1997), Mayberg (1997), and LaBar & LeDoux (1997), from which this overview is derived.

The neuroanatomy of emotion

Charles Darwin reintroduced the concept of a neurobiology of emotion into scientific discourse by asserting that some aspects of human emotional expression (e.g., laughing and crying, among others) are likely to be biologically determined, and probably genetically conserved across species. Darwin also suggested that the expression of emotions at least in part determines the development of a subjective feeling state that matches that expression ("he who gives violent gesture increases his rage"). This idea became better known as the facial feedback hypothesis, and although some limited support was provided by Tomkins (1962, 1963) and Laird (1974) almost a century after Darwin's first suggestion, this hypothesis is not generally accepted as an adequate account of emotional experience and expression.

James also developed a related idea predicated on the notion of visceral feedback, in which he suggested that peripheral physiological (particularly autonomic and visceral) changes provide input to the brain, and their perception determines emotional experience (1884, 1890 republished 1950). James did not pursue this hypothesis much beyond its original exposition, but the view was further elaborated by Lange (1887) and debated during the early-twentieth century by Cannon (1927). The point of debate appears to have focused on the lack of specificity between visceral events and emotions (different human emotions evoked by the same visceral events and vice versa), and concern that afferent visceral input to the brain is both too vague and too limited in breadth and depth of the information it conveys to adequately account for the specific and detailed quality of human emotions. These concerns led Cannon to conclude that the visceral feedback hypothesis is an inadequate account of emotions, and to suggest instead that emotions develop as a result of diencephalic (thalamus and hypothalamus) processing of sensory information that results in simultaneous reactions in the body (emotional expression) and information processing in the neocortex (emotional experience).

Papez (1937) and later MacLean (1949, 1952) further elaborated this view into the "limbic system" theory of emotion. This theory suggests that the hippocampus, amygdala, orbitofrontal cortices, septal region, thalamus, hypothalamus, and cingulate cortex form a "visceral brain" that mediates emotion and survival functions. In Papez' original formulation of the neurocircuitry of emotion (see Chapter 2), processing of emotionally relevant information begins with the entrance of multimodal sensory information into the hippocampus. From the hippocampus, information flows via the fornix to the mammillary bodies, at which point it continues into two parallel but separate pathways. One of these pathways leads to the hypothalamus, where emotional expression is generated via autonomic activity and the facilitation of automatic motor responses. The second pathway flows first to the anterior thalamus and then to the cingulate cortex, in which the conscious experience of emotion occurs. Information in the cingulate then flows back to the hippocampus, which permits modification of the system's responses to subsequently presented emotional information.

In their recent review, LaBar & LeDoux (1997) discuss the major criticisms of the limbic system theory of emotion. Most importantly, they note that the theory is flawed on both anatomical and functional grounds, largely as a result of its reliance on the hippocampus as a cornerstone of emotional processing. Although the hippocampus is clearly important for the processing of multimodal sensory stimuli and contributes to cognitive functions such as attention and memory, there is little evidence to support its role in emotional processing in the fashion suggested by Papez and MacLean. Instead, the amygdala appears to be much more essential to the processing of emotionally relevant stimuli, particularly with respect to the experience and expression of fear, and it may be only for this reason that the limbic system theory of emotion persists as an explanation of the neurobiology of emotion.

In their review of the neuroanatomy of limbic and subcortical areas, Mega et al. (1997) offer a modernized view of the limbic system based on an extrapolation of connectional anatomy performed in nonhuman primates. Their description emphasizes a selective distributed network approach to information processing that may more accurately inform us about the neurobiology of emotion. They outline two major paralimbic cortical-subcortical circuits based on connections with the amygdala/orbitofrontal cortices and the hippocampal/cingulate cortices.

The amygdala/orbitofrontal division integrates and processes information from cortical association areas and modulates visceral and motor responses to such information via projections to the brainstem, hypothalamus, and basal ganglia. The medial portion of the orbitofrontal paralimbic division appears to be highly connected to sensory association areas and the amygdala, and it facilitates entrance of visceral information into this circuit. Processing of this information is facilitated by motivational input from the infracallosal cingulate visceral effector region (see Figure 4.2). The lateral portion of this division is connected to the visual processing system in the inferior temporal cortex and to the auditory association areas in the dorsolateral temporal pole, and therefore serves as a gateway for highly processed visual and auditory information into the amygdala/orbitofrontal limbic division. The lateral orbitofrontal cortex is reciprocally connected to the supracallosal (anterior) cingulate region, which is itself connected to the dorsolateral prefrontal attentional system; these connections probably facilitate motivation towards and selective and sustained attention to emotionally charged (e.g., painful/aversive or pleasurable/rewarding) information that enters this division.

In short, the amygdala/orbitofrontal limbic division participates strongly in sensation (olfactory, gustatory, auditory, visual, visceral) based implicit information processing and responding, including regulation of visceral states and appetitive drives. In doing so, the amygdala/orbitofrontal limbic division facilitates what might be described as the "unconscious" aspects of emotional and social awareness, and generates much of the readily observable motor and visceral components of emotional expression.

The hippocampal/cingulate limbic division is primarily involved with the processing of multimodal sensory association area efferents that enter the hippocampus via the perforant pathway, from which the information appears to flow in the fashion outlined by Papez to the anterior and posterior cingulate. The posterior cingulate is involved in the consolidation of declarative memory and in associative learning and is reciprocally connected to the dorsolateral prefrontal cortex, which has been suggested to be involved in the working memory or "conscious" awareness and in the processing of information. In concert with these dorsolateral prefrontal influences, and via its inputs to the posterior parahippocampal and perirhinal cortices, the posterior cingulate modulates the flow of information through the perforant pathway and into the hippocampus in the fashion predicted by Papez (1937). In a sense, the hippocampal/cingulate limbic division provides a mechanism for the integration of cognitions into emotional information processing, and via its reciprocal connections to the amygdala/orbitofrontal division it could bring the "unconscious" emotional information from the amygdala/orbitofrontal limbic division into "conscious" awareness.

In their review, Mega et al. (1997) describe exactly this kind of reciprocal intersection of the amygdala/orbitofrontal and hippocampal/cingulate limbic divisions, and place the site of this intersection in the infracallosal cingulate. It is at this site that the efferents and afferents of both limbic divisions converge, thereby forming a selective distributed network that modulates and coordinates the state and responses of the internal milieu and externally directed attention mechanisms. The reciprocal connections between the two limbic divisions facilitate the development of emotions as we defined them at the beginning of this chapter, namely a state established by the relationship between the set of specific cognitions, motor responses, and somatic events that establishes subjectively experienced emotional feelings and observable emotional responses (Figure 5.2). Mega and colleagues note that the apparent role of the cingulate in the conscious experience of emotion is remarkably similar to that predicted by Papez, although the details by which this was accomplished are apparently much more complicated than he suggested, both with respect to the neurocircuitry involved and the neurochemical modulation of these circuits.

An additional element of the neuroanatomy of emotion deserves comment, namely the hemispheric asymmetry of emotion. In their seminal paper on this subject, Sackheim et al. (1982) reviewed reports of 119 cases of pathological laughing and crying in an effort to critically evaluate interhemispheric differences in the modulation of emotion. They noted that pathological crying is more than twice as likely to be associated with lesions of the left than the right hemisphere, while pathological laughing is more than three times as likely to be associated with lesions of the right than the left hemisphere, and that patients with episodes of both laughing and crying typically have bilateral lesions. They also note that patients undergoing right hemispherectomy for seizure control develop euphoria significantly more often than depression, suggesting that the left hemisphere substantially mediates the development of positive emotional states. They also describe the development of gelastic epilepsy (ictal laughing) as being predominantly associated with left hemispheric seizure foci, further suggesting the left hemisphere's role in the development of positive emotional states. The lateralization of dacrystic (ictal crying) epilepsy is less clear, although they note that the few available reports suggest a stronger association with right hemisphere seizure foci than with those on the left.

In summary, the left hemisphere apparently subserves positive emotion and the right hemisphere subserves negative emotion. Additionally, Sackheim et al. (1982) noted that female subjects tended to develop pathological crying with

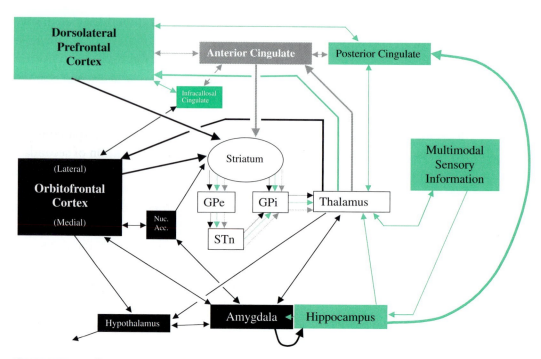

Figure 5.2 An illustration of the key elements and connections in the selective distributed networks subserving emotion and emotional regulation. Information enters the system via visceral and somatic afferents, sensory and multimodal association cortices, and neuroendocrine/neurohormonal mechanisms. The amygdala/orbitofrontal paralimbic division (ventral compartment), including the amygdala, hypothalamus, and orbitofrontal cortices (black) and the relevant subcortical connections to the striatum, globus pallidus (GP), subthalamic nucleus (STn), and thalamus (black arrows) establishes fundamental affective state or "tone". Based on integration of visceral, visual, auditory, olfactory, somatosensory information, this compartment subserves the automatically evoked or "unconscious" aspects of emotion. The hippocampal paralimbic division (dorsal compartment) includes the hippocampus, posterior cingulate gyrus, and dorsolateral prefrontal cortex (light green) and the relevant subcortical connections (light green arrows). This compartment interprets information from the ventral compartment, bringing emotional information into conscious awareness. The anterior cingulate-subcortical circuit (gray and gray arrows) is intimately connected to elements of both compartments (including an anterior cingulate-orbitofrontal connection not illustrated here) and modulates the activity of the system according to the individual's motivational state. In other words, this circuit assigns motivational valence to emotional information. The infracallosal cingulate (dark green) serves as a point of integration between the ventral and dorsal compartments.

left-sided lesions more consistently than males, who appear equally likely to develop pathological laughing with lesions to this side, suggesting a possible sex difference in the degree to which emotions are lateralized.

Several seminal studies of the emotional consequences of stroke by Robinson et al. (1983, 1984) and Starkstein et al. (1988, 1989a, b, 1990) also provide support for the hypothesis of hemispheric asymmetry in emotion. These studies suggest a stronger association of depression and pathological crying with left frontal stroke than right and a closer association of secondary euphoric/manic states with right frontal stroke. However, as Gainotti et al. (1993) and Gainotti (1997) note in the reviews on this subject, conflicting data on the relationship between the side of the lesion and its effect on emotional expression have hampered complete acceptance of the hypothesis of hemispheric lateralization of emotion. While not completely discounting this hypothesis, Gainotti has suggested that the role of the right hemisphere may be the generation of the subjective experience of emotion and the generation of automatic visceral and motor expression of emotion, while the role of the left hemisphere is more responsible for the regulation of and intentional control over emotional expression.

Although the neuroanatomy of emotion remains an area of controversy and one in need of additional exploration, our present state of knowledge suggests that:

(1) the neurobiological bases of emotional experience and expression involve a set of complex interactions between selective distributed networks involving paralimbic, subcortical, and cortical areas;

(2) the amygdala/orbitofrontal limbic division appears to be most closely associated with the generation of automatic visceral and motor components of emotional expression, and the development of unconscious (or, preconscious) emotional information;

(3) the hippocampal/cingulate and amygdala/orbitofrontal interact with the dorsolateral frontal-subcortical network via connections in the cingulate to bring emotionally relevant information (including visceral and motor responses) into conscious awareness;

(4) the right hemisphere is involved in generating, experiencing, and expressing negative emotions;

(5) the left hemisphere, and again perhaps mostly the left dorsolateral prefrontal area, is involved in the maintenance, regulation, and expression of emotion, and particularly positive emotion;

(6) both right and left hemispheric selective distributed networks involving the prefrontal cortices are necessary to inhibit the automatic visceral and motor expression of emotion mediated by more evolutionarily primitive limbic, diencephalic, and brainstem structures.

These modern views of emotional regulation complement that offered by Wilson in 1924. He suggested the existence of a "faciorespiratory" center involving the seventh and twelfth cranial nerves and the phrenic nerve capable of automating and coordinating affective expression upon receipt of input from the hypothalamus, thalamus, and subthalamus. He believed that the activity of this faciorespiratory center is subject to voluntary modulation by higher cortical centers, and that pathological laughing and crying resulted from lesions of the descending voluntary pathways that disinhibit the motor centers involved in emotional expression. Both views emphasize the importance of descending cortical inhibition of more evolutionarily primitive brain areas (diencephalic, brainstem, or both) in the regulation of emotion.

The neurochemistry of emotion

The major neurotransmitter systems involved in function of these frontal-subcortical and limbic-subcortical networks include dopamine, norepinephrine, acetylcholine, serotonin, glutamate, gamma-aminobutyric acid (GABA), and a number of neuropeptides including β-endorphin, enkephalin, vasopressin, and substance P, among others, all of which appear to play modulatory roles both within the networks described and with respect to each other. Although a detailed description of this neurochemistry is well beyond the scope of the present work, Figure 4.4 illustrates the major areas at which these neurotransmitters exert their effects. In this context, a few initial generalities about the neurochemistry of emotion can be made.

A relatively strong role for serotonin in the regulation of affective expression is suggested by the success of these agents in the treatment of major depressive episodes and pathological affect, particularly pathological laughing and crying and affective lability. Changes in serotonergic metabolites have been reported in depressed patients, as have changes in serotonin receptors in patients with depression following stroke. Affective regulation appears to require descending serotonergic afferents from the raphe nuclei to the faciorespiratory motor nuclei. Additionally, it has been suggested that the maintenance of euthymia following stroke may be related to a compensatory upregulation of right hemisphere serotonin receptors following injury to the left hemisphere.

Dopamine also appears to play a role in mood enhancement, possibly through its effects in the orbitofrontal and anterior cingulate cortices, and also in the modulation of reward mechanisms in the nucleus accumbens. Alleviation of affective dysregulation by dopaminergic agents suggests that dopaminergic modulation of frontal-subcortical, limbic-subcortical, and brainstem-neocortical circuits may be important in affective regulation. Additionally, reduction of affective dysregulation by agents with combined dopaminergic and noradrenergic, or serotonergic and noradrenergic properties and the effectiveness of predominantly noradrenergic agents in both primary major depression and depression following stroke suggest the importance of noradrenergic function in emotional regulation.

The effectiveness of carbamazepine in the reduction of irritability and rage (not associated with seizures) due to traumatic brain injury and of valproic acid in the reduction of these symptoms among patients with mental retardation and seizures suggests a possible role of GABA in affective regulation. Although it is unlikely that GABA alone is responsible for emotional regulation in any condition, this substance may facilitate and modulate emotional experience and expression even when the primary abnormality producing emotional dysregulation lies in another neurotransmitter system.

The role of acetylcholine in emotional regulation is less well understood, although such a role has been suggested for acetylcholine in depression and mania. Other neurotransmitters, neuropeptides, and neuroendocrine, and other neuroactive substances, including glutamate, paralimbic mu-opiate receptor agonists, corticotropin releasing factor and corticosteroids are also likely to feature significantly in the generation and regulation of emotions, although their roles in emotional regulation are not yet as well understood as those of dopamine, norepinephrine, and serotonin.

The neurobiology of emotional dysregulation

The selective distributed limbic-subcortical and frontal-subcortical networks rely on a normal balance of all of these neurotransmitter systems for the regulation of emotion, cognition, motor, and visceral responses. Although most clinicians are familiar with the putative roles of deficient serotonin and norepinephrine in depression, excessive norepinephrine in anxiety, dopamine and norepinephrine in manic and psychotic states, and acetylcholine in memory and mood states, these descriptions are oversimplified and do not adequately convey the complexity of the neurochemical regulation of emotion. It is very likely that many neurochemical aberrations can produce emotional dysregulation. At the present time, however, the literature suggests that disruption of normal neurochemical activity within certain regions of neuroanatomy described herein bears an association with certain types of emotional dysregulation.

For example, hypofunctioning of the left medial orbitofrontal cortex (that most closely associated with the amygdala and visceral responses) and left dorsolateral prefrontal cortex is associated with both primary depression and depression due to neurological disorders such as stroke and Parkinson's disease. The development of depression following left-hemisphere stroke may be a consequence of interruption of monoaminergic (norepinephrine and serotonin) pathways. Conversely, lesions of the right medial diencephalon, caudate, and orbitofrontal cortex are associated with mania, possibly due to the interruption of modulating neurotransmitter afferents.

Lesion of the hypothalamus, or disconnection of the diencephalon from descending cortical influence, may result in paroxysmal rage. Lesions of the amygdala may lessen the frequency or severity of these rage attacks, supporting the suggestion that the amygdala/orbitofrontal areas are indeed modulated by the hippocampal/cingulate and other frontal-subcortical circuits, without which the implicit emotional and visceral responses to internal or external stimuli may become excessive and uncontrolled. The production of emotional disturbances following disruption of the prefrontal-subcortical circuits suggests that other neurotransmitters involved in these circuits (e.g., glutamate, GABA, enkephalin, and substance P among others) may also have significant effects on the experience and expression of emotion.

Particularly relevant to this issue is Mayberg's recent (1997) exposition of a limbic-cortical dysregulation model of depression. Based on PET studies of transient induced sadness in healthy adults and major depression in psychiatric patients, an interaction between a network of dorsal structures (dorsolateral prefrontal, dorsal anterior cingulate, inferior parietal areas, and striatum) and ventral structures (ventral paralimbic, hypothalamic, subcortical, and brainstem) mediated through the rostral cingulate appears to be involved in the regulation of sadness. The studies included in this review suggest that sadness was associated with dorsal compartment hypometabolism and ventral compartment hypermetabolism. In a sense, these patients experienced an intense limbically-mediated affect and suffered a reduced ability to "think" their way out of it. The major difference between the depressed and normal groups was the persistence of these metabolic changes, with sustained changes present in the depressed group and transient changes in the otherwise emotionally healthy group.

In the depressed patients, a poor response to fluoxetine was predicted by more pronounced hypometabolism in the rostral cingulate, whereas a good response to treatment was associated with relatively elevated rostral cingulate metabolism and ultimately improvement in dorsal compartment metabolism and a reduction in ventral compartment hypermetabolism. These findings lend support to our discussion of emotion as divisible into sustained (mood) and transient (affective) states, each with subjective (dorsolateral prefrontal/cingulate mediated) and objective (amygdala/orbitofrontal, diencephalic, basal ganglia, autonomic) components. Additionally, these findings suggest a mechanism (disrupted interaction between neocortical and limbic/diencephalic/brainstem areas) by which emotional experience and expression may become partially or completely dissociated from one another.

Emotional dysregulation may therefore result from any significant disruption of the relevant frontal-subcortical, limbic-subcortical, or brainstem circuits, or by disruption of their connections to one another. Such disruptions may result from either damage to these areas by the multiple forms of injury and neurodegeneration already discussed, or by disturbances in the neurotransmitters upon which normal functioning of these areas is predicated.

Neuropsychiatric evaluation and treatment of emotional dysregulation

The literature reviewed suggests that emotional disturbances may develop in many neuropsychiatric syndromes as a result of injury to the complex selective distributed networks that generate, maintain, and regulate emotions. The task of understanding the relationship between a particular patient's neuropsychiatric illness and emotional disturbance is, however, not at all straightforward. The framework presented earlier offers a systematic method of comprehensively evaluating emotion in which both the experience and expression of affect are evaluated independently with respect to their duration, intensity, variability, contextual appropriateness (personal and social), and degree of voluntary control. Using this framework, when the presentation consists of a stereotyped, involuntary, uncontrollable, and nonspecifically provoked pathological expression of affect without a change in consciousness or motor automatisms (suggesting seizure) or a congruent alteration in affective experience, a diagnosis of pathological laughing or crying is most appropriate. When there is congruent and pathologic expression and experience of affect, a diagnosis of affective lability is most appropriate. When there is a persistent disturbance of the emotional baseline, then a mood disorder diagnosis is most appropriate. Occasionally, a patient will have both a mood disorder and affective disorder, as in the patient with both a post-stroke depression and pathological laughing and crying – although the baseline mood is depressed, episodes of pathological affective expression occur independent of any clear relationship to the underlying depression.

There are several implications of this understanding of emotion and approach to diagnosis for the treatment of emotional disturbances in neuropsychiatric disorders. First, offering patients a language with which to describe more precisely the type of emotional disturbance they are experiencing (mood disorder vs. affective disturbance) improves communication with their physician and caregivers. Second, understanding such problems in terms of their potential biological underpinnings can be used to address concerns of "weakness" or "poor character" and self-blame that many patients experience, or to which they are subjected by family and caregivers who do not understand emotional disturbances as neurobiological phenomena. Third, selecting the most appropriate treatment depends on an accurate understanding of symptoms. For example, a patient with a rapid cycling bipolar disorder is most appropriately prescribed a mood stabilizing agent such as lithium or an anticonvulsant. However, patients with affective lability are more likely to benefit from treatment with serotonergic or dopaminergic agents without concurrent mood stabilization – this approach is clearly not suggested for the treatment of a rapid cycling mood disorder, and indeed may significantly worsen this problem. Finally, a neuropsychiatric approach is essential in the further development of a meaningful neuroscience of emotion and improved treatments for emotional disturbances.

Summary

The neurobiological bases of emotional experience and expression involve a set of complex interactions between selective distributed networks involving the paralimbic, subcortical, and cortical areas. The amygdala/orbitofrontal limbic division appears to be most closely associated with the generation of automatic visceral and motor components of emotional expression, and the development of unconscious (or, preconscious) emotional information. The hippocampal/cingulate and amygdala/orbitofrontal interact with the dorsolateral frontal-subcortical network via connections in the cingulate to bring emotionally relevant information (including visceral and motor responses) into conscious awareness. The right hemisphere is involved in generating, experiencing, and expressing negative emotions, while the left hemisphere, and again perhaps mostly the left dorsolateral prefrontal frontal area, is involved in the maintenance, regulation, and expression of emotion, and particularly positive emotion. Both right and left hemispheric selective distributed networks involving the prefrontal cortices are necessary to inhibit the automatic visceral and motor expression of emotion mediated by more evolutionarily primitive limbic, diencephalic, and brainstem structures.

Given this perspective on the neurobiology of emotion, we suggest an approach to the evaluation of emotion that emphasizes both its temporal (mood = sustained emotional baseline, affect = transient emotional states) and phenomenological (duration, variability, intensity, appropriateness, degree of voluntary control of both expression and experience) components. The differential diagnosis of disorders of emotion should first include distinguishing between disturbances of mood and affect, and then further determining whether the disturbance is one of emotional expression or experience, or both.

6

Personality

Introduction

Personality is perhaps the most difficult aspect of brain–behavior relationships to describe, in part because personality is difficult to define and hence to study. While an intuitive definition of personality is appealing, namely those qualities that uniquely distinguish an individual from all others, the scope of this characterization is so broad as to defy detailed description. *Merriam-Webster's Dictionary* (1998) borrows from the traditions of academic psychology to define personality as "the complex of characteristics that distinguishes an individual or a nation or group, especially the totality of an individual's behavioral and emotional characteristics," thereby offering a set of parameters that constrain the boundaries of personality for both description and study. An alternative but complementary definition is provided by the American Psychiatric Association's *Diagnostic and Statistical Manual of Mental Disorders*, 4th edition (1994) or DSM-IV, in which personality is described as the "enduring patterns of perceiving, relating to, and thinking about the environment and oneself." This definition stresses the relative stability of patterns of cognition, emotion, and behavior, both over time and across a variety of contexts.

In many neuropsychiatric textbooks, personality is discussed in the context of frontal lobe function and is most often ascribed to the orbitofrontal cortex. This ascription is usually predicated on the time honored research method of lesion analysis, since dramatic (and sometimes dangerous) changes in the regulation of social behavior or "comportment" (such as empathy, nurturance, and the modulation of aggressive, sexual, and appetitive drives) may follow injury to this area. Because impairments in social behavior are often clinically described as a change in personality, the inference is that this circuit must therefore be the neural seat of personality. The case of Phineas Gage, mentioned in Chapter 4, has been much used for this purpose as an illustration of personality change due to frontal lobe injury.

The logic pairing these aspects of personality with orbitofrontal function is, in this example, understandable. However, it is neither valid nor sound to exclude arbitrarily the influence of other brain areas on personality and thus ignore other elements of personality such as motivation, intelligence, and such. While there is little doubt that orbitofrontal injury may produce dramatic and persistent changes in affective stability and social behavior, most definitions of personality suggest a "totality" of personal and interpersonal understanding and behavior, and therefore entail more than only emotional experience and social comportment. By extension, therefore, personality must involve more than orbitofrontal-subcortical circuitry alone.

For clinical purposes, "personality" may be considered a shorthand notation for a host of reciprocally interactive processes related to perception, basic and complex cognition, emotion, self-awareness and self-concept, social awareness and social skills. Changes in comportment may constitute one kind of evidence by which pathological changes in personality can be diagnosed. At the same time, many patients without overt changes in social behavior will nonetheless report profound alterations in personality following neurologic damage or illness. For example, patients with traumatic brain injuries, as well as their families, often report significant changes in motivation, trust or intimacy (paranoia), humor, language and performance skills, attention, or memory that fundamentally change their perception of and relation to themselves and their environment. When the relationship of such changes to overt social behaviors are subtle, usually without marked aggressiveness or disinhibition, affected patients might not be described by outside observers as having suffered a personality change. But brain injury patients and families will nonetheless often state that their biggest, ongoing problem is in accommodating to the personality changes that have developed as a result of such injury.

It is also important to be clear that personality is not equivalent to "sense of self" any more than it is equivalent to comportment. Consider the case of a formerly health conscious, hard working, "well-grounded" professional who suffers a severe traumatic brain injury affecting the anterior (dorsolateral) and medial (anterior cingulate) frontal cortices, right parietal cortex, and large areas of cerebral white matter. Among the deficits produced by his injuries are executive dysfunction, severely impaired motivation, anosognosia (failure to recognize one's impairments), and a general slowing and inefficiency of cognitive processing. When confronted by caregivers and family about the effects of his injury, he remains convinced (apathetically, in this case) that there is no injury, or perhaps only a trivial one, and persistently fails to see the need for physical rehabilitation. He also does not recognize the importance of working with the rehabilitation unit's social worker on discharge plans or future employability. The patient does not endorse a dramatic change in his sense of himself following his injury, but his unchanged self-appraisal is blind to the reality of his disabilities. In the eyes of observers, there has been a shocking change in personality: he seems both unaware of and unconcerned about his impaired health, social limitations, and his future. The patient is often bewildered by coaxing toward rehabilitation, repeated statements about the dim likelihood of his returning to work, and by the sadness of his family. The interpersonal dynamics that develop in such situations will inevitably change his pattern of relating to himself and his environment, even if he remains unable to understand why these changes occur.

The change in this patient fits the DSM-IV definition of Personality Change due to a General Medical Condition (Traumatic Brain Injury), Apathetic Type and would also possibly meet criteria for Dementia due to Head Trauma. While affective lability and behavioral disinhibition are not prominent features of his condition, their absence does not diminish the dramatic personality change that this man has experienced. Indeed their absence only highlights the fact that an enduring change in an individual's pattern of perceiving, thinking about, or relating to himself, whether or not that change is referable to orbitofrontal-subcortical circuitry, constitutes a change in personality. In this particular case, it is the profound impairments in motivation and cognition that are likely to be identified by family and caregivers as the basis for his personality change.

It is not our intent to offer a detailed discussion of all the philosophical and historical issues relevant to the concept of personality and personality change in this chapter. Instead, we will use this chapter to present a neuropsychiatric approach to understanding personality in terms of brain–behavior relationships that persist over time and across contexts. Although the content of our discussion here is somewhat speculative, we hope that it will stimulate interested readers to pursue further inquiry into this most important issue.

Personality

In all likelihood, personality has both genetic and environmental contributions. Twin studies suggest that genetics contribute 40–60% of the heritability of normal personality traits (Plomin et al., 1990; Livesley et al., 1993), a finding that has been consistently replicated and appears robust. The strongest genetic contributions to personality are often described as temperaments, or the set of inherited biases that determine the pattern of responses to emotional stimuli, and are the foundation upon which other aspects of personality are built. There are several models of temperament, each emphasizing different behavioral (Cloninger, 1987), regulational (Rothbart, 1991), and interpersonal (Rutter, 1987) dimensions. Buss (1991) suggests a model that emphasizes emotionality, sociability, and activity level, three dimensions with reasonably clear genetic heritability. Twin studies also suggest that social avoidance, cognitive style, impulsivity, and aggression each have relatively high genetic heritability, and that the presence of these traits in adult personality may be understood as being significantly influenced by genetic factors.

These genetically determined response biases, or temperaments, strongly influence the neurobiological parameters within which subsequent personality development occurs (Cloninger, 1986; Bouchard, 1994). For example, one theory alleges that genetic loading for relatively lower central nervous system dopamine activity may increase tendencies to asociality, restricted expression, or "deficit" (dysexecutive symptoms, anhedonia, impaired motivation) as seen in schizoid personality disorder. In such cases, the ability of either internal or external stimuli to generate affective responses of great magnitude may appear to be severely limited, and the individual may both experience and be observed to experience the environment as without much impact. Consequently, it seems reasonable to infer that such stimuli have a similarly limited impact on the development of patterns of relating to self and the environment. By comparison, genetic loading for increased dopamine activity might be associated with a tendency towards high or excessive reactivity to internal or external stimuli. This neurobiological state may distort and magnify the impact of the environment on learning by facilitating cognitive distortions or frank misinterpretation of stimuli, as in schizotypal personality disorder (Coccaro & Siever, 1995). Similarly, alterations in serotonergic activity have been suggested to affect tendencies toward impulsivity and aggression, with increased levels of serotonin inhibiting both spontaneous and induced impulsive and aggressive behaviors, while deficits or lesions in serotonergic systems may appear to increase such behaviors (as in idiopathic or acquired sociopathy, respectively). This line of thought suggests that in all cases stable neurobiological characteristics of the systems in the brain that serve emotion, cognition, and behavior fundamentally alter the course of personality development.

As can be inferred from the discussion, additional epigenetic determinants of personality development may derive from the interaction of temperaments, cognitive style, and the processes of learning produced by interaction with both external and internal (cognitive, emotional, somatic) environments. Here, cognitive style includes the set of abilities in perception, attention, language, memory, recognition, praxis, visuospatial skill, executive function, social intelligence (interpersonal style), and motivation possessed by an individual. The relative strengths or weaknesses in each of these areas may set limits on the manner in which external and internal stimuli are perceived, processed, responded to, and learned. The capacity for this kind of learning will probably affect the patterns of responding to self and environment that the individual develops.

While the interaction between temperament, cognitive style, and external and internal environment is unquestionably important, determining the types of environmental influences important to these interactions is very difficult. The influences of parents, peers, and early life stress (such as loss, rejection, abandonment, gain, reward, success, and so on) contribute to personality development. However, the wide range of variability in the neurobiological interaction between organism and environment makes generalizations about the effects of the environment on personality development extremely complex. Some of this variance, as suggested above, may be a consequence of temperamental and epigenetic constraints at the most fundamental levels of information processing in the brain (arousal, attention, and assignment of affective importance). Our tools for understanding the interaction of temperament, cognitive style, and the environment are very limited even in apparently well-studied individuals, making predictions about the impact of specific events on personality development frequently unsuccessful.

Although the means by which personality develops is not completely understood, the end product of this development is reasonably well established by young adulthood. Barring neurological injury or illness, personality appears to remain relatively stable throughout adult life. Efforts are ongoing to define those aspects of personality that constitute the means by which enduring patterns of relation to self and environment are formed.

Dimensions of personality and related neurobiology

Cloninger et al. (1993) developed the Temperament and Character Inventory in an attempt to quantify differences in components of personality. The instrument defines personality as the combination of temperament and character, with the latter term defined as the pattern of relationships with self and others that develops as a result of complex interactions between temperament and environmental factors. From this perspective, Cloninger describes three theoretical dimensions of character: self-directedness (responsible, goal-directed vs. insecure, inept), cooperativeness (helpful, empathic vs. hostile, aggressive), and self-transcendence (imaginative, unconventional vs. controlling, materialistic). Using this language, he offers a model of personality that includes eight general types: melancholic; dependent; schizotypal (disorganized); cyclothymic (moody); autocratic; organized; fanatical (paranoid); and creative. Used primarily for research, the technical descriptions of these eight types are not necessarily consistent with the more common descriptors in general psychiatry. For example, the term creative as used in this model refers to responsible, empathic, mature, and generative individuals, and does not carry the connotation of emotional instability and imagination commonly associated with creativity in other contexts.

The personality types described by this model have been studied with respect to their ability to characterize personality type systematically in persons with and without mental illness, and with respect to their ability to assign risk of mental illness (mood and psychotic disorders) according to personality type. The model provides modest predictive validity between personality type and psychopathology: melancholic individuals have the highest suicide rates, schizotypal (disorganized) individuals have the highest risk of psychiatric hospitalization and suicide attempt, while creative (enlightened) individuals offer the lowest risk of psychopathology. This approach suggests an alternative to conventional views of mental illness as a discrete disease state superimposed on an underlying personality and implies that psychopathology may represent an extreme on one or more continua of personality variables.

Approaching dimensions of function that characterize individuals (and their personalities) from a related but distinctly different perspective, Gardner (1983) offers a multidimensional model of intelligence. He suggests that intelligence is defined not only by executive functions associated with academic performance (verbal and mathematical), but also includes visuospatial, musical, motor (or, kinesthetic), interpersonal, and intrapersonal (or, self-reflective) abilities. In this model, an individual's "intelligence" is the product of the combined abilities from each dimension. For example, it is possible to have genius in some dimensions (such as verbal and logical–mathematical) but relative weakness in others (e.g., intrapersonal). As another example, an individual might have significant strengths in visuospatial and mathematical ability but be sorely lacking in verbal, intrapersonal, and interpersonal intelligences.

It is relatively simple to translate this multidimensional model of intelligence into one of personality, and translation that may be made clearer using the two examples above. The highly verbal and logical individual with impaired intrapersonal intelligence might easily be described as someone with a severely narcissistic personality. The second example describes someone more comfortable with images and numbers, and with relatively little facility for either interpersonal interactions or self-reflection, as might describe someone with a relatively schizoid personality. By expanding the notion of intelligence to include the interactive domains of cognition, emotion, and behavior, Gardner offers a model for understanding the neurobiological mechanisms of how an individual perceives, thinks about, and relates to self and how one behaves in the world. In essence, his is a model for the neuropsychiatry of personality.

When we use this model in terms of the brain–behavior relationships noted in the preceding chapters for the purpose of understanding personality, several important relationships emerge. Language provides an illustrative case in point. First, although language is generally regarded as function of (primarily) the dominant cortical hemisphere, the full range of language function is the product of extensive networking among the various frontal-subcortical circuits and the cortical language areas in both cerebral hemispheres. Understanding language, for example, requires intact dominant hemisphere networks to recognize and interpret syntax and meaning. At the same time, interpreting prosody, or the musicality and intonation of language, requires the involvement of non-dominant networks (Ross & Mesulam, 1979; Ross 1981; Starkstein et al., 1994). Prosodic interpretation facilitated by the non-dominant frontal lobe extends the understanding and expression of language beyond the literal meaning of words. Through the activity of the non-dominant hemisphere, we understand different meanings with different emphases and inflections ("You're going to *sing?*" vs. "*You're* going to sing?" vs. "You're *going* to sing?") and, from them, we interpret the inferred and abstract meanings of spoken and written language, particularly double meanings ("No, *really*, he's a *great* singer"). Adding a further dimension, the ability to interpret the non-linguistic cues accompanying spoken language often requires the integration of visual perceptual and associative functions with limbic-mediated affective responses to non-verbal cues. The next order of neural integration includes perceptual, limbic, language, and social intelligence (orbitofrontal-subcortical) circuits with executive and motivational circuits for the generation, organization, and execution of a response.

Theoretically, the pattern of information processing and integration across each of these neural domains proceeds according to "hard-wired" biases for affective responding (temperament) and for learned patterns predicated on the interaction of temperament and environment (character). As a consequence, therefore, neural stability tends to produce a relatively stable pattern of subjective and behaviorally expressed responses (personality). A continuum of differences in the relative strengths of the various brain functions in both hemispheres involved in language would be expected to produce differences in use and understanding of language among individuals, such as the ability to use language and narrative in self-reflection, the ability to understand or use humor, and to understand or make use of sarcasm in interactions with others. In other words, differences in intra- and inter-hemispheric language function should contribute to differences in the enduring patterns, or aspects of personality, that are language-dependent. Similar reasoning can be used to understand the neural bases of each of the seven domains of intelligence described by Gardner, and to synthesize them into a more complete understanding of personality.

Both of the models described in this section are explicitly deterministic. If personality is defined as an enduring pattern of perceiving, thinking about, and relating to self and the environment, and if these patterns are a function of a relatively stable neurobiological basis for responding and information processing, an individual's present mental state may be considered to be the direct result of a continuous and complex set of neurobiological cause-and-effects between the preceding brain state and new (external or internal) information. In this view, there are no uncaused events (every process is physically linked to the preceding event), although the causes may be opaque both to the individual experiencing their effects and to observers. It appears to follow logically from this neurobiological model that the opaque causes of behavior (described by psychoanalysts as the "unconscious" and by neuroscience researchers as the operations of basic cognition occurring on a level too fundamental and automatic for conscious appreciation) reflect essentially the same processes. Although theories of biological determinism are contentious, and rife with philosophical ramifications regarding free will and moral responsibility, examples like this one are of great value in grounding the neuropsychiatry of personality in neurobiology. This is particularly important clinically when building diagnostic schema and treatment plans that include the personality changes that accompany many neuropsychiatric illnesses.

Personality and neuropsychiatric illness

Although adult personality is relatively stable over time, understanding it as a product of the same neurobiology affected by other neuropsychiatric illnesses suggests that personality can at best be only *relatively* stable – personality is in all likelihood quite susceptible to change in the face of neuropsychiatric illness. The susceptibility of personality to change may be viewed as proportional to the complexity required to establish personality in the first place. As described in the introduction to this chapter, personality may be permanently altered as a result of injury to the brain. The processes by which injuries produce permanent personality changes should by now be clearer: by fundamentally altering the manner in which cognitive and emotional information is processed and behavioral responses are generated, neurological damage (including that produced by all manner of disease processes) alters the brain's ability to maintain previously established patterns of perceiving, thinking about, and relating to self and the environment.

It must also be noted that significant psychiatric disturbances, such as major depression, anxiety disorders, and substance abuse, may also alter adult personality, although more transiently than permanent neurological damage. While personality disorder may appear to predispose some patients to major psychiatric disorders, many patients in the midst of an active psychiatric disorder (e.g., major depression) believed to be superimposed on an accompanying personality "disorder" will be observed to undergo a resolution of that personality disorder (sometimes almost completely) when the major psychiatric disturbance itself resolves (Beck, 1999). Although transience challenges the notion that the observed changes are truly alterations of personality (on first inspection they do not seem "enduring"), many clinicians have witnessed the resolution of an apparent longstanding personality disorder in response to treatment of a subsyndromal depression, anxiety disorder, or alcohol dependence.

The same phenomenon has been described in terms of a changing pattern of ego mechanisms of defense (or coping styles) exhibited by individuals recovering from major depression (Akkerman et al., 1992, 1999; Albucher et al., 1998). Patients in the midst of a major depressive episode may exhibit a relatively stable and immature set of defensive styles, typical of patients with personality disorders. As they recover, the relative maturity (flexibility, adaptive ability) of the defenses increases, suggesting that outside the context of the major depressive episode affected patients may not necessarily exhibit stable patterns of relating to self and the environment characteristic of a personality disorder. By this account, personality changes positively with positive alterations in the underlying neurobiology (these issues are discussed in the next chapter).

If ostensibly stable and enduring aspects of personality may be amenable to change via pathological or therapeutic alterations in brain neurochemistry or structure, we must be circumspect about the conventional distinctions between major neuropsychiatric illness (DSM-IV, Axis I) and personality (Axis II). At a minimum, we should probably more often expect changes in personality to accompany major neuropsychiatric illnesses such as major depression, bipolar disorder, obsessive–compulsive disorder, traumatic brain injury, dementia, stroke, and should first try to understand why these features are part of the clinical presentation before diagnosing a personality disorder (which often results in rather different diagnostic and treatment formulations, if not also approaches by various caregivers).

For example, describing an impulsive, occasionally aggressive, and affectively labile traumatic brain injury patient as suffering from personality change due to the injury is likely to elicit very different responses from potential caregivers than assigning that same patient a diagnosis of borderline personality disorder. Further, the mutability of personality traits in the context of some of these illnesses should prompt caution with respect to concluding that difficult personality traits present during the acute phase of illness will necessarily complicate the long-term management of such patients. Even the troubling personality features of the traumatic brain injury patient described here may be significantly diminished by medications, environmental interventions, and the natural course of recovery from injury.

Our patients are probably best served when we consider all clinical neuropsychiatric phenomena, including personality, as the products of their underlying neurobiology. Any significant perturbation of this neurobiology may alter one or more aspects of cognition, emotion, and behavior and, consequently, the repertoire of relational patterns (personality) predicated on these functions. From this vantage point, the frequently difficult clinical interactions around patients with extremes of personality dysfunction, either with or without other signs of neuropsychiatric illness, may be understood as a sign of disturbed neurobiology that is not under the patient's immediate control. This can be reframed to the benefit of both patient and caregivers. In cases where aspects of personality have significantly complicated a patient's care (as in the case of an institutionalized patient with "acquired sociopathy" due to traumatic brain injury, who is resoundingly hated by the ward staff), describing the troubling clinical features in terms of their underlying neurobiology may provide an intellectual framework within which the involved caregivers and family may usefully isolate their own affect before approaching the patient and addressing the situations he creates. With the advantage of this perspective, clinicians can develop greater empathy for the patient's suffering as well as the intellectual detachment needed to perform a thorough examination and to construct a careful differential diagnosis. At the same time, caregivers and families can be educated regarding the nature of the problem. Appropriate treatments can be devised either to resolve the underlying cause or to devise strategies in the patient's environment to compensate for or manage the patient's behavioral problems.

Summary

This chapter explored our understanding of personality from the perspective of brain–behavior relationships, consistent with the approach developed throughout the first section of this book. Thinking now of clinical usefulness, we can summarize present knowledge briefly, as it might be applied in taking care of individual patients. (1) What we think of as personality is the final product of continuous and complex interactions among (a) limbic and paralimbic-mediated drive states; (b) cognitive processing of both internal and external stimuli; (c) continuous comparison between present and past states; and (d) a combination of genetic, epigenetic, and learned response determinants. (2) These interactions are parallel and reciprocal, operating not only in a bottom–up and top–down fashion as we have described in the preceding chapters, but also in a bottom–bottom and top–top manner. (3) Both superlative and profoundly deficient cognitive, emotional, and behavioral capabilities occur along continua of neurobiological functions. And, returning to the first observation above, (4) the specific and enduring patterns of cognition, emotion, and behavior that influence perceiving, thinking about, and relating to self and the environment define each individual's personality.

7

Psychological adaptation

Introduction: linking mind, brain, and psychological adaptation

The methods and mechanisms of human psychological adaptation have been much studied in recent years, most notably in the longitudinal reports of Vaillant and colleagues (Vaillant, 1977; Vaillant et al., 1986; Vaillant & Koury 1993). Studies of this nature have demonstrated, through empirical observation, that a hierarchy of psychological adaptive styles exists in human life. Of special concern in the present discussion is the observation that psychological adaptation, whether construed as ego defense mechanisms or as behavioral coping styles or in other terms, are linked to human physical health. Specifically, viewed in a long-term perspective, persons capable of adjusting to the crises of life in a flexible way that connects them to other people, often creatively managing the stresses they encounter, enjoy generally better health over the course of their life span. This is in contrast to those who, in adult life, are capable of only rigid, relatively uncreative defenses that serve often to drive others away.

The purpose of this chapter will be to offer a view of the ways in which the principal categories of psychological adaptations appear to be linked to the relative goodness of function of the components of the nervous system. Clinically, coping mechanisms describe a specific set of complex behaviors that can be observed reliably (Vaillant, 1977; Perry & Ianni, 1998) and that appear to be linked directly to the health of the brain. Acquiring clinical recognition skills with respect to coping mechanisms offers a practical method of viewing behavior with respect to brain function and impairment.

Teleologically, increasing the flexibility and creativity of adaptation to environmental (both internal and external) pressures suggests an obvious hypothetical advantage with respect to evolutionary pressures and demands on human beings over the eons. The more flexibly and more ingeniously organisms adapt to environmental threats, the more likely their health and preservation as a species will be. To some, therefore, it will come as no surprise that, as the ancient Greeks commented, a healthy mind and a healthy body occur together. Longitudinal study suggests that this is true both for the nervous system and for the other functions of the body that it monitors and mediates (Vaillant, 1979).

Clinically, however, it is important to recognize that a healthy mind requires a healthy body, including and particularly the nervous system. In order to function at one's best, all of the neural systems at the cortical level and below must be functioning in a reasonable, if not optimal, manner. This leads to the hypothesis that malfunction in the nervous system, specifically of the higher cortical and subcortical neural networks down through the structures of the brain stem, will, as a consequence of their dysfunction, limit the flexibility of adaptation that an individual may make. Put another way, a person whose brain becomes increasingly dysfunctional would be expected to demonstrate increasingly dysfunctional styles of adaptation to life.

In the clinical situation, therefore, the method of behavioral adaptation (ego defense mechanism or coping style) can be expected to offer a clue as to the possible dysfunction of one or another of the various systems and networks that constitute the human brain. Similarly, a documented dysfunction in one or another part of the brain should theoretically limit the ability of the organism to adapt to the psychological stresses of its environment, whether those are construed as emanating from within the organism or from outside of its physical boundaries. The clinician's ability and skill in recognizing more and less adaptive behavioral styles can offer a useful indication of the functioning of the higher centers of the brain, especially when a change in the style of psychological adaptation has occurred.

Clinical nosology of psychological adaptation

Before discussing this further, it will be necessary to provide a brief overview of the organization of human adaptational capabilities. We will do so using the terms articulated by Vaillant (1993) in his description of ego-defense mechanisms. To begin, one may usefully consider the ego as the conscious sense of one's self. The ego may be perturbed by a stress, either internally from its own conscious and unconscious drives, needs, and aggressions, or from the circumstances external to the human individual as when relationships with other people, physical illness, or other environmental stressors threaten one's sense of well being. When perturbed, the characteristic human response is normally one of increased anxiety: a sense of impending threat or disaster. This anxiety signals that a stress is present to which the person must turn his or her attention and begin to resolve; this type of anxiety is sometimes referred to as signal anxiety. As the anxiety climbs, the organism will follow the rule of Claude Bernard's *milieu interieur* and act in such a way as to maintain its own homeostasis. Speaking in biological terms, the physiologist Walter Cannon called this tendency to maintain homeostasis as the "wisdom of the cell," a phrase that George Vaillant has construed psychologically as "the wisdom of the ego." In order to cap the anxiety and adapt to its cause, the ego then constructs one or more coping styles that may be construed as ego-defense mechanisms, in the language of this line of research. Ego defense mechanisms are engaged primarily to gain control of the anxiety and, as a result, to begin an adaptation to the stress itself.

Although one must be careful to avoid the tendency to immediately ascribe value judgments to developmentally primitive defense mechanisms, it is certainly true that some coping styles are more adaptive than others. This may seem a truism to even the most casual observer of human behavior, but only in relatively recent times have the principles of science and empirical observation been applied to the assumptions underlying this simple statement. This body of work from several investigative sources, reviewed most comprehensively by Vaillant (1977), makes it clear that there is a hierarchy of possible styles of psychological adaptation. These range from very primitive inflexible responses, such as concrete denial of problems, through highly flexible and creative reactions such as humor, when one can laugh at oneself and one's predicament despite the adversity of one's circumstances.

Empirical study offers us the method of grouping the adaptive styles in four large categories, based on the nature of the response to stress clinically described. Table 7.1 lists a current vocabulary of these styles, construed in Vaillant's terms as defense mechanisms. The categories themselves are grouped along the hierarchical range from primitive to mature. For the present discussion, we will not consider examples of each defense mechanism, but refer the interested reader to book length discussions elsewhere (i.e., see Vaillant, 1993). To consider the relationship between brain function and adaptive style, we will focus on the larger domains of defense mechanisms and their application to neuropsychiatric assessment.

Table 7.1. The categories of coping styles (ego mechanisms of defense) and their putative association with various clinical states

Category	Response to crisis	Coping styles	Normal development	Associated clinical states
Primitive (psychotic)	The problem does not exist	Denial (concrete) Distortion/avoidance Psychotic projection	Early childhood	Decompensated major medical illness, bipolar disorder (manic or depressed), schizophrenia and other psychotic disorders, severe delirium, severe dementia
Immature (character or adolescent)	The problem exists but it's neither my fault nor my responsibility to address	Schizoid fantasy Passive aggression Neurotic projection Acting out Hypochondriasis	Adolescence	Mild to moderate delirium or dementia, chronic toxic states (e.g., alcoholism), personality disorders
Neurotic	The problem exists and it is my responsibility to address; however, I'm not fully able to integrate the affective and the cognitive components in a way that works towards a satisfying solution	Repression Intellectualization Displacement Dissociation Reaction formation	Adulthood	Mild acute depressions or dysthymia, generalized anxiety disorder, post-traumatic stress disorder, adjustment disorders, and much of the "normal" adult population
Mature	The problem exists and I am responsible for responding to it; I can use the affective and cognitive components of my responses to this problem to work together toward a solution that brings resolution and perhaps also helpful contact with others	Anticipation Altruism Humor Sublimation Suppression	Adulthood	Requires a relatively full and normal development and a central nervous system without active impairment

Primitive (psychotic) styles of adaptation

The first such group of adaptive styles are those referred to as primitive mechanisms when seen in the very young (children in their early years) or referred to as psychotic defenses when found in adults. The common strategy of adaptation in this class of mechanisms is to ignore the existence of any threatening stress whatsoever. One therefore finds that the stress is denied in a very concrete way (a refusal to acknowledge its existence), or distorted to such a great degree that acknowledgement of the stress itself, though not necessarily its consequences, is avoided (as when a person simply focuses on some other part of their life rather than face a particular difficulty). The third style in this group of defenses is to project the stress outward, again in a very concrete manner, and to believe that a stress (but not the actual stress) is being caused by some outside factor or person over which or over whom one has no control, as when a patient says the CIA or FBI caused his appendicitis.

Clinical examples of this range of coping styles are commonly seen in adults suffering from untreated schizophrenia or bipolar disorder. In the throes of a relapse of one's illness, the patient may ignore the presence of very real problems that require immediate attention (impaired judgment and insight), or perhaps delusionally misinterpret abnormal perceptions, minimize or deny their occurrence, or regard them as coming from a source other than one's own malfunctioning brain. In such cases, the primitive styles must still be considered as adaptations to the extent that they represent the individual's best effort to organize, understand, and communicate their experience within the limits of a dysfunctional brain. Though they do not serve to directly address or reduce the underlying stressor (deteriorating brain function resulting in relapsing illness), they do offer an attempt to translate profound anxiety or distress into a strategy that permits continued (if only very paranoid and fearful) existence. With appropriate medical treatment, improved or restored brain functioning may improve the patient's ability to make use of more flexible defensive styles and therefore a more adaptive manner of functioning. Descriptions of the course of patients with untreated major psychoses suggest that the ability to achieve highly adaptive psychological functioning is severely compromised when they go without medical treatment.

Immature (characterological) styles of adaptation

The next level in the hierarchy of defenses is that of the immature or adolescent defenses, so-called because they are seen normally in humans in their teen and early adult years. When these styles of coping with stress become psychologically entrenched in adults beyond the adolescent years, they are often referred to as character or characterological adaptive mechanisms (and typify the styles used by patients with character, or personality, disorders). The reactive stance, common to all of the coping mechanisms in the adolescent or character range, includes recognition of a stressor but disavows ownership or responsibility for the stressor and sometimes the response to it. The person has proceeded beyond ignoring the stress or threat common to primitive reactions, but has not yet apprehended the responsibility required to deal adaptively with difficult problems, stresses, or the anxiety they produce.

Coping styles at this level include a non-psychotic, less concrete form of projection in which others are blamed for one's own shortcomings; a passive/aggressive stance in which one's anxiety and anger are expressed indirectly or ineffectively through passivity or are directed against oneself; a hypochondriacal projection of anxiety into one's body or one's physical sensations; a retreat into a schizoid fantasy life in which real-world concerns become a secondary and less important part of existence; or a translation of the anxiety directly into action as a way of relieving the stress while avoiding conscious acknowledgement of the anxiety itself. As with the psychotic defenses, the immature defenses also represent the best adaptation to stress given the limited flexibility imposed by incomplete maturation or a decline in functioning – a perspective that obtains whether one views maturation and decline from a purely psychological or an entirely neurobiological perspective.

As a class, however, these adaptive styles do not locate the responsibility for responding to one's stresses as within oneself. Rather, they ascribe that responsibility to outside sources in ways that apportion blame to others for one's own distress, a process that serves to make others very uncomfortable. It is not hard to see, for example, why the victim of a punch by an "acting-out" developmentally delayed or a brain-injured patient may, because of the immature coping style and inability to recognize their role in and responsibility for mitigating recurrent use of such a style, regard the patient with dread rather than admiration. Similarly, the physician continually trying to find the cause for and provide relief to a histrionic patient with a hypochondriacal set of health concerns may also regard that patient's upcoming clinic visit with dread rather than eager anticipation. It is a small step to the observation that persons who drive others away will have a more difficult time than most in securing and making use of medical care – empirical study supports this contention (Vaillant, 1979; Hall et al., 1982).

Neurotic styles of adaptation

The third level of adaptive mechanisms are those referred to by Vaillant as neurotic defenses; he borrows an old term from depth psychology of the early twentieth century that refers to disjunction between thought and feeling. The neurotic styles are normally seen among adults, but do not represent the most flexible, most psychologically integrated form of adaptational responses to the various stresses of human life. At this level, the common theme among the specific styles is that the stress and/or one's response to it is consciously recognized and "owned" by that person. These adaptive mechanisms are progressed beyond the primitive ("no threat") and immature ("there is a threat but it's my fault or responsibility to deal with") stances of adaptation. In addition the person may identify that the problem to be faced includes a cognitive or intellectual component, engenders an affective or emotional response, or (more accurately) both.

The difficulty with the neurotic defenses is that the affective and the cognitive components of the adaptive response are not effectively integrated, hence the use of the term "neurosis." This is true, for example, in repression where the affective content is present in awareness and behavior, but the cognitive content is not appropriately paired with its associated affect. The inverse of this coping style is intellectualization, or isolation of affect, in which the cognitive component of the problem is present to consciousness, but the affective content is unavailable. Because of this lack of integration, the process of working through the stress and one's response to it toward a creative and adaptive solution is at least severely impeded if not altogether blocked. As a result, those using neurotic defenses often report feeling stuck in a behavioral pattern that is unpleasant or unhelpful, but nonetheless very difficult to change (sometimes referred to as the "repetition compulsion").

Other neurotic mechanisms include forming a diametrically opposed reaction to one's base (or unconscious) response ("convincing" oneself that a hated object is actually loved), displacing the problem to a less threatening object (directing one's anger at one's boss toward one's next door neighbor), or dissociating from the experience of the stress and one's reactions for brief periods of time. Persons using these adaptive mechanisms are aware of their psychological pain, but have a difficult time moving beyond the painful situation and their responses to it and towards a creative resolution. Nonetheless, such defenses continue to be adaptive in that they make anxiety and intellectual uncertainty tolerable and allow for other functions of a healthy life to be carried out, such as work and relationships with others. They do not, however, facilitate a sense of completed adaptation or of an adaptive response leading to a lasting resolution of the threat or one's reaction to it.

Mature styles of adaptation

Finally, the most adaptive coping mechanisms are described as mature. Building on the stances of the previous three groups, the mature coping styles include recognition of the threatening or stressful problem, ownership of the response to it, and recognition of *both* its affective and cognitive components. Mature coping styles then go further by facilitating the integration of affect and cognition and permitting one to work through the stress and one's responses to distress in a way that engenders a sense of genuine mastery and that may even be of service to other people.

Examples of this include being able to express the feeling and the thought content of a painful situation in a humorous way that includes oneself as part of the joke. Another option is to take the emotional and the intellectual content from the problem faced and build some activity or other effort that is aimed at assisting others with similar problems – altruism. This is distinguished from the neurotic defense of reaction formation, in which someone actually wanting help him or herself addresses that unmet, and therefore, distressing need by trying to serve others – also known as pseudoaltruism – which when thwarted reveals its limited flexibility by leaving the person with no other adaptive strategies with which to address this stress. Instead, the altruistic person is genuinely fulfilled by such service and, if for some reason performing this service becomes impossible, the altruistic person is sufficiently flexible (mature) to cope effectively using other strategies as well.

Suppression, another mature style, permits one to temporarily forestall addressing a stress or one's immediate reactions to it in the service of continuing with one's tasks or other immediately pressing problems. Unlike the primitive defenses that altogether ignore the problem (denial), immature defenses that put the problem in someone else's hands (projection), or neurotic defenses that repress but never address the problem directly, suppression is a temporary postponement after which one does examine and directly address the problem and works toward a solution.

Sublimation, in this nosology, refers to combining the thought and the feeling components of one's response to the problem into a production, such as a work of art or literature or other human creative act, such that the experience of and reactions to the stress are genuinely addressed and resolved. This style, as with many of the mature defenses, may also facilitate connections with and benefits for others since the work or sublimated expression is often shared with others.

The last of the mature defenses, anticipation, uses the earliest reactions to real or potential stresses as a signal to begin addressing it, often well in advance of any timed outline in which a response is required.

As in the other levels of adaptive styles, the mature mechanisms limit the anxiety created by the stressful problem or situation. Mature coping styles, in contrast to the others, provide genuine resolution of the problem and one's reactions to it, satisfaction and mastery of both, and often serve to engage other people as willing helpers in the effort of adaptation. This group of coping styles might be expected to provide, and have been empirically associated with, the best outcomes in terms of physical health as well as in social and psychological health (Vaillant, 1977; Vaillant & Koury, 1993).

The neuropsychiatry of psychological adaptation

To develop a neuropsychiatric perspective on successful and less successful coping styles, several preliminary considerations are warranted. The first of these is recognizing the simultaneous development of brain and behavior over the course of normal human development. As noted above, the primitive defenses are those characteristically seen in young children. As mothers and most pediatricians will attest, a toddler's insistence on avoiding, or even denying the existence of, a pressing problem (e.g., a dirty diaper) is not considered entirely abnormal for that stage of development. As cognitive faculties develop and toddlers begin to understand better the world around them, their capacity to respond to stresses in their world becomes increasingly grounded in reality and somewhat more flexible – at least in as much as it permits them to begin to acknowledge the stressors and to generate responses that are related to those stressors, even if ownership and responsibility remain externalized.

Parents of adolescents will attest to the "normal" (or, at least not developmentally unexpected) passive/aggression, acting out, hypochondriasis, and projection that, for a time, transform many otherwise mundane daily stresses into seemingly catastrophic events. This age is marked developmentally by the development of increasingly abstract and complex thought, social awareness (or at least self-consciousness), and integrative abilities as well as a progression towards leaving the comfort of parents and moving to an independent life. Growing through this time of adolescent adaptation, most adults eventually arrive at the point of recognizing painful affects and difficult cognitive complexes of thought and engage in the necessary adaptation or work of integrating them. As this development proceeds further, acquisition of increasingly mature defense mechanisms occurs naturally.

A second consideration in this area are the preliminary studies suggesting that the development of adaptational styles may be influenced, and perhaps in some sense constrained, by genetics (MacKinnon et al., 1990). Studies of this nature are very preliminary and require replication; however, they present the very interesting possibility that the development of one or another of the various general styles of adaptation to life may be rather more concretely predicated on neural systems and networks than has been openly acknowledged up to the present time.

The third consideration is that of clinical experience in which the flexibility of psychological adaptation appears to vary as a function of brain health, and that certain of the various coping styles already reviewed tend to be associated with pathological or non-pathological states. While systematic studies of this statement in a large number of persons have yet to be accomplished, we offer the following vignettes as illustrations of this phenomenon.

A 27-year-old woman was referred to the neuropsychiatry clinic for evaluation and treatment of non-epileptic seizures. The patient's development had proceeded normally until she sustained a severe traumatic brain injury at age 16. This injury produced significant cognitive impairment (Full Scale IQ = 82, with prominent problems in executive function and verbal learning), major depression, and complex partial seizures with intermittent secondary generalization (left frontal origin). She was treated with carbamazepine and fluoxetine in the first year following her injury with fair control of her seizures (about one per month) and remission of her depression. Although she completed high school at age 19, she was unable to consistently maintain employment due to her cognitive impairment, seizures, or both. As a result, she was unable to become financially and socially independent from her mother and grandmother, with whom she lived. As a result of her anger and frustration over her perceived loss of future independence, the relationship with her family was, at best, highly fractious.

She eventually married, permitting her to leave the home. She had two children and remained at home as a full-time homemaker; she received support and assistance from her family only when she requested it, and enjoyed a sense of accomplishment and success as a mother and homemaker. Her seizure disorder remained under control with carbamazepine; intermittent relapses of her depressive disorder were successfully treated with brief (about one-year) courses of selective serotonin reuptake inhibitors.

Her husband initiated an extramarital affair about three months before the patient came to neuropsychiatric attention. He eventually filed for divorce and insisted that the patient and their children move out of their home. Without the ability to seek out other supports or to creatively garner resources that might permit her to remain independent, the patient reluctantly returned to living with her mother and grandmother. It was at this time that the patient began having "seizures" with increasing frequency.

These spells were inconsistent in presentation, sometimes involving whole body tonic–clonic movements but with preserved level of consciousness and ability to appropriately interact with her environment. Within two months, the patient was having as many as 40 of these spells per month, and was being taken to various emergency rooms at least weekly. Video-EEG monitoring documented that these spells were not of epileptic origin. She was subsequently referred to the neuropsychiatry clinic for evaluation.

The patient reported a litany of additional symptoms that suggested the presence of a recurrent episode of major depression. At the time of consultation, although she could acknowledge her unhappiness, she was not able to engage in an inquiry into the possible relationships between her unhappiness, the recent stressors in her life (loss of marriage, loss of independence, humiliation at having to return to living with her mother and grandmother), and the development of her pseudoseizures. Indeed, direct discussion of the pseudoseizures by the referring neurologist had generated an angry and markedly distressed reaction towards him (akin to "how dare you call me crazy"), and most attempts at such during the initial consultation met with a similar response. Her principal concern was to treat the "seizures," as she felt they were responsible for all of her present problems.

The patient presented with a complex combination of significant brain dysfunction, both chronically and acutely. Her chronic intellectual impairment and emotional (mood) dysregulation placed some limits on the flexibility of her adaptation to life, particularly as regards her independence. As she had never fully resolved the conflicts between her desire to be cared for, her wish to become independent, and the genuine challenges that she faced in so doing, she had, at best, remained "stuck" in this neurotic conflict. Her marriage had permitted her to become relatively independent from her family. However, her marriage and move away from her family merely displaced her dependency needs onto a more acceptable object (her husband), and facilitated her repressing awareness of the original and underlying conflict; neither of these adaptations resulted in any real resolution of her conflict over her dependency/individuation issues.

When these neurotic-level psychological adaptations were thwarted by her husband's decision to divorce her and demand that she move out of their house, and by the subsequent stresses these events imposed, her distress and anxiety became intolerable. She began developing a recurrent major depression, perhaps fueled not only by these stresses, but also by her rather tenuous neurobiological state. As this depression developed, her defense style shifted to a rather more immature level, most obviously evidenced by pseudoseizures. While this immature defense style (in this nosology, pseudoseizures are a form of a hypochondriacal – or somatically focused – defense) is indeed highly maladaptive, it served several much needed adaptive purposes.

First, the development of pseudoseizures re-directed her anxiety regarding her several losses and sense of failure or "defectiveness" onto an emotionally "safer" object, her body, which she already regarded as defective. Second, the causes of the pseudoseizures and their relationship to her feelings were unknown to her, thereby permitting disavowal of any role or responsibility for the pseudoseizures and a useful misattribution of her distress and other affects to the pseudoseizures themselves (rather than their causes). Third, their occurrences permitted gratification of her consciously unacceptable dependency needs through the more acceptable avenue of attention to her seizures.

Several studies have documented such regressions in defensive style during major depression, and note that treatment of the major depression often results in a return to more adaptive levels of psychological functioning (Mullen et al., 1999; Akkerman et al., 1992, 1999; Kneepkens & Oakley, 1996). With this in mind, the first task of treatment was to address the recurrent major depression using the same methods that had proven successful previously, namely treatment with a selective serotonin reuptake inhibitor. The patient was started on sertraline 50 mg per day; this dose was increased to a maintenance dose of 100 mg over the following six weeks. By the end of two months, her pseudoseizures had declined in frequency to a rate of approximately one per week. Noting that this treatment had not produced a full recovery, additional treatment strategies were needed.

The patient's baseline cognitive functioning presented a particular challenge in treatment; dynamic therapy aimed at developing a conscious understanding of the conflicts driving her regression was severely limited by her verbal learning and executive impairments. Since her procedural learning was relatively better preserved, a course of therapy aimed at identification and rehearsal of more effective coping strategies was developed.

The patient was first helped to identify activities and situations that she found relaxing and enjoyable under usual circumstances. These included painting, reading, watching television, playing the piano, and walking. A hierarchy of enjoyable activities was developed, and a schedule for daily involvement in one (or more) of them was developed.

Concurrently, the patient began a journal to document the events of her daily life, the use of the various activities, and her emotional state at the beginning and the end of each day. This was needed not only as a compensatory strategy for her declarative memory impairments (which made discussion of the week's events and stresses in therapy otherwise impossible), but also as a means of encouraging her to use a more adaptive coping style (intellectualization) in the service of improved health. She was encouraged to enlist the opinions and observations of her family in a daily fashion and to include their observations in her journal; although this met with some resistance initially, she came to experience her discussions with them as collaborations rather than dependencies, and over time began to value, rather than revile, these interactions.

Over time, the patient began to identify patterns in her daily life that were either emotionally helpful or emotionally distressing, many of the latter being routinely associated with a pseudoseizure. Because this examination was also coupled with identification of strengths, skills, and recognition of her ability to (at least occasionally) more effectively cope with everyday stress, she became better able to tolerate the idea of a connection between negative events, her emotional reactions, and the pseudoseizures. By then reinforcing the use of emotionally helpful activities when faced with negative events or intense negative affects, the pseudoseizures gradually ceased by the end of the first year of treatment.

This case illustrates several issues in the neuropsychiatry of psychological adaptation. First, acute stressors (biological, psychological, or social) can cause a rapid decline in the level of adaptive functioning. The development of persistently less mature and significantly maladaptive coping styles in a patient who generally functions at a relatively higher level may reflect the development of a neurobiological disorder, psychological conflict, severe social stressors, or some combination of these. In this case, all of these factors were operative: the patient was experiencing a major depressive episode, psychological conflict regarding dependency needs and worthlessness, and multiple social losses and conflicts. Second, the presence of alterations in underlying neurobiology (in this case neuropsychiatric disturbances and seizures due to a traumatic brain injury) may reduce the threshold for such psychological regressions, resulting in an increased likelihood and greater severity of such. Third, a defensive style may be improved by prompt treatment of underlying neurobiological disorders such as major depression. Finally, patients with neuropsychiatric disorders may present particular psychotherapeutic challenges, for example cognitive impairments limiting the use of more traditional "talk" therapies. Nonetheless, a creative therapist may be able to use patients' remaining strengths to facilitate a return to the best possible level of psychological adaptation of which they are capable.

A similar interaction between brain dysfunction and the regression of coping mechanisms can be seen in the second case.

A psychiatric resident informed her supervisor that she had been called to see a 60-year-old male patient on a medical unit who carried the provisional diagnosis of depression. When she interviewed this patient, she found "a very nasty old man." She went on to describe a patient with severe chronic obstructive pulmonary disease who was obstreperous in his relationship with the nurses and with the medical house staff. He constantly blamed the house staff for their ineptitude in his case, and occasionally refused minor medical procedures such as blood drawing. At interview he was irritable and demanding, and belittled the psychiatry resident while also asking him to finish the interview and leave as soon as possible. His medications included prednisone, 30 mg daily, which was used to treat an acute exacerbation of his lung disorder. While he refused to cooperate with a complete cognitive exam, he was able to attend to the interview and maintain his concentration insofar as his irritability would allow. His speech was goal directed and coherent. There was no evidence of hallucinations, and although he did not appear frankly delusional he was least suspicious of, if not overtly paranoid about, his caregivers and their abilities.

In this case, the resident (aided by her supervisor) suppressed her own angry response to this patient in the service of carefully considering a differential diagnosis for his irritability and maladaptive coping strategies (ones that threatened to alienate the people attempting to care for him). The patient's maladaptive coping strategies included a form of neurotic projection in which he viewed others as having a serious problem (ineptitude) rather than acknowledging both medical problem that threatened his health and his own inability (or ineptitude) to control the affects that he was experiencing. The specter of an elderly patient employing a coping strategy more characteristic of an adolescent prompted a search for one or more causes for his emotional dysregulation (irritability), mild paranoia, coping strategies inconsistent with his stage of development, and also the possible relationships (psychological and neurobiological) between these problems and his medical illness and treatment.

At the top of the differential was the possibility of adverse effects of the prednisone used to treat his pulmonary disease. This medication is well known to produce emotional disturbances and sometimes frank psychosis when administered in relatively high doses. The patient's emotional symptoms may be best understood as those of substantial affective dysregulation, manifest as irritability and anger, due to treatment with corticosteroids. It appears that the severity of the patient's affective disturbance interfered with his ability to engage with his physicians and consultants in efforts to understand his condition, his treatment, or his reactions to these stressors. Although the patient's basic cognitive abilities seemed relatively unaffected by his condition, he also developed suspiciousness; this severely restricted his ability to engage in any discussion of his medical condition and neuropsychiatric symptoms, his extremely intense affects, and to understand the relationship between these factors (which was, presumably, not consciously known to him).

In this context, one of medication-induced acute loss of emotional regulation and restriction of cognitive abilities, the patient's behavior was most usefully understood as a loss of his usual adaptive coping styles – in other words, a biological disturbance yielded a concurrent psychological disturbance, in this case a psychological regression. Because discontinuing the corticosteroids was not medically acceptable, the consultants recommended treatment with a haloperidol 0.5 mg twice daily targeting his mild paranoia and excessive irritability. On follow-up examination 24 hours later, the patient was much less irritable and even affable and cooperative during his interaction with the psychiatry resident. At this point he exhibited a much greater degree of patience as well as an ability to apprehend and to value the concerns of the medical staff and their recommended treatments. He was still able to voice many questions about his medical care, but had given up the stance that the medical staff was incompetent or otherwise trying to hurt him.

This case illustrates the intimate relationship between psychological defense mechanisms and the relative functioning of the brain itself. In this instance the steroid doses were sufficient to impair the usual complex cognitive abilities of the patient and to drive his affect to an overwhelming level of uncontrollable intensity. Unable to use his usual and more mature coping styles to integrate cognitions and affects of this nature, a regression to a more "characterological" coping style occurred. While in this mode of coping, unacceptable and overwhelming affects were projected onto others, both prompted by and in support of his mildly distorted cognitions, and fostered a stance in which his own internal distress was managed by attributing responsibility for it to others. When the unwanted effects of the exogenous steroid were pharmacologically attenuated, brain function improved and his adaptive strategies return to their more usual and developmentally appropriate level. In cases such as this, acute regressive shifts in adaptive strategies may serve to indicate deterioration of normal brain physiology.

Summary

When considering styles of psychological adaptation and brain function, we may think of two parallel hierarchies that are interconnected. Behaviorally, the clinician can observe the hierarchical construction of coping styles that vary from primitive to highly flexible and mature. Simultaneously, there is a relative hierarchy of central nervous system functioning that begins in very primitive functions in the brain stem and moves rostrally to a series of complex interconnections. While studies of early development and longitudinal studies of adult development argue that brain functioning and adaptive abilities are functionally connected, we have only hypotheses at present to suggest that in more acute settings, such as that of the clinical encounters described above, we can use observations of changes in adaptive functioning as indicators of brain dysfunction. Much work needs to be done in sorting out the details of the relationship between these clinical phenomena and the neurobiology upon which they are predicated. Until such work affords clearer principles that bridge these two conceptual frameworks, we may still find the perspective offered by an understanding of psychological adaptation useful in the practice of any area of medicine, and especially neuropsychiatry. To that end, a few practical principles are offered here.

First, ascertain the coping level at which the patient appears to be functioning: primitive; immature; neurotic; or mature. One clue is the perspective and opinions of those with whom the patient interacts: do others regard him or her as ill (psychotic); a big pain (immature); somewhat "quirky" or plagued by various "hang-ups" (neurotic); or admirable (mature)? While identifying very specific defenses demonstrated by patients is often interesting, at the end of such interpretations it is often more useful to have determined the larger category that best describes the patient's general style of adaptive functioning.

Next, ascertain whether there has been a shift (acute, subacute, or chronic) in adaptive style. This information is often most usefully garnered via interview of family members or others who know the patient well.

Construct a differential diagnosis that seeks to relate the patient's current adaptive style to biological (medical, neurological, psychiatric, substances, and toxins), psychological (psychodynamic or other developmental issues), and social stressors – especially if they are new to the patient or are perceived as different by those in his or her life.

Where acute changes in adaptive strategies suggest the possibility of an underlying medical disorder, the approach for evaluation should mirror that for delirium (described in Chapter 12). Relatively subtler and slowly progressive declines in adaptive functioning from a previously acquired baseline should suggest the possibility of a more insidious medical (especially medication-related), neuropsychiatric (e.g., dementia, depression), or substance (e.g., alcoholism) problem. Where psychological explanations for maladaptive strategies are the best available, they should be addressed by a psychotherapist. Importantly, many forms of psychotherapy, including cognitive–behavioral, psychodynamic, and psychoanalytic therapies, may all be helpful towards the development of more adaptive coping styles.

If one views the patient's current coping styles as the best available adaptive strategy given his or her present biological, psychological, and social context, suggesting that he or she simply "stop it" or "do something else to deal with it" entirely misses the point that the patient is doing his or her best – to do otherwise will almost certainly encourage further regression. In the service of maintaining the highest possible level of function at all times, it may sometimes be necessary to appeal to the adaptive aspects of an otherwise maladaptive coping style; for example, offering the hypochondriacal patient a return appointment and further follow-up rather than a psychological interpretation of the presenting symptom or an unnecessary medical or surgical intervention. While so doing, the patient's ability to make use of related but more adaptive defenses can be encouraged and reinforced in psychotherapy.

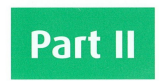

Part II

A neuropsychiatric approach to evaluating the patient

8

Neuropsychiatric evaluation

Introduction

The practice of neuropsychiatry requires familiarity with brain–behavior relationships and facility with the language and skills of both neurology and psychiatry. In the preceding chapters we have offered an approach to understanding brain–behavior relationships that we find clinically useful. In this approach we attempt to understand the basic elements of cognition, emotion, and behavior in terms of their relationship to both structural and functional neuroanatomy. While our approach is necessarily incomplete, given both the limitations of current knowledge and our own efforts to be concise rather than comprehensive, we find that these basic concepts do usefully guide the clinical interview and examination, development of the differential diagnosis, and the construction of a treatment plan.

How one understands brain–behavior relationships strongly influences the types of information one seeks during an evaluation, both during the interview and in the collection of collateral information. If problems in impulse control, problem solving, insight, and judgment are regarded as signs of disrupted frontal-subcortical circuitry, the history will focus on a search for developmental or acquired causes of such disruptions. These might include traumatic brain injury, stroke, metabolic diseases, neurodegenerative disorders, white matter disease, or primary neuropsychiatric disorders that involve these areas (e.g., schizophrenia, mania). Although impaired impulse control and problem solving may be ascribed to personality pathology or immature ego development (i.e., "acting out"), it is also important to evaluate even these phenomena in terms of their possible neural substrates to ensure that all possible causes of such problems are considered.

From this understanding of brain–behavior relationships – that mental events are brain events – the neuropsychiatric evaluation combines the neurological and psychiatric interviews and examinations in order to develop a comprehensive body of clinical information from which to ascertain diagnoses and develop treatment plans. The history section inquires about present and past neuropsychiatric and medical problems and their treatments, if any, assesses the course of development, and the family history and social context in which the presenting problems are occurring. The examination includes the relevant portions of the general physical examination, complete neurological and mental status examinations, and is particularly attentive to subtle cognitive, emotional, behavioral, and motor (e.g., primitive reflexes) pathology. Laboratory procedures will vary depending on the differential diagnosis supported by the history and examination, but frequently involve neuroimaging, electrodiagnostic testing, neuropsychological testing, and a variety of biochemical laboratory assessments. The results of these various evaluations are viewed as offering complementary information sets to be used together to provide the best possible understanding of the signs and symptoms of neuropsychiatric conditions.

As a result of combining the neurological and psychiatric examinations, a neuropsychiatric evaluation is frequently quite lengthy and labor intensive, and may require several evaluation sessions to complete. Additionally, other professionals such as referring physicians (generally psychiatrists, neurologists, or primary care specialists), neuroradiologists, electroencephalographers, neuropsychologists, physiatrists, physical, occupational, or speech therapists must often be called upon to collaborate during the evaluation process, either via provision of collateral information or performance of additional assessments. Consequently, the neuropsychiatric evaluation is most appropriately considered to be a multidisciplinary task guided by a professional with expertise in brain–behavior relationships.

A complete description of all aspects of the neuropsychiatric evaluation is well beyond the scope of the present work. In this chapter, we assume that readers have a basic familiarity with the elements of the history taking and with physical, neurological, and psychiatric examinations. We have therefore intentionally avoided a lengthy description of each element of the neuropsychiatric evaluation. Instead, we offer an outline of the neuropsychiatric evaluation in tabular form (Tables 8.1–8.5), within which we highlight a few aspects of the examination that may be relatively unfamiliar to practitioners outside neuropsychiatry and behavioral neurology. It is our hope that clinicians may copy this outline and use it as a guide (or reminder card) in their clinical practice. We have found this practice useful in our teaching clinics, not only as a teaching tool but also, more practically, as a reminder to ourselves

Table 8.1. Essential elements of a neuropsychiatric history

Evaluation section	Essential elements	Items of particular interest
History	Chief complaint, history of present illness, and symptom description	Symptoms should be described in terms of their quality, intensity, duration (both onset and course), relationship to precipitating factors, response to palliative efforts, and context (appropriate, appropriate but excessive or deficient, or inappropriate). Neuropsychiatric symptoms may be usefully clarified and quantified with scales such as the Neuropsychiatric Inventory or Neurobehavioral Rating Scale. Specific problems may also be more fully and accurately assessed using scales such as the Delirium Rating Scale, the Galveston Orientation and Amnesia Test, the Overt Aggression Scale, and the Apathy Evaluation Scale, among others
		Collateral history from medical records, family, friends, caregivers, and other records should be sought as the patient's ability to provide accurate information may be affected by the presenting neuropsychiatric condition
		Include screening questions for paroxysmal events (e.g., seizures, stroke, other "spells," etc.). Be particularly aware of "atypical" features such as unusually early or late onset, unexpected associated features (e.g., movement disorders or neuropsychological impairments in "primary" psychiatric illnesses), unusually rapid or slow course of illness, or treatment-resistance
	Medical, surgical, neurological, psychiatric, and substance history	Inquiry into past psychiatric and substance history should not rely solely on qualitative terms (e.g., "No, I've never been depressed'). The clinician should ask the patient to describe their understanding and use of such terms in order to avoid misunderstandings regarding important parts of the history, especially when inquiring about conditions whose labels are used commonly in lay conversation and whose referents may be quite different than that understood by clinicians (e.g., depression, "petit mal" seizures, "migraine" headaches, etc.). Where possible, use formal criteria (e.g., DSM-IV, CAGE questions, etc.) to structure the inquiry and to more rigorously evaluate the patients' qualitative descriptions

Table 8.1. (*cont.*)

Evaluation section	Essential elements	Items of particular interest
	Trauma history	Inquire about concussions and other "mild" injuries in detail, including mechanism of injury, loss of consciousness, impairment in memory for the event (post-traumatic amnesia), or any alteration in mental status at the time of the injury ("dazed and confused"). Any such injury may be significant if the patient experiences a marked decline in functioning (cognitive, emotional, behavioral, motoric, etc.) as a direct result of the injury. The significance of injuries in childhood is often minimized by patients and should be investigated more thoroughly in light of a change in developmental course following the injury (e.g., marked change in school or social performance)
	Medications and medication history	Present and past medications, including dose, duration of treatment, and response or adverse effects should be noted. Medication allergies and reactions (e.g., rash, blood dyscrasias, movement disorders, etc.) should be noted. Environmental exposures (e.g., exposure to toxic substances) should also be assessed. Substance use, abuse, and dependence must also be assessed, if not done earlier. Also, information regarding use of herbal remedies and supplements, vitamins, minerals, and other over-the-counter medications should be obtained, as many possess significant psychoactive agents
	Developmental history	Include prenatal, birth, preschool, and school history. Timing and achievement of developmental milestones should be determined. Learning disabilities and strengths should also be noted, including any participation in special education programs. Manner and quality of interaction with peers should be noted
	Handedness	A variety of formal questionnaires and scales to assess handedness are available. About 90% of the population is left-hemisphere dominant, resulting in right-handedness. Of the 10% who appear to be left-handed, about half are still left-hemisphere dominant, at least for language. Asking a patient to pantomime or perform real tasks (see Mental Status Examination chapter), which eye is used to

Table 8.1. (*cont.*)

Evaluation section	Essential elements	Items of particular interest
		look in a telescope, and which foot is used to kick a ball will usually reveal handedness preference. Note that these procedures will sometimes reveal mixed handedness (e.g., right hand, left foot, left eye)
	Social/cultural history	Include assessment of education, employment, military, relationship, and legal history, including past or present litigation. This assessment should determine the patient's highest level of functioning, the temporal stability of that functioning, and the pattern of any decline in functioning
		Also determine the patient's and family's understanding of current problems, the nature of self-prescribed treatments they may have already tried, and their willingness to accept medical treatment. If prescribed treatments can be safely added to self-treatments some patients may better accept them, and compliance with prescribed treatment may be enhanced
	Family history	Include questions about medical, neurologic, psychiatric and substance problems, even if not formally diagnosed or treated. Again, use formal criteria (DSM-IV) to structure the inquiry and to determine the validity of any qualitative terms used by the patient or family
	Review of systems and symptoms	This should be viewed as an expanded and detailed consideration of the history of present illness. Structured reviews and symptom inventories (e.g., Neuropsychiatric Inventory, Neurobehavioral Rating Scale, Overt Aggression Scale, Apathy Evaluation Scale, etc.) should be used routinely to document both the extent and severity of current problems and also to establish both a qualitative and quantitative baseline from which to evaluate treatment effectiveness. Where possible, self-report quantitative scales such as the Symptom Checklist 90 – Revised (SCL-90-R) and the SF-36 Health Survey may offer a time-efficient method of comprehensive review of symptoms and symptoms that more fully informs the evaluation and establishes a quantitative baseline against which the effects of treatment can be measured

Table 8.2. Essential elements of a neuropsychiatric examination

Evaluation section	Essential elements	Items of particular interest
Examination	Physical examination	Vital signs, including heart rate, respiratory rate, blood pressure, height, and weight
		General examination for evidence of development anomalies, trauma, physical signs of substance abuse (e.g., "track marks") or withdrawal, or other signs of medical illness
		Specific examinations relevant to the neuropsychiatric presentation (e.g., auscultation of carotid arteries, cardiac examination, etc., in a patient with suspected vascular dementia; abdominal examination in a patient with alcohol dependence)
	Elemental neurological examination	Cranial nerves examination, including:
		I – olfaction, use items such as coffee grounds or cinnamon
		II – visual fields, visual acuity, and funduscopic examination
		III, IV, VI – extraocular movements (up, down, and lateral gaze)
		V – facial sensation
		VII – facial motor ability
		VIII – hearing and vestibular function
		IX – gag reflex (test on each side of the posterior pharynx)
		X – palatal elevation (deviates to intact side)
		XI – sternocleidomastoid and trapezius motor strength
		XII – tongue protrusion (deviates to affected side)
		Motor examination, including:
		tone, or resistance to passive manipulation
		bulk
		abnormal involuntary movements (e.g., tics, tremors, chorea, etc.)
		strength – including assessment for pronator drift
		Sensory examination, including:
		pin-prick
		temperature

light touch

vibration

proprioception

Coordination examination, including:

finger-to-nose (look for ataxia, dysmetria, tremor, etc.)

fine finger movement (repeated thumb–finger opposition)

rapid alternating movements (repeated palm–back of hand)

heel-to-shin (place heel below knee and move up and down shin)

Gait examination, including:

station – including assessment for the presence of Romberg sign

walking – including tandem, toe, and heel, and arm swing; assess turning

Reflex examination, including:

deep tendon reflexes in face (jaw-jerk) and all extremities

plantar responses

assessment for Hoffman's sign (flick distal phalanx of middle digit of hand – if this

produces flexor contraction of the thumb, sign is positive)

primitive reflexes (see Table 8.3)

Mental status examination   General and cognitive (see Table 8.4 and the Mental Status Examination Chapter)

Table 8.3. Primitive reflexes and pathological responses

Primitive reflexes and pathological responses[a]	Examination maneuver	Normal response	Abnormal response	Comment
Glabellar	Tapping 10 times on the glabella (area just above and between eyebrows)	No blinking	Partial or full blinking in response to each tap	If response extinguishes within three taps, response should be noted but not necessarily considered abnormal when it occurs in the absence of other pathological responses
Snout	Light tap on patient's lips; alternatively, and to determine the presence of any asymmetry of response, tap above the upper lip just lateral to the filtrum on each side	No movement	Lips pucker	May be normally present in 30% of persons 60 years or older
Suck	Gloved knuckle is placed between patient's lips	No movement	Sucking motion	Performing this examination on aggressive patients is not recommended
Rooting	Stroke patient's cheek	No movement	Head turns toward side being stroked	
Palmomental	Stroke palm from lateral aspect of hypothenar eminence to thenar eminence	No movement	Ipsilateral mentalis (chin) muscle contracts	May be normally present in 20% of persons 30 years or older and in 50% of persons older than 50 years

Sign	Maneuver	Normal response	Abnormal response	Comments
Grasp	Place two fingers in patient's hand and stroke across palm or along fingers	No grasp	Patient grasps fingers	An alternative abnormal response is for the patient to reflexively extend the wrists and fingers – this is referred to as an avoidance response
Self-grasp	Examiner uses patient's hand to stroke patient's contralateral ulnar surface	Strokes ulnar surface	Grasps forearm	
Nuchocephalic	Patient stands with eyes closed and examiner sharply rotates patient's head and torso.	Head rotates with torso	Head does not rotate with torso	Similar to a doll's eyes response using the torso and head
Gegenhalten	Examiner passively manipulates patient's extremities	Patient relaxes and does not resist manipulation	Patient is unable to permit passive manipulation and offers a "counterpull," or an increasing resistance to manipulation	Roughly translates from German as "stop movement," and is suggestive of frontal lobe dysfunction; may be more akin to dyspraxia (can't integrate command to relax limb with execution of the task) than to other primitive responses

Note:

[a] Although often referred to as "frontal lobe" signs, the abnormal responses elicited by these maneuvers may occur when elements of the frontal-subcortical circuitry are disrupted. These responses are relatively insensitive markers of frontal-subcortical pathology. However, the presence of two or more severely abnormal responses (suck, rooting, grasp, self-grasp, any unilateral response) or three or more mildly abnormal responses (glabellar, palmomental, snout, or bilateral responses) is highly specific for frontal lobe (including frontal white matter and subcortical connections) dysfunction from any cause (e.g., Alzheimer's disease, traumatic brain injury, frontal neoplasm, or stroke)

Table 8.4. Essential elements of the mental status examination[a]

Mental status examination	Essential elements	Specific items requiring assessment	
General	Appearance and Behavior	Arousal	
		Dress, grooming, and hygiene	
		Facial expression	
		Posture, motor activity	
		Attitude toward the examiner	
	Speech	Quantity	
		Volume	
		Tone	
		Rate	
		Rhythm	
	Thought Process	Structure (organization)	
		Style	
	Thought Content	Perception	
		Interpretation of environment	
		Themes and concerns	
		Lethality	
	Emotion	Mood	
		Affect	
Cognitive	Arousal	Level of arousal	
	Attention	Selective	
		Sustained vs. distractibility	
		Alternating or multitasking	
	Language	Fluency (verbal and written)	
		Repetition	
		Comprehension (verbal and written)	
		Naming	
	Memory	Immediate	Verbal
		Recent	Visual
		Remote	Procedural
	Praxis	Limb-kinetic	
		Ideomotor	
		Ideational	
		Constructional (visuospatial skill)	

Table 8.4. (*cont.*)

Mental status examination	Essential elements	Specific items requiring assessment
	Recognition	Visual
		Auditory
		Tactile
	Complex Cognition	Executive function
		Social intelligence
		Motivation

Note:

[a] Refer to Chapter 9 for a more detailed description of the elements of this examination.

when both examining patients and dictating reports on the often lengthy neuropsychiatric evaluation.

Lengthier and more detailed descriptions of the neuropsychiatric evaluation are offered elsewhere. Interested readers may find additional useful and detailed information in Taylor (1999), Strub & Black (1997), Mueller & Fogel (1996), Filley (1995), Trzepacz & Baker (1993) and Ovsiew (1992).

Three other major components of the evaluation, namely the mental status examination, neuroimaging, and electrodiagnostic techniques, are presented in detail in the following three chapters. Because the mental status examination is to neuropsychiatry what the stethoscope is to cardiology, its importance to the neuropsychiatric evaluation cannot be overstated; hence, we offer a detailed review of this examination in Chapter 9. Clinicians new to the fields of neuropsychiatry and behavioral neurology may not be familiar with some elements of the examination needed in neuropsychiatric practice, so we have made considerable efforts to be inclusive in our description of this portion of the neuropsychiatric evaluation.

We have also dedicated chapters to electrodiagnostic techniques (Chapter 10) and neuroimaging (Chapter 11) to provide a basic introduction to the method and language of both. As with our previous analogy, electrodiagnostic and neuroimaging techniques are as fundamental to the neuropsychiatric evaluation as are the electrocardiogram and chest X-ray to cardiology, and any clinician interested in neuropsychiatry should have at least a passing familiarity with them. Additional aspects of the history, examination, and laboratory diagnostic procedures that are relevant to the evaluation of specific neuropsychiatric problems are presented in additional detail in Part III.

Table 8.5. Laboratory procedures commonly used in the neuropsychiatric evaluation[a]

Evaluation section	Commonly performed procedures	Items of particular interest

Laboratory procedures	Neuroimaging	Structural imaging
		    computed tomography (CT) – best in acute/emergency situations
		    magnetic resonance imaging (MRI) – best study if anatomic (especially white matter) detail is needed
		Functional neuroimaging
		    functional MRI
		    diffusion-weighted MRI
		    magnetic resonance spectroscopy (MRS)
		    single-photon computed tomography (SPECT)
		    positron emission tomography (PET)

	Electrophysiologic assessment	Electroencephalography (EEG)
		    standard EEG
		    digital EEG
		    ambulatory EEG
		    quantitative EEG (QEEG)
		    evoked potentials (EP)
		    event-related potentials (ERP)
		Magnetoencephalography (MEG)
		    magnetic source imaging (MSI)
		    magnetic evoked fields (MEF)

	Neuropsychological testing	Specific question(s) must be included in the referral for neuropsychological testing. Usefulness of such testing depends, at least in part, upon the referring clinician's ability to frame the specific clinical issue to be addressed
		Diagnostic evaluation using clinical evaluation and standardized tests, including:
		    fixed batteries (e.g., Halstead-Reitan, Wechsler Adult Intelligence Scale)
		    flexible batteries (e.g., Luria-Nebraska)
		    projective testing (e.g., Rorschach, Thematic Apperception Test)
		    personality assessment (e.g., Minnesota Multiphasic Personality Inventory)

Table 8.5. (*cont.*)

Evaluation section	Commonly performed procedures	Items of particular interest
		reliability and validity scales to assess effort and possible malingering
		Determination of relative neuropsychological strengths and weaknesses is useful for:
		diagnosis – suggested by typical patterns of performance
		treatment planning – capitalize on strengths, compensatory strategies
		tracking treatment effectiveness
		medicolegal issues
	Blood work	Selection of tests is best determined according to the differential diagnosis established by history, examination, and other laboratory procedures, as described in Part III of this book. Screening tests have relatively low yield when performed indiscriminately
		Renal and hepatic panels and complete blood count are appropriate before initiating some medications (e.g., tricyclic antidepressants, mood stabilizers)
	Lumbar puncture	Should be performed expeditiously whenever a central nervous system infection is suspected
		Generally, lumbar puncture is only otherwise indicated when a specific etiology is being pursued (e.g., multiple sclerosis, central nervous system lymphoma, etc.), in high risk groups with altered mental status (e.g., AIDS, oncology patient, etc.), or when other diagnostic tests have failed to reveal a cause of neuropsychiatric impairments
		Lumbar puncture may be useful for the diagnosis of normal pressure hydrocephalus (gait and mental status may transiently improve immediately following this procedure) and pseudotumor cerebri (relief of headache following procedure)

Note:

[a] Selection of tests should be predicated on the differential diagnosis established by the history and examinations described in Tables 8.1–8.4.

9

The mental status examination

Introduction

The mental status examination (MSE) is a systematic assessment of an individual's quality of mental functioning, and consists of a series of systematic and hierarchically organized observations and questions. The MSE is, of course, only one part of a more comprehensive clinical examination, and findings of the MSE are best interpreted in this larger context. For example, impairment of language such as non-fluent aphasia often occurs with deficits in other aspects of neurological function, such as right hemiparesis, and together may quickly lead the clinician to a diagnosis of dominant hemisphere injury (i.e., stroke). However, patients will sometimes demonstrate abnormalities of mental function without clear abnormalities on general physical or neurological examination. In such cases, the examination will often be described as "non-focal," though with acknowledgement of an "altered mental status." Although some aspects of the MSE may at first seem mysterious and of uncertain significance, when performed by a clinician experienced in its administration and interpretation, the MSE can provide a series of observations capable of detecting localizable brain dysfunction. This chapter will convey the message that abnormalities on the MSE should be regarded as evidence of localized dysfunction referable to injury of either specific structures or specific networks of structures in the brain.

The MSE is sometimes criticized as being qualitative rather than quantitative and relying heavily on the subjective administration and interpretation of the examiner. Studies have shown, however, that the results of the MSE are comparable in validity and reliability to other parts of the physical examination, such as auscultation of the lungs or heart, palpation of the abdomen, or assessment of reflexes. In all such aspects of clinical examination, the skill of the clinician's examination and interpretation of findings is paramount. Though all can provide only qualitative data, each provides useful diagnostic information that the wise clinician will not wish to ignore.

In a sense, the MSE is a stethoscope for listening to brain function and is the primary clinical tool for examining and understanding cognition, emotion, and behavior.

In understanding and using the MSE, it is important to recognize that in most cases *the overall pattern of findings* on the examination provides the key to developing the differential diagnosis, although in some relatively rare cases a single abnormal finding will be sufficiently specific for this purpose. The task for the clinician is to be comfortable performing the examination and remain, at the same time, cognizant of the cognitive, emotional, and behavioral data being observed so that any abnormal findings may be properly understood and used to direct the MSE towards greater degrees of specificity.

In addition to obtaining valuable diagnostic information, the MSE serves several other purposes. It is during the general MSE that the clinician listens to the patient's concerns (or the lack thereof in some cases), simultaneously hearing not only what is said but also how it is said, whether spontaneously or in response to the examiner's questions. The astute clinician, hearing certain patterns of impairment in communication or memory early in the interview, begins to formulate the differential diagnosis, and pursues questions in a manner that both acknowledges and supports the patient's strengths and while facilitating further examination of deficits. When it is clear that structure is needed to help the patient communicate concerns, the MSE can provide a useful framework that will reassure both the patient and the clinician.

The MSE may also provide a measure of the severity of the patient's condition, document a baseline of functioning for future reference, and guide treatment planning. For example, the cognition of a patient with a delirium due to pneumonia will change as the pneumonia progresses or resolves. Much as the clinician charts the course of pneumonia by auscultation and percussion of the chest, so may the severity of the accompanying delirium be monitored by the MSE.

The MSE is an essential component of clinical neuropsychiatry. It is through this examination that the history is further explored and confirmed, that diagnostic and treatment decisions are made, and that the effect of treatment is assessed. Although the MSE has limitations in quantification of cognitive impairment, when performed in a thorough and thoughtful manner the importance and utility of information obtained through the MSE cannot be overstated. This chapter will outline the MSE as structured in Table 9.1 and describe the concepts and techniques needed for its performance.

Table 9.1. Essential elements of the mental status examination

Mental status examination	Essential elements	Specific items requiring assessment	
General	Appearance and behavior	Arousal	
		Dress, grooming, and hygiene	
		Facial expression	
		Posture, motor activity	
		Attitude toward the examiner	
	Speech	Quantity	
		Volume	
		Tone	
		Rate	
		Rhythm	
	Thought process	Structure (organization)	
		Style	
	Thought content	Perception	
		Interpretation of environment	
		Themes and concerns	
		Lethality	
	Emotion	Mood	
		Affect	
Cognitive	Arousal	Level of arousal	
	Attention	Selective	
		Sustained vs. distractibility	
		Alternating or multitasking	
	Language	Fluency (verbal and written)	
		Repetition	
		Comprehension (verbal and written)	
		Naming	
	Memory	Immediate	Verbal
		Recent	Visual
		Remote	Procedural
	Praxis	Limb-kinetic	
		Ideomotor	
		Ideational	
		Constructional (visuospatial skill)	

Table 9.1. (*cont.*)

Mental status examination	Essential elements	Specific items requiring assessment
	Recognition	Visual Auditory Tactile
	Complex cognition	Executive function Social intelligence Motivation

The general mental status examination

The general MSE consists of a series of observations and questions that assess the patient's appearance, behavior, manner, content of thinking, and emotional state. The beginning portion of the MSE is entirely observational – it is possible to perform and report a detailed general MSE on a patient who refuses to participate in the examination. The patient's appearance and behavior, attention, speech, thought process, thought content, and emotion are all observable outside the strict interaction of an interview, and can be documented as such. In fact, for the safety of the consultant called to see the "non-participatory" patient, this information may be invaluable. For example, one might choose to have a security officer present when examining the hyper-aroused, disheveled, glaring, tense, and growling patient, who appears visibly distracted and upset by internal auditory and visual stimuli, disorganized in both thought and behavior, frightened of and possibly paranoid about the examiner, and extremely irritable and angry. By contrast, one might feel more comfortable interviewing alone a patient who is curled up under their bed sheets in the fetal position, avoiding eye contact, whimpering softly, not engaging with the examiner, and crying. In neither case is any information directly obtained by interview, but from these observations comes a wealth of clinical information that can guide the interview, the differential diagnosis, and decisions about potential interventions. This section will provide a framework within which to observe mental state, and offer a language for describing such observations.

Appearance and behavior

The examination begins with the patient's appearance and behavior. The purpose is to describe the manner in which the patient attends to and engages with both self and environment. The first task is to define and describe the patient's level of consciousness. *Arousal,* or *level of consciousness,* is a function of the activity of the reticular formation, including brainstem and thalamic components and their projections throughout the rest of the brain. Clinically, several levels of arousal are often described: alertness; somnolence; lethargy; obtundation; stupor; semi-coma; and coma. Although definitions have been offered for each of these terms, clinical use of each term (both between different clinicians and within the various interviews of a single clinician) does not always follow its formal definition, and such descriptions can be quite confusing. Additionally, patients may sometimes be hyper-aroused, as in some deliria and in mania. Consequently, we echo Strub & Black (1985) by suggesting that the use of any qualitative term should be accompanied by a brief description of (1) the level of stimulus (verbal, physical, and/or noxious physical) necessary to arouse the patient, and (2) of the patient's behavioral response (becomes alert, meaningfully engages, responds unintelligibly, withdraws, and/or does not respond) to the stimulus. For example, a patient would be most helpfully described as "somnolent: aroused easily to verbal stimulation, while aroused the patient was fully engaged in the interview, and gradually returned to sleep upon conclusion of the examination." This type of statement provides a clear picture of the patient's ability to respond to and engage with the environment.

Physical appearance includes the patient's dress (e.g., casual, formal, unusual, naked), grooming (e.g., neat, meticulous, disheveled, use of make-up), and personal hygiene (e.g., clean, dirty, malodorous). Observations of these aspects of appearance inform the examiner about the patient's ability or willingness to attend to self-care and to conform to social norms. Patterns of unusual self care or neglect may be used to support (in conjunction with data from the remainder of the examination) certain diagnoses, as in the patient with chronic schizophrenia who wears three woollen coats in August, under which he is naked, dirty, and malodorous, or the patient with a right hemisphere stroke producing hemi-neglect whose left face is unshaven and left hemi-body is undressed and unwashed.

Similarly, observations of *facial expression* (e.g., smiling, crying, staring, glaring), *posture* (e.g., upright, supine, tense, fetal), and *motor behavior* (e.g., calm, retarded, catatonic, agitated, fidgety, tics or abnormal movements) provide information about the patient's emotional state and ability to engage with the examiner. In some cases, this information will also suggest a certain line of inquiry and guide the development of the differential diagnosis. For example, a flat expression, slightly stooped posture, and little spontaneous movement save a 3–5 Hz resting tremor of the face and hands in an elderly patient immediately suggests parkinsonism, and should prompt further examination with the differential diagnosis of this problem in mind.

Attention

Attention refers to the patient's ability to focus on a specific stimulus without being distracted by extraneous (external or internal) stimuli. In the general MSE, an initial assessment and comment on attention is necessary, at least with regard to the patient's ability to engage in the interview and examination, since an inability to attend will affect the way in which the subsequently assessed elements of mental status are interpreted. When attention is disturbed, the quality of the disturbance is important to note, as it may support specific items in the differential diagnosis. For example, the patient may be excessively distracted by noise or movement in the hallway or in the examination area, which might suggest either mania or delirium. Similarly, the patient may appear to be distracted by visual or auditory stimuli not evident to the examiner, which might suggest a delirium, dementia, or a psychotic disorder. Further, the patient may be inattentive to stimuli on one side of the body only or in one field of vision, which might suggest hemi-neglect as seen in some strokes. Additional assessments to characterize selective and sustained attention problems can be performed during the cognitive MSE.

Speech

In the strictest sense, speech refers only to the motor capacity for oral articulation, and generally that associated with language. It is, however, distinct from language, which is the cognitive process by which the world is given declarative representation and that permits symbolic communication with other individuals. Speech is also distinct from voice, the laryngeal function of phonation. Disorders of speech (dysarthrias) may or may not be associated with disorders of voice (dysphonias) or language (aphasias). In the general MSE, the pattern of speech is observed. It is particularly important to note when a severe dysarthria is present, as the presence of such should raise concern for a host of significant neurological problems that may involve either central or peripheral nervous systems, or both.

In most primary psychiatric disorders (e.g., depression, mania, schizophrenia) the capacity for articulation is relatively normal, but additional information can be obtained by noting other dimensions of speech. The quantity (e.g., talkative, silent, commenting spontaneously or with prompting), volume (e.g., normal, soft, loud), tone (e.g., forceful, dramatic, shouting, mumbled), rate (e.g., normal, rapid, slow), and rhythm or prosody (e.g., normal, monotonous, oddly accented) are also useful descriptors of speech that may help guide formation of the differential diagnosis. For example, a description like "does not speak spontaneously, but when prompted speaks softly, slowly, and monotonously" would likely suggest problems in frontal functioning – perhaps schizophrenia or an apathetic syndrome, or less likely a mild non-fluent aphasia. Contrast this with a description like "speaks spontaneously, and in general in a conversational manner, with normal volume, tone, rate and rhythm, but intermittently makes singular, loud, shouting, rapid and oddly accented vocalizations of a profane or derogatory nature," which might suggest a vocal tic as in Tourette's syndrome.

Thought process

Thought process refers to the sequence, logic, coherence, and relevance of a person's thought as it leads to selecting and achieving cognitive, emotional, or behavioral goals. Describing thought process can be challenging for many students, in part because the language used in this portion of the examination is technical and employs many terms-of-art (jargon). As a means of introducing this technical terminology, it may be helpful to divide the thought process operationally into two major components: structure (or organization) and style. While it is not useful to establish an inflexible dichotomy between these two aspects of thought process, framing thought process in this fashion may be useful in the examination, description of findings, and formulation of contribution of such to the differential diagnosis.

The structure or organization of thought refers to the logic and relevance of thoughts to internal or external cues. To use an architectural analogy, structure characterizes the way thoughts are built, both logically and simply like the single open space of a post-modernist apartment or in a highly illogical and disturbed fashion like the drawings of Escher.

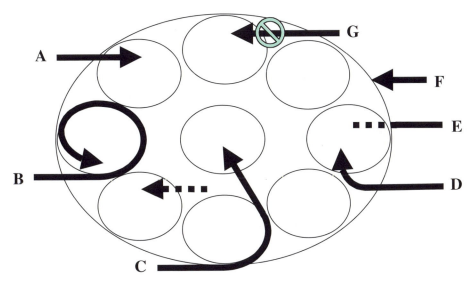

Figure 9.1 A diagram to illustrate the structure of thought as described in the general mental status examination. **A**, goal-directed; **B**, circumferential; **C**, tangential; **D**, circumstantial; **E**, loose; **F**, incoherent or "word salad;" **G**, thought blocking.

Structure

To make the language used to describe thought process understandable, we offer a diagram that illustrates the structure of thought (Figure 9.1). This diagram is like a master blueprint for thought, with the large circle representing the entire edifice (the brain) and each smaller circle representing a specific room (idea or thought) within the edifice. At any given time there are a number of ideas contained within the brain. In response to the appropriate internal or external cue, the most relevant one is accessed and used to generate either a verbal or nonverbal response.

In most circumstances, thoughts are *goal-directed* (Figure 9.1-A), meaning that in response to a specific cue, a direct, appropriate, and meaningful response is generated. In our architectural analogy, after the instruction to walk into the kitchen, the person chooses the most direct pathway and indicates when the kitchen has been entered. A somewhat less organized structure of thought is *circumferential* thinking (Figure 9.1-B), in which unnecessary detail and initial indirection occur before an ultimately appropriate and meaningful response is reached. In our analogy, after being asked to walk into the kitchen the person explores every room in the house before finally entering the kitchen and giving an indication to that effect. *Tangential* thinking exemplifies less organized thought (Figure 9.1-C), in which initial movement toward a response is ultimately directed inappropriately and the intended (or requested) goal is not reached. In the analogy, although there is initial movement toward the kitchen, the patient walks instead into the adjacent dining room, indicates that the dining room has been reached, and never moves on to the kitchen.

A similar structure of thought is *circumstantial* (Figure 9.1-D), in which the patient responds to a cue both with unnecessary detail and indirection and a failure to reach the appropriate and meaningful response. This seems almost a combination of circumferential and tangential thinking – after being instructed to go to the kitchen, the patient explores and reports on every room along the way before finally getting stuck in the dining room. Alternatively, circumstantial thinking is also used to refer to an evasive manner of thought (intentional or not) in which the direct, appropriate, and most meaningful response appears to be avoided. For example, a paranoid patient may never quite answer a question directly, but instead offers a series of indirect answers that together provide circumstantial evidence from which the actual answer can be inferred. Using our analogy, when asked "are you in the kitchen?" the patient might respond, "I was in the dining room." Repeated questions might elicit answers such as, "I did walk in the hallway," "I am not in the living room," "The kitchen has white walls," and so on. From these answers, a practiced interviewer might be able to infer the answer to the original question, though perhaps only after recognizing that the responses given are not merely tangential but circumstantially related to the desired response.

Even less organized is *loose thinking* or *loose associations* (Figure 9.1-E) in which a cue elicits an apparently unrelated response. This is like asking the patient to go to the kitchen and hearing that he is playing baseball in the backyard. To the interviewer, and sometimes also to the patient, the manner in which the response is generated may appear genuinely mysterious, as if the patient has simply been transported to the wrong thought. It may be more likely that a rapid series of tangential responses occurred, perhaps out of the conscious awareness of the patient, such that the response seems without obvious relation to the cue, but is in fact distantly related to it in a manner unique to the patient's associations. Experienced interviewers practiced at listening to the content of thought associations can often infer and articulate both the cognitive and affective content of the patient's concerns, and sometimes even reconstruct the logic of the associations with the patient.

Incoherence, sometimes referred to as word salad, (Figure 9.1-F) is a severe form of thought disorganization in which the patient responds to a cue with meaningless connections or severely disordered syntax and semantics. This structure of thought is really a lack of structure, and may be viewed as a severe form of loose associations. In our analogy, the patient claims to be simultaneously present in several rooms. Severely disorganized patients with schizophrenia or mania may demonstrate this style of thought, and patients with fluent aphasias (or *jargon aphasia*) may appear superficially similar. Incoherence should be taken as evidence of a severe disturbance in thought, language, or both, and should prompt a thorough neuropsychiatric assessment.

Finally, the structure of thought may also be characterized as *blocked* (Figure 9.1-G). This, again, is a lack of structure: the patient is unable to reach the desired response to a cue, and appears to lose the task altogether. In the analogy, when asked to go to the kitchen, the patient stops at the front door, sits down, and may not clearly recall the original instruction. This impaired structure of thought has been called "derailment," suggesting that the patient's train of thought has been more than simply misdirected; it has been taken off the tracks and stopped altogether. Blocked thought is evident in some patients with severe prefrontal dysfunction: those with anterior cingulate-subcortical circuit pathology with diminished motivation and those with impaired dorsolateral prefrontal-subcortical circuitry who cannot generate and organize thought spontaneously. Such thought blocking may sometimes be observed among patients with schizophrenia, Parkinson's disease, frontal lobe tumors or strokes, traumatic brain injury, and other disorders disrupting frontal-subcortical circuits.

Style

Within different thought structures, the patient also demonstrates a style of expression that further characterizes thought process. Style of thought is normally amenable to change, such as interruption or redirection, if circumstances so warrant. When style is abnormal, it often follows a characteristic pattern such as pressure, flight of ideas, echolalia, perseveration, substitution, neologism, circumlocution, and clanging.

When a patient presents *pressured thoughts*, he appears unstoppably driven to expression. This results in speech that is typically difficult to interrupt or redirect. For example, some patients with mania, once started on a thought, will continue with that thought despite efforts by the interviewer to the contrary. Some liken this to a steamroller moving down a hill – once it starts rolling, there seems no way to stop it. It is the driven quality, and not the speed of thought, that defines pressure. Recalling the systems subserving the sort of complex cognition involved in thought process, pressured thinking may reflect overactivity of the anterior cingulate-subcortical circuit resulting in excessive and interminable motivation to develop and communicate thoughts.

By contrast, *flight of ideas* describes an abnormal style of thought in which one idea is quickly followed by another, and another, and so on. In contrast to patients with pressured thinking, patients with flight of ideas alone can be interrupted and redirected, even if these actions by the interviewer serve only to start such flights of ideas in a new direction. The rapid velocity of thought defines flight of ideas. The phenomenon may reflect overactivity of the dorso-lateral prefrontal-subcortical circuit, providing excessive generation of thoughts and, in a sense, abnormally heightened verbal or behavioral fluency. Often pressure and flight of ideas occur together, making examination of the patient by direct questioning extremely difficult. In such cases, it seems not unreasonable to infer greater degrees of brain dysfunction, and using the model we have offered one might imagine excessive (or at least dysregulated) prefrontal activity.

Echolalia refers to the seemingly automatic repetition of words or phrases spoken to the patient. Echolalia may occur without the patient comprehending what is said (discussed further in the subsequent section, "*Language*"). Although most often seen in patients with schizophrenia or mania, it may also be a feature of aphasic patients, particularly those with transcortical aphasias. Recalling that the circuit for repetition is relatively distinct from those for fluency and comprehension, all of which are typically functions of the dominant hemisphere, we may better understand why hypofunction of both the frontal and temporoparietal association cortices in the dominant hemisphere might predispose so-affected schizophrenic patients to echolalic responses.

Perseveration, when used in the strictest sense, refers to the repetition of a single word or short phrase and an inability to shift from this to a new thought despite redirection or interruption by the interviewer. This may be seen in patients with frontal lobe injuries producing dysexecutive function. Perseveration is also used in psychiatry to describe a pattern of persistence with a theme, as when all elements of the interview inevitably lead back to "the CIA is after me". We might again infer problems with dorsolateral prefrontal-subcortical circuitry and may observe perseveration in either sense of the word in patients with neuropsychiatric disorders such as dementia, schizophrenia, or obsessive–compulsive disorder.

A *substitution* is an incorrect or an unintended use of a word during expression of a thought. The substitution may sometimes rhyme with or be phonetically similar to the correct or intended word. Substitutions are common among patients with fluent aphasias, and may also be seen in patients with mania or schizophrenia. When substitutions result from language disturbances, they do not appear to be intentional and may go unnoticed by the patient. Although *parapraxes*, or "slips of the tongue," are often taken as a psychologically different problem in style of thought, they too may be interpreted as substitutions in this context. Whether these substitutions indeed have intrinsic meaning or instead simply represent misfirings of closely associated linguistic areas in the temporal or frontal cortices is unclear and debatable. Nonetheless, parapraxes may have meaning when either the speaker or the listener choose to interpret them further, and regardless of meaning ascribed to them they should be noted as part of the style of thought.

Neologisms are new words created while expressing a thought. As an example, a manic patient describes the food he is eating as "fantastalicious," combining fantastic and delicious into a single new word. Although the word origin may be relatively obvious in this example, in some cases neither the phonemic nor the semantic roots are clear. When this occurs, the language errors are described as abstruse neologisms. A deficit in the associative (comprehension) or productive (fluency) aspects of language function, or in both, might be inferred, although the exact nature of the dysfunction by which neologisms are produced is not entirely understood.

Circumlocution is the style of talking around a word, often offering semantically or functionally related words in an effort to communicate the same meaning despite difficulty in offering the intended word. For example, when shown and asked to name a piece of chalk, a circumlocution might include identifying it as "that stuff you use to write on a blackboard" or "you know, its that white powdery stuff that you write with . . . they use it in schools." While conveying some relevant and related concepts about the intended referent, circumlocutions fail to succinctly communicate using the most appropriate word or name. Not surprisingly, this is a relatively common finding in patients with language disorders, particularly those with transcortical sensory aphasias.

Finally, *clanging* is a style of thought in which the person produces a series of rhyming words, often from substitutions and neologisms, and often while beset by flight of ideas. This style of thought can be seen in manic patients or among patients with schizophrenia with severe thought disorganization. Although the neurobiological underpinnings of this style of thought are not well understood, our approach suggests either some dysfunction of dorsolateral prefrontal-subcortical activity and/or excessive activity between such frontal-subcortical pathways to associative language areas producing a series of rapid associations to phonemically similar words and an inability to appropriately terminate the generation of such associations.

Thought content

Thought content describes the ideas, themes, and experiences expressed by the patient. Thought process is "how" thought proceeds, and thought content is "what" that thought is about. In the general MSE, the task is to observe in some detail what the patient appears to be thinking about, either by virtue of the content of verbalizations or by inference based on nonverbal behavior (e.g., responding to nonverbal stimuli). Assessment and description of certain aspects of thought content (e.g., delusions, hallucinations, specific anxieties, lethality) is a requisite component of any MSE. Consequently, we will briefly describe these aspects.

Delusions are erroneous beliefs that usually involve a misinterpretation of perceptions or experiences and that are held firmly despite evidence to the contrary of the belief (e.g., fixed false beliefs). For example, a man is brought to the emergency room by his wife because he is convinced, wrongly she believes, that he is being watched by the Central Intelligence Agency (CIA). When asked by the examiner why he believes this is happening, he states that for the last two weeks a black car has been parked on the street in front of his house. Hearing this for the first time herself, his wife then tells him that the car belongs to their new neighbors who moved into the house next door two weeks ago. In response, the husband replies, "Well, then the neighbors must be working for the CIA." Further descriptions of the neighbors occupations are interpreted by the man as "cover stories" used to conceal their surveillance of him. In other words, despite evidence to the contrary, the patient maintains his false belief and misinterprets new information in a manner that supports his delusion. In some cases it will not be clear whether the ideas are merely overvalued eccentric ideas, or fantasies, and in such cases ascribing a delusional quality to them is not appropriate. Instead, such ideas may be most fairly described using terms that state the conviction with which they are believed and maintained despite questioning or even contradictory evidence.

Persecutory delusions are the most common type, and typically involve beliefs about being tormented, followed, tricked, spied upon, or subjected to ridicule. Referential delusions are also common and include beliefs that gestures, comments, printed media, broadcasts on radio or television, or other events are directed towards or are about the patient. Grandiose delusions involve beliefs about power, intelligence, social role, beauty, or other "remarkable" qualities or abilities. Somatic delusions are somewhat less common, and are focused on a fixed, false belief about a somatic problem, usually some kind of disfigurement or infestation, as in a delusion of parasitosis. Religious delusions generally include belief that one has an extraordinarily special relationship with God (one is a messiah, angel, messenger, prophet, shaman or other) or that one is God or some other kind of singularly god-like figure. As noted above, such delusions are sometimes especially difficult to distinguish from culturally held religious beliefs, and must be assessed and interpreted with respect to the social, cultural, and religious context of the patient.

The American Psychiatric Association's *Diagnostic and Statistical Manual of Mental Disorders*, 4th edn (1994), referred to as DSM-IV, also describes bizarre delusions. A delusion is bizarre if it is not only fixed and false, but also clearly impossible, not understandable, and does not derive from ordinary life experience. The DSM-IV gives the example of believing that a stranger has removed one's internal organs and replaced them with someone else's organs without leaving a scar. In general, such bizarre delusions involve an impossible loss of control over mind or body, or conversely involve unbelievable powers of mind or body, or other impossible events. For example, patients may report thought withdrawal (thoughts being pulled from one's head as if by physical force), thought insertion (thoughts placed in one's head by an external force like cards being put in a card file), or thought broadcasting (internal thoughts are loud enough to be "heard" by others).

A cautionary note is in order when making attributions about the presence of delusions. First and foremost, no psychiatrist should ever function in a professional capacity as an arbiter of social norms. Various political entities, especially in recent history, have employed psychiatrists in this way, to the detriment of everyone concerned. This is especially dangerous with respect to the practice of medicine – if the psychiatrist is actually, not merely perceived as, a functionary of the state, there can be no basis for the trust needed to form the healing relationship between physician and patient.

How then may the clinician approach the patient whose thought content is clearly abnormal? Consider the case of a middle-aged police lieutenant who confides to a colleague that the U.S. Federal Bureau of Investigation (FBI) has put threatening voices in his head using a micro-transmitter implanted by his family physician during a routine ear check. His colleague brings this to the attention of the police officials who then relieve the lieutenant from duty and require a psychiatric examination. Several simultaneous approaches are useful in determining whether the lieutenant's thought content is abnormal and qualifies as a delusion.

First, on its face, the story carries both a persecutory quality and a science fiction content that suggest a wide gap between *content* and reality. If the FBI is truly interested in a minor police functionary, they would likely use standard, legally accountable, techniques to demonstrate their concern. Has the patient notified his family, hired a lawyer, or otherwise taken steps to substantiate and remedy his concern? If so, what was the result? If not, what explanation does the patient give for his inaction?

Second, does the patient's *social context* support his belief or does it find the belief foreign and unsubstantiated? In the lieutenant's case, his fellow police officers immediately recognize that the belief is out of the ordinary and potentially dangerous. They engage their standard procedures for dealing with an illness and send their colleague for diagnostic evaluation. While the police officials are themselves engaged in observing others closely, they recognize that the lieutenant's concerns are outside of the appropriate social framework. Similar contextual comparisons are necessary when evaluating other aberrant beliefs, especially political or religious concerns.

Third, and generally most telling, the clinician should ask *how* the erroneously held beliefs came to the patient's attention. In this case, the lieutenant concluded that the FBI was watching him when he inferred that the threatening voices inside his head could only be due to an outside source and that the FBI was the only agency technically capable of arranging this. Because he hears voices, he understood that a micro-transmitter was necessary. The only opportunity for implanting such a device would have been during his yearly physical exam. To the examiner's knowledge, such transmitters do not exist, the physician was providing the same service he had done for the previous 10 years and a follow-up examination reveals no foreign body or other abnormality in either auditory canal. The *way* the belief came about rests only on the patient's inferences, follows a very concrete thought process, can't be verified independently, and bears no logical relation to more likely ways of delivering threats.

Fourth, and finally, when offered alternative explanations that counter the belief, such as that others suffering depression often encounter such beliefs, the patient quickly denies that this applies to him and holds ever tighter to the original content.

From this evidence, the most reasonable conclusion is that the lieutenant suffers from a delusion, a symptom requiring a careful assessment and differential diagnosis. The clinician has organized the differential after recognizing thoughts in which: (1) content varied dramatically from likely reality; (2) there was no corroboration when compared to the patient's social context; (3) the history of how the belief came about undermined the credibility of its content; and (4) the patient could not entertain the possibility of an alternate or contradictory explanation. Careful attention to these concurrent approaches will assure clinical science and avoid a stance of social arbitration.

Perceptual disturbances, including illusions and hallucinations, are also part of thought content. *Illusions* are misperceptions of real external stimuli, for example seeing a human face in the face of a clock. *Hallucinations* are subjective sensory perceptions in the absence of relevant external stimuli, for example seeing a face hanging in midair. Illusions and hallucinations may occur in any sensory modality (visual, auditory, olfactory, gustatory, or tactile) and although they may sometimes be misinterpreted to the point of delusion such misinterpretations are not a necessary element of illusory or hallucinatory experiences. Patients may be perfectly aware that their perceptions are erroneous, and retain insight into the nature of the experience as illusory or hallucinatory. For example, a grieving person sees a face in the air that resembles the dead relative, but does not believe that the person is present and watching her every movement. Another classic example is the patient who recognizes that the snakes crawling out of the sport coat hanging in the closet signal the beginning of delirium tremens and the need to get to a hospital quickly.

Although illusions and hallucinations are not pathognomonic of any specific condition, some clinical trends are worth noting. In general, isolated visual hallucinations should be considered manifestations of an underlying medical or neurological dysfunction, such as delirium, until proven otherwise. Although patients with psychiatric problems such as schizophrenia or mania with psychosis may experience visual hallucinations, they usually also have auditory hallucinations. Persistent visual hallucinations, however, should prompt a thorough neuropsychiatric evaluation in any patient, with or without psychosis.

Auditory hallucinations are much more common than visual or other hallucinations in primary psychiatric disorders like schizophrenia, psychotic mania or depression. They often take the form of voices, and are usually perceived as distinct from one's own thoughts. The experience of hallucinatory voices may be a running commentary about oneself, an ongoing conversation among several voices, or commands to perform certain, often self-injurious, behaviors.

Tactile hallucinations are most common as isolated phenomena in intoxication or withdrawal states, as in formication, or the sensation of worms crawling under one's skin. They may also occur with hallucinations in other modalities as a part of either psychiatric or neurological illnesses. Isolated olfactory and gustatory hallucinations are most often seen as auras of complex partial seizures although, again, they may be part of multi-modal hallucinatory experiences in psychiatric or neurological conditions.

Anxiety symptoms should also be noted as a part of thought content. The most common include obsessions, phobias, general anxiety, and compulsions. Obsessions are recurrent, uncontrollable thoughts, images, or impulses that the patient considers unacceptable or alien. Phobias are persistent, irrational fears, accompanied by a compelling desire to avoid the feared object. General anxiety refers to apprehensive anticipation of future danger or misfortune accompanied by a feeling of dysphoria or somatic symptoms of tension; although this is an emotional state (as defined in Chapter 5), it is still most common in psychiatry to inquire and describe anxiety and its referents at this point in the examination. Compulsions involve repetitive acts a person feels driven to perform in order to produce or prevent some future state of affairs, although expectation of such an effect is unrealistic. Although they may be associated with a variety of anxious conditions, we most often consider them in the context of obsessive–compulsive disorder. Although compulsions are really behaviors rather than cognitions, because most patients will associate them with some thought content it is convenient to note compulsions in this same section of the examination.

Dissociation is broadly defined as a disruption in the usually integrated functions of consciousness, memory, identity, or perception of the environment, and is therefore best described in the context of thought content. Specific types of dissociation include depersonalization (experiencing oneself as either "out of body" or simply not oneself) or derealization (experiencing the environment as having an unreal or surreal quality). Other related phenomena include *déjà vú*, or the experience that one's current environment has been previously experienced when it has not (mistaking unfamiliar for familiar), and *jamais vú*, the experience that one's environment is novel when it is not (mistaking familiar for unfamiliar). All of these experiences may be seen in either psychiatric or neurological illnesses, and have most often been attributed to temporal lobe pathology (and particularly schizophrenia and partial complex epilepsy of medial temporal origin) when observed in either category of illness.

Finally, *lethality* issues (thoughts of suicide and homicide) should also be noted in the assessment of thought content. Assessment of suicidal ideas should include quality (passive wish to be dead, active desire to kill oneself), intent, plans (such as wrist cutting, overdose, shooting), and ability to perform the act (for example, access to weapons). Homicidal thoughts should be similarly assessed. It is generally considered standard practice also to inquire of safety plans, emergency contingencies, and insight into the likelihood of acting (planned or impulsively) on such ideas. The evaluation of lethality requires care and diligence, and is described in much more detail in other standard psychiatric textbooks (e.g., Kaplan et al., 1994).

Emotions

In the context of the general MSE, emotions refer to feeling states and are described using the terms mood and affect. As discussed in Chapter 5, some authors suggest using mood to describe the patient's reported emotional state, and using affect to describe the observer's impression of the patient's emotional state. We suggest using mood to refer to the patient's sustained (days to weeks or longer) emotional baseline and affect to refer to more transient (minutes to hours) emotional changes that occur on top of the baseline mood (Figure 9.2). This method of conceptualizing and describing emotion seems both more consistent with the current nosology of mood and affective disorders (especially that in the DSM-IV) and, we believe, also offers the possibility of acquiring more accurate clinical information regarding both subjective (patient report) and objective (expressed and observable) emotional changes over two different time domains. In clinical neuropsychiatry, this distinction is a very important one as the treatments of mood disorders are not necessarily the same as those for disorders of affect.

For example, patients with frontal injuries will often describe "mood swings." When pursued in further detail, these mood swings do not appear to involve mood (a sustained change in emotional baseline) at all. Instead, these patients state that their emotional baseline is really rather neutral (sometimes euthymic), but that with little or no provocation they become inappropriately enraged or sad for a relatively brief period of time, after which they return to their neutral emotional baseline. This pattern is better referred to as affective

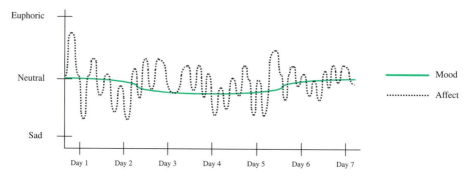

Figure 9.2 A diagram of the distinction between mood and affect. Mood, as shown by the solid line, varies only slowly over the course of the week depicted. By contrast, affect varies more quickly, though as mood decreases (become more sad) there is a relative restriction of affect. If lower mood states were further depicted, the range of affective variability would be even more restricted.

lability, as it describes a disturbance in the regulation of moment-to-moment emotion. The implications of this distinction are quite different, as mood swings are often treated with mood stabilizers such as lithium or anticonvulsant medications, whereas affective lability is (in the context of traumatic brain injury or Parkinson's disease) often treated with psychostimulants (e.g., methylphenidate, dextroamphetamine) or selective serotonin reuptake inhibitors. In a patient with mood swings due to bipolar disorder, prescribing either of these latter treatments without concurrent administration of a mood stabilizer may have disastrous results (e.g., medication-induced mania or rapid cycling).

Both mood and affect should be assessed objectively (clinician observation) and subjectively (patient report). Mood may be described using traditional clinical terms such as euphoric, irritable, depressed, or euthymic, and this approach is generally accepted. It is also useful to describe both mood and affect in everyday terms (e.g., happy, sad, angry, disappointed), which are more often used by patients. When there are discrepancies between the patient's apparent mood and their report of it, this should be noted as it may have diagnostic import. Occasionally, patients with *alexithymia* (without words for feelings) will be encountered, and these patients will appear to be genuinely unable to describe their emotional state. Similarly, apathetic patients will sometimes describe a lack of feeling though they may appear superficially "flat" or "depressed." In both cases, there may be a complex disturbance of frontal-subcortical circuits that challenges categorization or even recognition of distinct emotional states.

Discrepancies between affective appearance and feeling may also occur, as in patients with pathological crying and/or laughing (also known as pseudobulbar palsy). Some of these patients will appear profoundly sad or hysterical with very little or no provocation, as described above, but will report a dissociation of their appearance from their conscious experience of affect. This condition is distinguished from affective lability, in which such episodes include a change in both experienced and expressed affect.

The cognitive MSE

The purpose of the cognitive examination is to assess a broad range of cognitive functions, from basic to complex. In contrast to the general MSE, most of the cognitive examination requires direct interview and examination. As outlined here, the format follows the organization of cognition presented in chapters 3 and 4 – the elements of the examination are ordered according to relatively increasing complexity. As noted in those chapters, performance on more complex tasks is at least in part dependent on relatively normal performance on the more basic tasks.

A cautionary note about administration and interpretation of the examination findings is warranted before beginning this discussion. Although the hierarchical model of cognition has merit, it is extremely difficult to assess a singular aspect of either basic or complex cognition because in reality processing and responding to any stimulus involves simultaneous processing of that stimulus at multiple cognitive levels. Additionally, and as discussed in Chapter 4 (Complex cognition), the processing of information is not only simultaneous at different levels but also highly reciprocal between them. Consequently, even a relatively simple task of basic cognition such as attention using the verbal letter vigilance task (responding only when the letter "A" is spoken by the examiner) involves processing at more complex levels of cognition. In this case, the task requires sufficiently intact language to comprehend the task, praxis to execute the type of response indicated by the instructions, and prefrontal activity to generate the appropriate response at the appropriate time. In other words, influence travels both up and down the hierarchy as it is usually depicted.

Given this problem in administration and interpretation, it is important to remember that impaired performance on any single task must be considered in the context of the entire cognitive MSE. In the end, it is the *overall pattern of findings* that are used to make determinations about cognitive strengths and deficits. Performing more than one task for each area of cognition offers a better chance of accurately determining the areas in which cognition is impaired. Given this cautionary note, the elements of the cognitive MSE presented here are organized according to the area of cognition with which they are most strongly related.

Arousal

The cognitive MSE begins with an assessment of arousal. As discussed in the general MSE, arousal is described in terms of the level of consciousness. This requires briefly describing the stimulus necessary to elicit a response from the patient, the nature and duration of the response, and the behavior that follows when the stimulus is discontinued.

Attention

Attention refers to the ability to focus on a specific stimulus, sustain that focus, and remain free from distraction (external or internal) while the focus is sustained. Attention appears to require the operation of a complex network including the reticular formation, the hippocampus, the thalamus, the frontal lobes, the right parietal lobe, and the numerous interconnections among these structures. As in the general MSE, assessment should first include general observations about the patient's ability to attend to self and environment. Attention may be further assessed using digit span (digit repetition), the random letter (letter vigilance) test, serial subtractions, and double simultaneous stimulation.

The digit span (digit repetition) task is a useful test of attention and freedom from distractibility. The patient is first asked to repeat a list of single digits in the same order as spoken by the examiner. Digits are dictated at the rate of one per second, and with as little inflection as possible (avoiding grouping of the digits into telephone-style number groups). Increasingly larger sets of digits (usually beginning with a set of three) are offered until the patient fails to repeat the set correctly. The task is then performed with the patient repeating the digits in the reverse order as that dictated by the examiner (i.e., "1-2-3" is repeated as "3–2-1"). Normal performance on this task is 7 ± 2 in the order dictated, and 5 ± 2 in reverse order. Although the reverse order portion of the task is typically performed, Strub & Black (1997) have suggested that the reverse order digit span task is sufficiently dependent on other aspects of cognition (and especially executive function) that impaired performance on only this part of this assessment should not be taken as evidence of impaired attention alone.

The random letter (letter vigilance) test is, as its name suggests, a test of sustained attention or vigilance. In this task, the patient is instructed to signal, either verbally or nonverbally, each time the examiner says the letter "A" in a long random list of letters. The average person should complete the task without errors. Errors of omission (failing to respond when the letter "A" is spoken) suggest impaired vigilance, and errors of commission (responding to letters other than "A") suggest either impulsivity (usually orbitofrontal impairment) or perseveration (impaired dorsolateral prefrontal function). Any errors on this task should be taken as evidence of attentional impairment. Several written versions of this task are also available including symbol, number, and letter cancellation tasks.

The serial subtraction task is included on the mini-mental state examination (MMSE), and is one of the more familiar tests of sustained attention. In this task, the patient is asked to count backwards from 100 by sevens, and normal performance requires completing five serial subtractions. Alternatively, the patient may be asked to spell the word "WORLD" backwards, with normal performance (correct spelling in reverse) suggesting normal attention. From a practical standpoint, it is common practice to administer either (or both) tasks during the MMSE and to incorporate the higher of the two performance scores into the overall score on the MMSE. Conceptually, it is important to be clear that both versions of this task are more than tests of attention alone, and errors may reflect premorbid intellectual capability, education, calculating or language abilities, and/or cultural biases attendant to ethnic or socioeconomic status, as well as or instead of indicating a disturbance of attention. Consequently, when errors are made on these tasks it is important to assess further attention using the previously discussed tasks.

Double simultaneous stimulation is a test of directed attention, a lateralized function organized so that each hemisphere can attend to the contralateral hemispace. The patient is first touched unilaterally, with each side tested for intact sensation. Then bilateral (double) simultaneous stimulation is applied. Normal patients will report experiencing the simultaneous stimuli, while patients with impaired attention (usually due to parietal injury) will fail to report experiencing the stimulus on the side of the body contralateral to the injured hemisphere during delivery of simultaneous stimuli. Impairments on this test suggest the possibility of hemi-neglect, are most common on the left side of the body, and should prompt a search for parietal pathology.

Language

Language is the verbal or written representation of thought that permits symbolic communication with other individuals. As noted in the general examination, it is to be distinguished from speech (the motor capacity for the oral articulation) and voice (the laryngeal function of producing sound by phonation). Language should be assessed early in the cognitive MSE, as deficits may make subsequent evaluation of some other aspects of cognition extremely difficult, if not impossible. The important elements of language that should be specifically assessed include fluency (verbal and written), repetition, comprehension (verbal and written), and naming.

Figure 9.3 (adapted from its counterpart in Chapter 3) is a schematic diagram for assessment of language – the gross anatomic relationship of the above functions, and the patterns of language disturbance that result from disruption of those functions. The accompanying table identifies several of the classic aphasia syndromes and the patterns of language disturbance produced by lesions to specific parts of the language pathways.

Assessment of language begins with fluency, which refers to the ability to produce spontaneous speech without undue word-finding pauses or failure in word searching. Proper function relies on an intact motor cortex, including the motor association areas and Broca's area (Brodmann area 44). Non-fluent speech is characterized by reduced phrase length (maximum of five words or less between pauses) and incorrect grammatical structure (agrammatism). It is assessed throughout the course of the examination, with observation for word-finding difficulties, substitutions, or neologisms. Fluency may be more specifically assessed with a word list generation task. The patient is instructed to list aloud in 60 seconds as many words as possible within a given category (e.g., animals, fruits) or beginning with a certain letter (e.g., F, A, S). Normal function is characterized by production of 18 or more items per category or 12 or more items per letter. Although this test is primarily dependent on language, it may also be affected by impairments in complex cognition (dysexecutive function or impaired motivation). Writing should be further assessed by asking the patient to produce a writing sample. This sample should include a simple sentence, and should be evaluated based on its construction (proper grammar and syntax) and meaningfulness (even if rather banal). Sentence writing, perhaps even more so than spoken language, requires consideration of the patient's level of education and literacy; deficit, if present, should be assessed not only in absolute terms (e.g., agrammatisms or neologisms) but

Type of aphasia	Fluency	Repetition	Comprehension	Naming
1. Broca's	Impaired	Impaired	Normal	Impaired
2. Wernicke's	Normal	Impaired	Impaired	Impaired
3. Conduction	Normal	Impaired	Normal	Impaired
4. Transcortical Motor	Impaired	Normal	Normal	Impaired (mildly)
5. Transcortical Sensory	Normal	Normal	Impaired	Impaired (mildly)
6. Mixed Transcortical	Impaired	Normal	Impaired	Impaired
7. Global	Impaired	Impaired	Impaired	Impaired
8. Anomic	Normal	Normal	Normal	Impaired

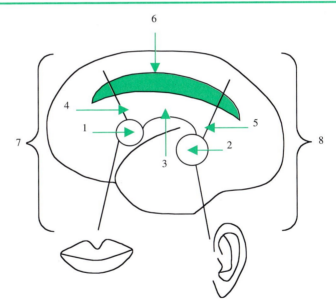

Figure 9.3 Schematic representation of language areas, their connections, and the classic aphasia syndromes associated with damage to these areas.

also with regard to whether the quality of writing represents a change from the patient's usual level of performance. Decreased verbal and/or written fluency is usually indicative of dominant (usually left) frontal lobe dysfunction, be that dysfunction of motor association cortex needed for language (Brodmann areas 46 and 47), Broca's area, dorsolateral prefrontal cortex (middle and superior frontal gyri), anterior cingulate gyrus, or some combination of these.

Repetition is a linguistically and anatomically distinct function and, as its name suggests, it is the ability to repeat language correctly. Proper function depends on the integrity of Wernicke's area, Broca's area, and the arcuate fasciculus connecting these areas. It may be spared or involved exclusively in certain types of aphasia as when its preservation in isolation results in echolalia. Repetition is assessed by asking the patient to repeat material of increasing difficulty and length, beginning with monosyllabic words and then proceeding to complex sentences. Agrammatical phrases, such as "no ifs, ands, or buts," are important test stimuli, as the patient with impaired comprehension will have great difficulty elaborating a partially understood agrammatical stimulus into a correct response. Normal performance is errorless, and isolated impairment of repetition is usually an indication of white matter pathology (as in conduction aphasia).

Comprehension refers to the ability to understand spoken (or written) language. Proper function relies on the integrity of the sensory (temporoparietal and parietal) portion of the dominant hemisphere, including Wernicke's area (Brodmann areas 22, 41, and 42, and possibly 39 and 40). It must be tested in a structured fashion that does not rely solely on the patient's ability to respond verbally, since comprehension and fluency deficits may occur simultaneously. The assessment of comprehension should begin with simple stimuli, and employ pointing commands and yes/no questions. Pointing commands should not be the only assessment method used (nor commands such as that on the MMSE – "Take this piece of paper in your right hand, fold it in half, and place it on the table") because impairment may suggest problems in comprehension, praxis (integrating comprehension and execution), or both. When yes/no questions are used, it is important to alternate between questions requiring either response, to reduce the likelihood of perseveration obscuring interpretation of the examination. As this portion of the assessment continues, the test stimuli should be made increasingly complex, moving from yes/no questions to true/false questions, and then to complex questions. An example of this latter task is asking the patient to respond to a brief story like, "A lion and a tiger are fighting. The lion is killed. Which one is alive?" Additionally, the patient's ability to read and respond appropriately to sentences of increasing complexity should also be assessed. As noted above, a screening question for impaired comprehension (as that suggested on the MMSE, noted above) may abbreviate the examination somewhat if the patient's response is entirely normal. However, since impairment on this task may reflect aphasia, apraxia, or both, any degree of impaired performance on this screening question should prompt a more assiduous assessment of both comprehension and praxis.

Naming is the ability to identify objects verbally in one's environment. It is a diffuse cortical function that depends on the integrity of a large number of association areas including the frontal-subcortical circuits needed to manipulate information appropriately in the sensory association areas. It is one of the earliest acquired and most basic language functions, and is almost invariably disturbed to some degree in all types of aphasia. It is best assessed by confrontation naming, where the examiner points to a variety of objects and asks the patient to name them. The ability to name objects from several categories and to name parts of objects (for example, the eraser on a pencil, the stem on a watch, the index finger on the hand) should also be assessed. Individuals with impairment of this language function will often have more trouble naming parts of objects and may have greater difficulty naming objects from one category than from another. Additionally, impaired naming should be distinguished from impaired recognition – when a patient is unable to name a visually presented object, the same object must be presented using other sensory modalities (such as tactile, auditory, or olfactory) before the naming problem is definitively ascribed to an aphasia rather than an agnosia.

Memory

Memory is the mental process that permits encoding and retrieval of experiences and perceptions. It depends on a large number of brain structures as discussed in Chapter 3. Memory is clinically assessed along three dimensions: immediate, recent, and remote.

Immediate memory, or registration, may be assessed using the tests of attention described earlier in this section, or by the registration task suggested by the MMSE. In this task, the patient is asked to repeat three items immediately after their presentation. When testing registration (and also recent memory), it is useful to provide three relatively complex items: two concrete (visualizable) objects with parts (such as apple pie, red Cadillac, or fire engine), and one abstract item (such as honesty, truth, or beauty). The utility of these items is related to the relatively greater effort required to associate the concrete objects consistently with their respective qualifiers (that is, red with Cadillac, apple with pie), and the tendency of inattentive and amnestic patients to transpose the qualifiers and items inappropriately (e.g., red apple is repeated instead of red Cadillac). Additionally, use of an abstract item is important because of its intrinsic lack of features that might facilitate association and encoding using multiple sensory modalities (e.g., visualization). Where concrete objects may be remembered using cross-modal associations (like sound, sight, and touch), this is not as easily done for abstract items. Normal performance is without error on the first repetition. Any difficulties with this task should prompt a more thorough assessment of attention. Importantly, if these items are to be used to assess incidental memory (spontaneously acquired recent memory) then the patient should not be warned that they will be asked to recall the items after a few minutes nor otherwise prompted to rehearse repetition of the registration items.

Recent memory is a more complex function, and most easily assessed in two ways. First, questions about orientation to person, place (building, floor, city, state, country), time (day, date, month, year, season), and situation (personal information, current events) are asked. Orientation may be thought of as recent memory for the patient's "who, where, when, and why." Normal performance on this test is errorless. When impairments occur, most recently acquired information (time, situation, place) is typically lost first. With increasingly severe impairment, memory for personal information (date of birth, place of origin, and in very severe cases even name) may also be affected. Loss of orientation to person rarely occurs without significant anterograde memory disturbance, as evidenced by disorientation to situation, time, and place. Isolated loss of memory for past information (retrograde amnesia), particularly for personal identity, in the absence of the ability to remember new information (anterograde amnesia) should be considered very unusual, and may suggest a more "psychological" memory disturbance, such as psychogenic amnesia or a dissociative state.

While orientation is a function of recent memory, it should not be the sole assessment of this function or of mental status more generally. Among delirious patients, disorientation is not invariably present, leaving a large number of delirious patients unrecognized if only orientation tests are used to assess mental status. If the patient makes errors on orientation, the correct answers should be given, repeated, and the patient should be asked to recall these answers several minutes later. Failure on this recall indicates impaired new learning and predicts problems on additional recent memory tasks. The pattern of errors on orientation is also useful to note: delirious patients will often mistake the unfamiliar for the familiar ("this [hospital room] is the factory I work in"), whereas psychotic patients will often mistake the familiar for the unfamiliar ("I am on Mars"), although certainly there are many exceptions to these observations.

New learning ability should also be assessed, and follows naturally from the assessment of immediate memory. The patient is asked to recall the previously presented items (apple pie, red Cadillac, and honesty) about five minutes after they were presented. As noted above, patients should not have previously been instructed to remember these items, as this may encourage rehearsal of a task intended to assess incidental memory. Patients with normal memory are expected to recall all items at five minutes. When errors are made, it is first useful to offer semantic prompts that may permit recall by association (for example, "a type of all-American desert," "a very large and brightly colored car," "a quality possessed by people who tell the truth"). When semantic cues do not facilitate recall, this should be noted, and then specific recognition cues should be provided (for example, "Was the item an apple pie, cherry tart, or ice cream sundae?"). It is useful to note the pattern of impairment. In general, problems with recognition suggest an encoding problem (e.g., a pattern more suggestive of cortical impairment, often hippocampal), whereas memory helped by either associative or recognition prompts suggest relatively intact encoding but impaired retrieval (e.g., a pattern more suggestive of frontal-subcortical dysfunction, including that caused by either subcortical or white matter pathology).

Recent memory (new learning) also may be assessed using a variety of visual tasks. In the context of the office-based cognitive MSE, perhaps the easiest of these is a hidden-objects task. In this task, the examiner hides several (usually 4 or 5) objects around the office with the patient watching. Several minutes are allowed to elapse, after which the patient is asked to retrieve the objects. If the patient is unable to retrieve all the objects, the examiner asks the patient to name the remaining hidden objects. This is a simplified version of a visual memory task included in the Rivermead Behavioral Memory Test. Another visual memory task involves the reproduction of several pictures by memory. In this task, the patient is shown several cards with simple designs or figures. After several minutes, the patient is asked to reproduce these designs or figures from memory. This is a simplified version of the Rey-Osterrieth Complex Figure Test of visuoconstructional and visual memory abilities. With both types of visual memory testing, interpretation of errors must take into account not only similar encoding and retrieval aspects of memory, but also any problems with praxis (ideomotor, ideational, or constructional) and recognition that are subsequently discovered upon further examination.

Finally, remote memory may be assessed by asking the patient to recall events of a personal and historical nature. When information regarding personal history is included in the assessment, it must be verifiable by collateral sources such as the hospital record, family or caregivers. Performance on recall of historical information (for example, "When was World War II?," or "Who wrote *Romeo and Juliet*?") must be interpreted in the context of the patient's intelligence, education, and social experience.

Praxis and visuospatial abilities

Praxis refers to the ability to integrate comprehension of a task with execution of that task. It requires the patient to have intact comprehension and immediate memory (hence its placement at this point in the cognitive MSE) and also the motor capacity for execution of the task. In other words, one cannot fairly ascribe apraxia of the right hand to a patient with a peripheral nerve injury that produces complete paralysis of the right upper extremity. Visuospatial abilities also depend on the ability to integrate sensory (parietal and occipito-parietal) with motor functions. Loss of visuospatial praxis is usually regarded as a sign of non-dominant parietal lobe dysfunction, while loss of motor praxis (e.g., limb-kinetic or fine motor, ideomotor or single task, and ideational or performance of sequential tasks) is more suggestive of dominant hemisphere frontal lobe pathology.

Praxis is assessed using commands along each of the above dimensions. For example, asking the patient "Show me how you brush your teeth," "Show me how you comb your hair," or "Show me how you button your shirt," should yield appropriately executed pantomimes, imitated actions, or actual performances on command. Impairment in performance of these tasks may suggest either limb-kinetic or ideomotor dyspraxia. For example, when asked to show how to blow out a match, the patient blows but does not pantomime holding a match or instead blows out a finger. The distinction between dyspraxia and apraxia is really a matter of clinical judgment, with the latter usually reserved for qualitatively describing severely impaired or failed execution of any portion of task either on command or even spontaneously. As in previous chapters, use of such terms should be followed by a brief description of the performance to which it refers.

In general, pantomime is a more complex function of praxis than imitation, which is in turn more sensitive to impairment than actual task performance on command. Therefore, in many cases of cortical dementia, pantomime will be impaired before either imitation or actual performance, following the usual pattern of loss of more complex function before loss of more basic function. Also, performance on command is more complex than spontaneous performance, and some patients with impaired praxis during the examination may demonstrate relatively better praxis under everyday conditions. Such observations should not be taken as incontrovertible evidence of malingering, but instead should suggest the possibility of dyspraxia or apraxia to commanded tasks.

Ideational praxis may be assessed by asking the patient to complete a series of tasks in a specified sequence, and is most commonly assessed by using the three-step command suggested on the MMSE (i.e., "take this piece of paper in your right hand, fold it in half, and place it on the table"). This task can be used as a screening tool for both ideational and ideomotor praxis, as it is generally the case that normal ideational praxis is predicated on normal ideomotor praxis. It may also be useful to increase the complexity of the task if one is to perform a single screening assessment; we find it useful to ask patients to "touch your right hand to your left ear after you point to the ceiling." In this command we assess not only ideational and ideomotor praxis, but also include a temporal qualifier and a screening tool for right–left confusion. Inability to perform this task should prompt reassessment of its constituent elements: ideomotor praxis ("show me your hand"); right–left confusion ("show me your *right* hand" and "point to your *left* ear" as separate commands); and temporal sequencing ("point to the floor after you point to the ceiling"). Using this method, one may not only assess praxis along several dimensions but also screen for right–left confusion. The presence of the latter suggests the need for further evaluation for a Gerstmann syndrome (right–left confusion, finger agnosia, acalculia, and agraphia), a problem most commonly associated with dominant (usually left) parietal lobe lesions.

Visuospatial ability is routinely assessed using design copy or construction and, in contrast to the problems noted above, is generally regarded as being more heavily dependent on right, not left, parietal lobe function. In design copy, the patient is instructed to copy two- and three-dimensional designs and to draw a clock. On the MMSE, two interlocking pentagons provide the design for copying. Correct performance on this task requires that each polyhedron have five sides, five corners, and that they overlap by only one corner from each

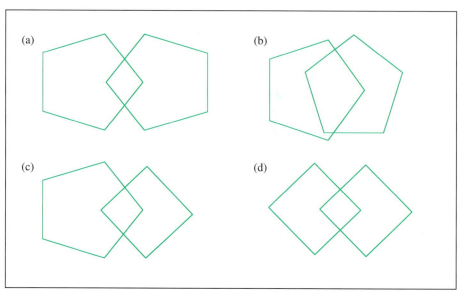

Figure 9.4 Construction design using interlocking pentagons. (a) Illustrates the figure to be copied; (b–d) illustrate various errors of increasing severity.

(Figure 9.4). Responses are graded as poor (unrecognizable), fair (moderate distortion or use of one or two squares instead of pentagons), good (mild distortion or two pentagons but with two overlapping corners), or excellent (perfect).

A more complex constructional task incorporates a three-dimensional element to the design, as in a cube (Figure 9.5). Performance on this task is also rated as poor (unrecognizable), fair (moderate distortion or loss of three-dimensionality), good (mild distortion), or excellent (perfect).

Another frequently used task of visuospatial ability is the clock-drawing task. This is relatively more complex than either of the previous tasks and does have some advantages over them both. In this task, the patient is instructed to draw a circle and then place numbers in the circle as would appear in the face of a clock. Once the clock is drawn, the patient should be instructed to place the hands in the clock to one of several positions requiring correct interpretation of the numbers and also proper positioning of the hands. Clearly, this method of screening requires more than visuospatial skill alone; however, and like the example for ideomotor praxis given previously, if the patient is unable to perform the task without error, task and performance can be deconstructed into their constituent elements for more detailed assessment.

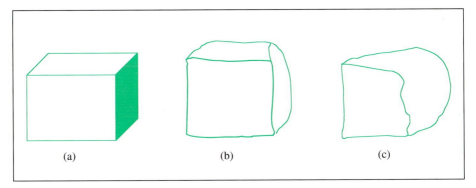

(a) (b) (c)

Figure 9.5 Cube design for copy task. (a) Illustrates the figure to be copied, (b) illustrates a cube without three-dimensionality (moderate) and (c) illustrates a severely distorted cube (poor).

The first portion of this task requires visuospatial construction skills similar to that in the previous tasks, but additionally requires the ability to generate and execute a plan for the placement of the numbers in the correct order and position (reflecting the influence of dorsolateral prefrontal-subcortical function on design copy). A variety of distortions may be produced, ranging from complete failure to generate the design (constructional apraxia), moderate distortion of the circle (constructional dyspraxia), misplacement of the numbers (dysexecutive function, either poor planning for frankly incorrect placement or impulsivity/stimulus bound behavior for placement on the stated, rather than intended, number), mild distortion of one or both elements of the design (dyspraxia), or some combination of these. Additionally, this design is somewhat more sensitive to hemispace neglect, in which the numbers (typically those on the left) are not placed in the appropriate space or are omitted entirely (Figure 9.6).

The second portion of the task, placement of the hands to read "ten past eleven," requires comprehension, problem solving, visuospatial ability, and freedom from distraction (impairment which is referred to as stimulus-bound behavior). The wording of this portion of the task includes numbers that appear on the clock, of which the meaning of one of them, i.e., "ten", is actually represented on the clock by the number "2." Consequently, the task requires understanding the command, associating the number "ten" with its intended rather than its literal meaning, processing the visuospatial information that allows placement of the hands on the clock, and resisting the stimulus-bound impulse to point the hand indicating "ten past" at the "10" (Figure

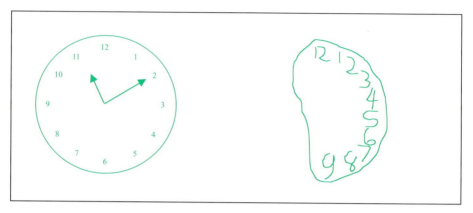

Figure 9.6 Clock drawing task. On the left is the figure drawn correctly, and on the right is an example of a severely distorted clock with evidence of both poor motor planning and left-sided neglect.

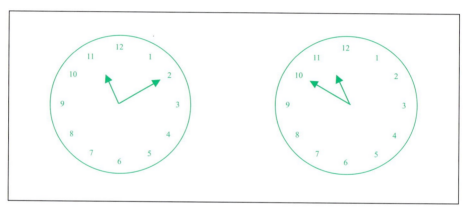

Figure 9.7 Clock drawing task. On the left is the correct figure, on the right is an example of a stimulus-bound response (patient asked to place the hands to read "10 after 11").

9.7). An analogous task may be constructed using "five after nine" if the task is to be repeated again in the same patient. This version of the clock-drawing task is fairly complex, and is used by some clinicians as a brief cognitive screening tool by itself. Because the task requires sustained attention, normal comprehension, written repetition, ideational praxis, and executive function, some regard the clock-drawing task as an expeditious method of broadly (although superficially) assessing cognition. With that in mind, systematic scoring methods are available for interpretation of clock drawing performance.

Recognition

As discussed in Chapter 3, recognition refers to the ability to identify an object in a specific sensory modality. Impairment of recognition in a single sensory modality is an agnosia. It is important to be clear that recognition is predicated on normal language function, and especially naming. Language permits encoding of declarative, symbolic representations of objects; when the neural networks subserving such encoding are impaired, patients may have difficulty recognizing objects regardless of the sensory modality in which they are presented. By contrast, an agnosia involves difficulty recognizing an object in a single sensory modality, despite the ability to understand the task and to name the same object when it is presented in another sensory modality. Consequently, when a subject demonstrates impaired naming on the language section of the cognitive MSE, it is important to present the same objects in other modalities in order to ascertain whether the problem is indeed one of naming or is instead a problem in modality-specific recognition (agnosia).

The examination of recognition is relatively straightforward, but does require that the objects used in the examination have properties that permit them to be identified when presented in each sensory modality independent of the others. For example, a piece of blackboard chalk has a distinct appearance, smell, and feel and is useful for testing recognition in each of these three senses. Coffee grounds, paper clips, a traditional (or analog) watch capable of making a ticking sound are all also useful objects for this task. If a patient is unable to identify the object using one sense, the object should be presented again using another single modality. Failure to identify multiple objects in a single sense (for example, vision) with preserved identification of these same objects using other senses suggests an agnosia. Detailed descriptions of the various agnosia are provided in Chapter 3 (Basic cognition).

Complex cognition

Complex cognition is highly dependent on more basic cognitive functions. Consequently, in the examination of any patient, basic cognition should be examined and understood prior to examination and interpretation of performance requiring complex cognition. When impairments of one or more aspects of basic cognition are present, it is important to determine whether any additional impairments in complex cognition are out of proportion to that expected from dysfunction in basic cognition alone. This is often very difficult to determine at the bedside or in the consultation office, and for this reason any uncertainty with regard to the relationship between impairments in basic and complex cognition should be regarded as a very strong reason for ordering formal neuropsychological testing.

As noted in Chapter 4 impairments in complex cognition may also adversely affect performance on tasks of basic cognition. A good example may be taken from our discussion of the clock drawing task, in which accurate construction of the clock not only requires intact visuospatial abilities, but also abstract reasoning (as when "ten past" means put one hand pointing toward the two), motor planning, and ability to inhibit impulsive (or stimulus bound) responding. As another example, the aberrations of thought process described in the general MSE may result from disruptions of frontal-subcortical circuitry, and may produce tangential or loose associations, perseveration, thought blocking, or other major neuropsychiatric phenomena. However, clinically similar disturbances may also result from language dysfunction alone. Therefore, it remains essential to have assessed basic cognition thoroughly before ascribing the clinical phenomena to a disturbance in complex cognition. As a final cautionary note, the patient's intelligence, education, and social environment must be considered when interpreting performance on this portion of the examination.

Assessment of complex cognition is one of the most interesting sections of the cognitive MSE, and many aspects of this portion of the examination are familiar elements of the more commonly administered psychiatric MSE. We will make efforts to relate the techniques described in this section to the frontal-subcortical circuitry upon which they are most dependent. Useful areas of assessment include fund of knowledge, word list generation (in the setting of otherwise fluent language), alternating sequence tasks, the Luria hand tasks, calculations, pattern recognition tasks, abstraction, insight, and judgment or problem solving. Word list generation was discussed in the *Language* section above, and will not be repeated here. Additionally, social intelligence and motivation have been described in some detail in previous chapters, and the latter is discussed again in Chapter 15 (Diminished motivation and apathy). For brevity, we refer readers to those sections of the book for additional details on these elements of complex cognition, but will emphasize here that we consider the assessment of these areas to be an important part of the evaluation of complex cognition and that formal methods (e.g., Apathy Evaluation Scale, Neuropsychiatric Inventory, etc.) should be used when impairments in these areas are suspected.

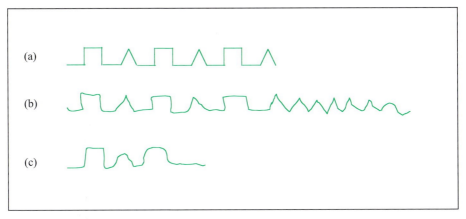

Figure 9.8 Alternating sequence task. (a) Illustrates the example pattern, (b) is an example of perseveration on one element of the task, (c) is an example of impaired generating ability and motor impersistence.

Fund of knowledge refers both to the patient's store of knowledge and the ability to access, retrieve, and report that knowledge on command. Standardized questions assessing fund of knowledge, organized in sets of increasing difficulty and complexity, are available. At the bedside, inquiry includes assessment of historical (presidents, authors), geographical (location of places on a map, distances), and factual (scientific facts, number of weeks in a year) knowledge. It has been suggested that the dorsolateral prefrontal cortex and the mediodorsal nucleus of the thalamus are particularly important for retrieval of remote memories. These structures, and the networks in which they participate, organize semantic associations through heteromodal and sensory association cortices. Consequently, even when these association cortices (e.g., auditory, visual, tactile) are intact, and the associative "engrams" in these areas are stable, they may not be accessed easily when the frontal-subcortical circuits are damaged. Additionally, retrieval of memories is in all likelihood also dependent on anterior cingulate-subcortical circuitry to provide sufficient motivation to retrieve information, either spontaneously or on command.

Alternating sequence tasks assess the ability to shift between conceptual sets. To assess this ability, the patient may be shown a brief written pattern of alternating letters or symbols (Figure 9.8) and instructed to copy and continue it. A common error on this task is difficulty generating the pattern, which may reflect dorsolateral prefrontal-subcortical and/or anterior cingulate-subcortical circuit dysfunction, and particularly of the dominant (left) hemisphere.

Alternatively, the patient may persist with the task but perseverate on elements of the pattern or persist in repetition when termination is appropriate (as when the end of the page is reached). This impairment may reflect dorsolateral prefrontal-subcortical (perhaps of the indirect basal ganglia pathway) dysfunction or may be more lateralized to right frontal pathology.

The *Luria hand tasks* (developed initially by the Russian neuropsychologist, A. R. Luria) are a series of sequential hand movements that test the ability to copy and persist with a motor task. The fist-edge-palm task is one example of these tasks, and is easily used at the bedside. The patient is instructed by the examiner to copy hand movements, and the interviewer then proceeds to tap on the table or bed in a series that proceeds first with a fist, then the edge of the hand, then the palm of the hand. The patient should repeat this sequence and is asked to continue doing so. Normal performance is at least five complete repetitions without error. Mistakes on this task are similar to those on the alternating sequence task, typically consisting of motor impersistence or perseveration. Our interpretation of these mistakes is also similar to that listed above, involving dysfunction of (most likely dominant hemisphere) dorsolateral prefrontal-subcortical circuits in the case of motor impersistence and possibly nondominant dorsolateral prefrontal-subcortical dysfunction in the case of perseveration. Again, impaired performance may also develop as a consequence of diminished motivation due to anterior cingulate-subcortical circuitry. As with other tests of complex cognition, interpreting problems on this task as evidence of impairment in this area is contingent on being able to demonstrate relatively normal basic cognition, especially comprehension and praxis.

Calculation requires the ability to manipulate mathematical knowledge, and has often been ascribed to dysfunction of the left hemisphere (including posterior structures such as the left parietal lobe/angular gyrus/heteromodal cortex) and also perhaps of the dorsolateral prefrontal-subcortical circuit. Calculation is best assessed by testing basic arithmetic (addition, subtraction, multiplication, and division) both verbally and graphically. One useful test is to provide an increasingly difficult series of addition problems, as in $7 + 6$ (simple), $13 + 9$ (single digit carryover), $22 + 15$ (double digit without carryover), and $37 + 45$ (two digit carryover). A common practice to use monetary calculation (e.g., number of quarters in $1.75, or number of nickels in $1.00). However, many people will perform better when tested in this fashion, perhaps because the calculation is aided by concrete associations (money) not available when performing abstract calculations alone and because the associations may be influenced by greater motivation. This dichotomy in performance is useful when patients demonstrate impaired calculation – one may regard impairment in both general mathematical and monetary calculations as a more severe impairment (acalculia) than impairment in only one of these two areas.

Pattern recognition is a simple form of abstraction, in that it permits the association of two or more objects or events with one another. Pattern recognition (even if only implicit) is the basis of both classical and operant conditioning. While this aspect of complex cognition requires the ability to identify the association of objects or events, it does not necessarily entail the ability to make more abstract generalizations from recognition of such associations. One may be able to recognize the co-occurrence of two events without understanding the nature of the relationship of their pairing. For example, a young child may learn that his four-legged furry companion is a dog (let's say it's a cocker spaniel) and recognize other dogs appropriately when they are similar enough to this pattern. However, this same child may over-generalize the pattern to include some cats and may not recognize other dogs as such (for example, a chihuahua). The fact that they possess some degree of pattern recognition is not sufficient for abstraction, though it is a necessary prerequisite for this more complex cognitive ability.

The assessment of pattern recognition may be performed using verbal, graphic, or behavioral (procedural) test stimuli. When assessing pattern recognition verbally or graphically, patterns of letters or numbers are presented, after which the patient is first asked to identify whether there is a pattern used in the presentation, and (if so) to then describe the pattern in words. For example, one might tell the patient to answer the following arithmetic problems: "$1+1=(2)$, $2+2=(4)$, $4+3=(7)$, $7+4=(11)$, $11+5=(16)$, $16+6=(22)$, $22+7=(29)$. At the end of this sequence, the patient is asked, "What would the next problem be?" (the answer is "$29+8=37$"). Next, the patient is asked "What was the pattern in this series of problems?" (Each addition is created by adding the next integer in sequence to the sum of the preceding problem). Some patients may be able to produce the next problem correctly but not be able to articulate the pattern; we have seen this pattern more commonly in patients with relatively milder forms of dysexecutive function, and generally regard this pattern of performance as supportive of such. If the patient is entirely unable to recognize the pattern verbally, the same pattern should be presented graphically (written down) to see if this facilitates recognition. As with other tests of executive function, interpretation of performance should take into consideration the patient's education and baseline math skills.

As an alternative to a verbal or written pattern recognition task, a behavioral (or procedural) task may be used. One such example is a variation on the classic ball-and-cup trick of many street performers and magicians. In this assessment, the examiner holds out both hands palms up, with a paper clip in one. The examiner asks the patient to point to the hand containing the paper clip. The examiner then closes both hands and places them behind his or her back. Both hands are then brought out front again, this time with both hands closed. The patient is asked to guess which hand holds the paper clip. After the patient makes a guess, both hands are opened, revealing the location of the paper clip. The patient is told that this procedure will be repeated several times, and asked to indicate the hand in which they believe the paper clip is held before the examiner reveals its true location. The examiner shifts the paperclip from hand-to-hand (during each movement of the hands behind his or her back) in a pre-determined pattern (for example, right–right–left). After several repetitions of presenting the paper clip in this fashion, the patient is then asked to indicate the pattern of location/presentation of the paperclip. Most patients will recognize these patterns, and impairment often suggests problems in dorsolateral prefrontal-subcortical (executive) function.

Abstraction is the ability to make complex associations from or among objects or concepts, to organize observations and associations into themes and generalities, and then to interpret them beyond their apparent or literal meaning (as in double meaning, inference, sarcasm, and satire). Assessing abstraction occurs throughout the interview as the patient communicates the history of present illness, interprets the cause and nature of their problem, and reasons through the treatment alternatives and strategies. The opening question of the clinical interview may make difficulties with abstraction immediately apparent. Many patients with traumatic brain injury, Alzheimer's disease, or schizophrenia will respond to the question, "What brought you in today?" with an answer like "My father's car," or "The Number 10 bus from downtown." These are concrete responses to a question that is asking more about the reason for their visit to the clinic than the mode of transportation that brought them. Abstraction is specifically assessed by asking the patient to interpret similarities and proverbs. When evaluating the ability to interpret similarities, the patient is asked to explain what two overtly different objects or ideas have in common, or to offer a description of the way these objects are essentially similar to one another. Abstract responses organize the objects or ideas into a common category, while concrete responses are those that note only a similar

Table 9.2. Examples of prompts used to assess similarities along with examples of common abstract and concrete responses

Prompts	Concrete response	Abstract response
Apple and orange	Round Have seeds Eat them	Fruit
Table and chair	Have four legs Sit at one and eat at the other Can sit on them	Furniture
Sun and moon	Round In the sky Give light Orbit the earth	Part of the solar system Celestial bodies
Painting and poem	Written on paper Need a pen to make them	Works of art Express feelings
Fly and tree	Fly lives in/flies to a tree One is small and one is big	Living things Things in nature

function or characteristic. Table 9.2 gives some examples of responses to similarities.

Proverbs are commonly used phrases or sayings that convey a message beyond their literal meaning, and are therefore often used as test stimuli for the assessment of abstraction. Assessment of proverb interpretation may be performed in two ways. In the first method, the clinician presents a few commonly used proverbs to the patient and asks whether he or she has previously heard each saying. When a familiar proverb is found, the patient is asked, "Tell me what people usually mean when they say that." In this test of interpretation of familiar proverbs, the patient may offer a concrete response, an abstract response, or both. This is particularly useful when common use of the proverb is itself only partly abstract, as in the following example. Although most people have heard the saying, "The grass is always greener on the other side of the fence," a patient might respond with a concrete response "Well, that grass is greener," or "They must water their lawn a lot." Although a common interpretation of this proverb is "People tend to think things are better somewhere else," this itself is only a partially abstract, or semi-abstract, response. A more fully abstract interpretation might be "Although people tend to think things

Table 9.3. Examples of prompts for use in the assessment of abstraction using proverbs, with examples of possible responses

Prompt	Concrete response	Semi-abstract response	Abstract response
A stitch in time saves nine.	One stitch is less than nine.	It takes less time to sew one stitch than nine.	It is easier to fix a problem when it is small.
People who live in glass houses shouldn't throw stones at others.	Throwing stones will break the glass.	Some things are very vulnerable to damage.	You shouldn't criticize others because you are also vulnerable to criticism.
Don't judge a book by its cover.	The book's cover is green.	There is more inside the book.	To understand something, you need to look beyond superficial appearances.
Even monkeys fall from trees.	Monkeys fall out of trees.	It's pretty hard to keep climbing.	Even experts make mistakes.
Rome wasn't built in a day.	Rome took a long time to build.	In general cities take a long time to build.	Big projects take time.

are better elsewhere, it usually turns out that they are pretty much the same as where they are now." Some patients may provide both the partially abstract and abstract interpretations, noting that while people often intend the partly abstract response, the saying is more appropriately used to convey the abstract meaning.

It is also useful to ask the patient to interpret the meaning of an unfamiliar proverb. This requires the patient to derive a meaning for a novel idea in front of the examiner. The patient should be encouraged to state the logic behind the interpretation offered, since this may provide additional information about his ability to abstract. Similarly, if a concrete interpretation is offered initially, the patient should be asked if there is another way to understand it, or what meaning it might have for people. This also provides information on the thought process guiding the patient's responses. Table 9.3 provides examples of proverbs for use in either version of this test.

Abstraction is also used in understanding humor, particularly that involving word play (as in sarcasm and satire) and situation comedy. These types of humor require the observer to take in the literal meaning, understand the covert meaning, and recognize the disparity between them that forms the crux of the joke. Interestingly, many patients with problems in abstraction also have difficulty understanding humor, or may have a tendency to find humor where and when others usually do not.

Abstraction is a very complex cognitive function, and is heavily dependent on bi-hemispheric function, frontally and elsewhere. Right and left temporoparietal areas are required for language and prosody (rhythm and inflection) recognition, respectively. Left dorsolateral prefrontal-subcortical circuitry is required for further association, interpretation, and organization of information. Anterior cingulate-subcortical circuitry is required for motivation to proceed with interpretation, and orbitofrontal-subcortical circuitry is needed to compare the emotional valence, social context, and personal and social appropriateness of information and potential responses. Right frontal lesions have been associated with alterations in humor, specifically the development of a rather concrete and sometimes latently hostile sense of humor, historically referred to as *Witzelsucht*, a German word roughly translated as "addiction to trivial joking." Clinically, these patients often fail to understand language-based humor, responding instead to violent slapstick routines such as those of the Three Stooges or children's cartoons. Further, such patients are sometimes prone to be inappropriate in their expression of humor, either with respect to its content or social context. Although it is difficult to be more certain of the nature of such interhemispheric interactions, it appears clear that the capacity to abstract both language and events operates most completely when both the posterior and anterior portions of the right and left hemispheres are functioning properly.

Insight is the ability to assess information accurately about oneself and one's role in generating his or her own life circumstances and problems – in other words, insight is the capacity for accurate self-reflection and self-appraisal. This ability is assessed throughout the course of the examination by observing the patient's ability to recognize his or her own illness, problems, skills, and limitations. It is likely that insight requires a broad array of cognitive skills, including abstraction, and may be impaired to varying degrees in psychiatric disorders and neurological disorders. It is also likely that there are inter-individual differences in this ability between otherwise normal persons, and has even been suggested by Gardner (1983) to represent a specific domain (an intrapersonal domain) of intelligence.

Because insight requires the integration of knowledge about self, environment, time and circumstance, it is heavily dependent on intact function of all areas of the brain from which this information is derived or processed, even though it is often discussed in the context of the operation of frontal-subcortical circuits. Consequently, disturbances of insight may develop following a broad range of injuries: cortical, subcortical, white matter, or a combination of these.

For example, many patients with schizophrenia, and in particular those "hypofrontal" patients with prominent negative symptoms, often have severely impaired insight with regard to their own problems and the actions of others. As a result, they may not recognize their illness and may interpret the actions of others in a paranoid fashion. Patients with posterior ("receptive") aphasias after temporoparietal stroke may appear similarly paranoid. However, in so affected stroke patients the lack of insight facilitating such paranoia likely results from impaired language comprehension and tertiary associative information needed for input to the prefrontal areas, rather than from primary pathology in the frontal lobes.

Another example is the patient with *anosognosia*, a profound unawareness of neurological deficit, most commonly manifesting as left hemi-inattention or left hemi-neglect. This problem usually results from infarction of nondominant (usually right) parietal areas, and appears to be most strongly related to the inability to integrate ongoing information about the body and visuospatial cues into a comprehensive working-image of the self. Consequently, these patients are not able to provide frontal-subcortical circuits with the information needed to develop insight into their deficits, and in fact often behave as though their deficits do not exist.

Judgment and problem solving require the ability to integrate information about the self, the environment, time and circumstance into adaptive behavior, and are two of the most truly complex aspects of cognition. Although judgment and problem solving are both commonly assessed by presenting the patient with a practical problem requiring a solution (as in the fire-in-the-theater scenario, or the stamped-addressed-envelope-on-the-street problem), these cognitive functions should be assessed throughout the examination. The patient's ability to reason throughout the interview, to understand the rationale for interview and the questions they are asked, and to translate that understanding into behavior that will serve to get their needs met all require good judgment and problem solving. Assessment of these abilities is particularly important with respect to determining a patient's ability to provide for his or her own needs independently, to consent to treatment, and to make other decisions competently.

However, the interview alone should not serve as the only arena in which judgment and problem solving are assessed. Some patients will present with apparently intact intelligence and abstract problem solving skills, but demonstrate impairment in putting that abstract knowledge to use in everyday life. For example, a patient may be able to understand the significance of criminal behavior, the potential consequences of such behavior for both victim and perpetrator, and the reasons that laws exist to deter against and punish criminal behavior, yet find themselves repeatedly committing acts for which they are arrested. Damasio (1994) notes that some patients may appear to possess good judgment as assessed by abstract or intellectual problem solving in the examiner's office, yet their behavior suggests a profoundly impaired ability to translate that intellectual understanding into real-life situations that require its application.

This problem has been extensively described in patients with orbitofrontal-subcortical circuit dysfunction, either through injury (e.g., the patient Phineas Gage we discussed in Chapter 4) or various neurochemical derangements. This is the type of "social intelligence," or social judgment, that we described in Chapter 4: the ability to understand oneself and one's social context; to integrate the emotional valence and survival value of that social context with one's intellectual understanding of personal needs and the social context; and to develop behaviors that are capable of meeting one's needs, including sometimes delaying gratification of those needs. As Damasio (1994) has suggested, it is likely that reasoning is the highest level of cognitive function, and requires the successful integration of both cognition and emotion to produce the complex cognition needed to meet the demands of everyday life.

Summary

The MSE is a systematic evaluation of a broad range of general mental and cognitive functions. While some illnesses are defined by a single abnormality on the examination (as in Wernicke's aphasia due to stroke), most neuropsychiatric problems involve impairments in multiple domains of cognition. The pattern of deficits and strengths revealed by the MSE, along with clinical history and physical examination, provide information about brain function and facilitate the development of the differential diagnosis. Although it will not always be practical to perform all of the specific assessments discussed in this chapter, our hope has been to provide a wide and relatively detailed set of tools for the examination of patients with neuropsychiatric problems and to offer a framework that correlates the procedures and findings on MSE with our approach to understanding brain function.

10

Clinical electrophysiology

Introduction

Over the last 70 years, clinical electrophysiology has become increasingly sophisticated, widely used, and diagnostically helpful. Electroencephalography (EEG) is a clinical electrophysiological technique that is often used in neuropsychiatric evaluation and research. Although seizure disorders and various forms of encephalopathy are the most common clinical indications for EEG, in recent years the application of this and other electrophysiological techniques has broadened to include the evaluation and study of many neuropsychiatric problems.

EEG, magnetoencephalography (MEG), evoked potentials, and event-related potentials all measure brain activity and may provide complementary sets of information. However, they represent fundamentally different approaches to studying brain activity and, at present, the latter three techniques are generally regarded as tools for neuropsychiatric research. By contrast, standard EEG is frequently used in clinical neuropsychiatry and the relatively recent development of digital and quantitative techniques for EEG recording and analysis is facilitating increasingly detailed interpretation of clinical electrophysiological data. Clinical interpretation, however, requires substantial training and experience with EEG, and for clinicians with no specific training in this area, the meaning of EEG reports may not be immediately understandable in terms of the problems with which patients present. While a brief discussion cannot serve as a definitive resource either on EEG technology or interpretation, this chapter will provide a brief review of a few basic principles of clinical electrophysiology and a discussion of the role of electrodiagnostic techniques in the neuropsychiatric evaluation.

Electrophysiology and recording

EEG electrodes detect the surface electrical activity of the brain. EEG records both radially and tangentially oriented electric currents generated by the neural tissue underlying them, although radially oriented currents are detected much more reliably. Radially oriented currents are those in which orientation is directed from within the head out towards the surface of the scalp, as if drawing a line from the center of the head to the scalp that depicts the radius of the skull. Tangentially oriented currents are those that have an orientation tangential to the scalp surface that overlies them. The large neurons in the cortex are oriented such that current flows up and down the six cortical layers, whether that cortex is on a gyral or a sulcal surface. As a result of their cortical organization, the orientation of neurons on gyral surfaces produces radial currents, while those on sulcal surfaces produce tangentially oriented currents.

Sweat, scalp, muscle and connective tissue, skull, dura, and cerebral spinal fluid (CSF) all act as insulation with respect to the external detection of electrical currents produced by the brain. These tissues significantly attenuate and diffuse cortical electrical activity before it reaches the scalp. Consequently, the EEG is best able to detect cortical potentials that are generated relatively close to the recording electrodes, namely those generated at the gyral cortical surfaces. Although inferences can be made about deeper sources in some research paradigms, in general the standard clinical EEG is most useful as a tool for detecting superficial cortical potentials. It is not very useful as a tool for recording deep (for example, medial temporal) potentials without the use of special techniques such as sphenoidal or nasopharyngeal electrode placement, intracranial depth electrodes, or intracranial electrode grid placement.

As a result of dipole orientation and signal strength, localizing cortical potentials using standard clinical EEG is challenging. A substantial amount of the cortex produces tangentially oriented currents to which EEG is relatively insensitive. Further, attenuation and diffusion of both radial and tangential cortical signals over the scalp severely limits precise localization of abnormal electrical activity. Although these limitations do not invalidate EEG's utility as a diagnostic tool, they should prompt one to remain relatively cautious about overinterpreting EEG results. For example, it is entirely possible for a standard clinical EEG to fail to detect a tangentially oriented (sulcal) or deep (medial temporal) epileptogenic focus, giving the appearance of an "absence" of pathology where in fact there is a significant abnormality present.

Traditional methods of EEG interpretation are also sometimes criticized as highly susceptible to recording and display artifacts, excessively subjective and dependent on the skill of the electroencephalographer, and imperfect in their ability to provided quantitative data either for clinical or research purposes. In light of these problems, digital EEG and quantitative EEG (QEEG) have been developed over the last decade as a means of overcoming these problems with standard EEG. Both of these relatively newer techniques involve computerized acquisition of EEG data, and the latter offers the ability to perform detailed and quantitative data analyses. For example, QEEG can quantify the amount of activity occurring at any frequency (power), the synchronization of activity between brain areas (coherence), the phase relationship of different areas of brain to one another, and the symmetry of activity between brain areas or even specific electrodes. Additionally, with high-density EEG (that is, 32-, 64-, 128-, or 256-channel recordings) complex mathematical algorithms are available for enhanced localization of activity in both spatial and temporal domains. At present, QEEG is neither widely available nor routinely used in clinical neuropsychiatry and is generally considered a research technique with significant clinical promise. We will not consider QEEG in detail here, but the principles discussed in the following sections pertain to both standard and to QEEG techniques.

Similarly, evoked potential (EP) and event-related potential (ERP) are electrophysiological techniques that measure brain activity at specific frequencies and in relation to specific stimuli or cognitive activities. In the evaluation of some traditionally "neurological" disorders (e.g., optic neuritis) evoked potentials may be diagnostically helpful when they define abnormalities in the latency (which suggests delayed nerve conduction time, as occurs with demyelination) or amplitude (as occurs with loss of cortical neurons) of the electrical response to the stimulus to which the patient is subjected. In some neuropsychiatric disorders, the middle- and late-latency cortical potentials (those occurring 30–400 milliseconds after a stimulus) may be abnormal in latency, amplitude, or both. However, such findings generally appear to reflect brain dysfunction nonspecifically. For example, the auditory P300 (a late-latency cortical potential) appears to reflect attentional processing and may be abnormal in many neuropsychiatric disorders. As a result, auditory P300 recordings are of little use diagnostically in clinical neuropsychiatry, because abnormalities support only the presence of brain dysfunction rather than suggesting its specific cause.

As more is learned about the neurobiology underlying specific EP and ERP events these techniques may become more clinically useful. For example, if auditory P50 abnormalities can be consistently found to reflect relative cholinergic deficits, then such abnormalities may suggest treatment strategies using cholinergic agents in the various clinical syndromes where such EP abnormalities occur. For the present, however, with regard to neuropsychiatric disorders EP and ERP are most appropriately regarded as research techniques.

Magnetoencephalography (MEG) detects the magnetic fields produced by summed cortical electrical dipoles in the brain. This technique is more sensitive to tangentially oriented currents than EEG, and is susceptible to attenuation of signal only by virtue of the distance of the recording device from the source of activity (i.e., it is not susceptible to signal attenuation by bone, blood, or scalp). As such, it is a technology complementary to EEG, and it may be used with EEG to perform a more detailed assessment of brain electrophysiology.

While the lack of attenuation due to soft-tissue signal attenuation is a significant advantage over EEG, magnetic field strength falls off at a rate of $1/r^2$ from its source; since the strength of the magnetic fields produced by the brain is very small, recording these fields from the surface of the head and in the context of the very large ambient magnetic fields of the earth presents a formidable technical challenge. While the technology presently available to meet this challenge does so superlatively, both the equipment and its routine operation is quite expensive and analysis of MEG data requires a very high level of engineering and scientific expertise. Largely as a result of its cost, the highly specialized expertise required for implementation and data analysis, and the relatively small number of research labs applying this technology to the study of neuropsychiatric disorders, as yet MEG has not been universally accepted for use in clinical neuropsychiatry. It has become increasingly used in some pre-surgical seizure localizations and for pre-surgical somatosensory brain mapping, though. The potential for increased application of MEG to the study and clinical diagnosis of neuropsychiatric disorders does exist and should be intensively further explored. However, we will focus the remainder of this chapter on the most widely accepted and clinical useful electrophysiological technology: EEG.

Electroencephalography

EEG methods are standardized to facilitate improved reliability of both recording and interpretation, particularly with respect to the detection and approximate localization of abnormal electrical activity. In most clinical settings, electrodes are placed on the patient's scalp according to the 10–20 International System of Electrode Placement (Figure 10.1). In this system, a series of electrodes are placed around the patient's head, using the nasion (the space between the eyes immediately above the bridge of the nose) and the

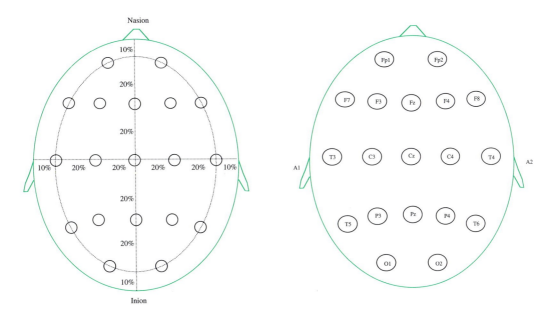

Figure 10.1 The 10–20 International System of Electrode Placement. On the left, the head is labeled with a circumferential line running through the nasion and inion, another running over the top of the head in the sagittal midline from the nasion to inion, and a third running over the top of the head (coronal midline) from one pre-auricular point to the other. Sagittal midline electrodes are placed above the circumferential line by a distance equal to 10% of the length of the sagittal midline, and spaced apart by 20% of the length of the sagittal midline as they converge up to the central point. Coronal midline electrodes are placed in similar fashion. Circumferential electrodes are spaced apart by 10% of the distance of the circumferential line created by the most frontal (Fp1 and Fp2), most occipital (O1 and O2), and lateral temporal (T3 and T4) electrodes. The rest of the electrodes are placed in lines running sagittally and coronally as defined by these placements. On the right is the 10–20 system with labeled electrodes, including the A1 and A2 reference electrodes.

inion (the occipital protuberance) as anatomical reference points to define a series of lines and distances according to which the electrodes are placed. First, a circumferential line at a level defined by the plane of the nasion and the inion is drawn around the head. Second, a line passing through the vertex (midline) and another line passing from the ear-to-ear through the vertex (central line) are drawn. Third, the lengths of the midline and central lines are measured. These lines and their lengths are then used to determine the electrode placements in a series of relationships based on increments of 10% and 20% off these reference lines (see Figure 10.1), hence the designation of this system as the "10–20" system. The purpose of placing electrodes in such an arrangement is to permit a relatively standardized and repeatable recording of brain electrical activity in a given patient, between patients, and among EEG laboratories.

As stated above, while EEG records both radially and tangentially oriented potentials, radial potentials make up the majority of those reflected in the EEG data acquired by standard clinical assessments. On the paper or computer-based display of recorded potentials, when current is moving towards an electrode (towards the scalp) it will be recorded as a positive (upward) deflection on the display. When current is moving away from an electrode (away from the scalp), it will be recorded as a negative (downward) deflection. Historically, paper records reflected the reverse of this relationship (e.g., positive current produced a downgoing tracing) but most laboratories are moving to adopt the more intuitive tracing representation of activity described here (positive = uP, negative = dowN).

Of course, speaking of positive and negative potentials is relative and only meaningful when comparing the potential differences between two electrodes. Two electrodes located at some distance from one another are needed to detect relative "positive" and "negative" charge differences between them, and since diffusion and attenuation of charge across the scalp surface makes it very difficult to detect small absolute potential differences between two closely spaced electrodes. To facilitate making finer comparisons between cortical electrodes, two additional electrodes are placed at the ears, creating electrical "references." The current measured at any given electrode can then be compared not only to that measured at others on the scalp, but also to that at the "reference" electrode (ear), which is ideally not detecting any significant cortical currents. That being the case (more or less), the cortical electrical activity reflected on the scalp is not detected (or at least not strongly detected) at the reference electrode, thereby creating a relatively large potential difference between the electrodes that can be reasonably easily amplified and displayed as an EEG tracing.

Once electrodes are placed and reference electrodes are established, the manner in which the recordings at the electrodes are examined with respect to one another can be systematically changed. Paired electrode signals are compared to one another, and these comparison pairs are referred to as channels. The most common arrangements of electrodes include the referential montage (each electrode compared to a reference electrode) and bipolar montage (each electrode compared to an adjacent electrode). Through these different

Table 10.1. Major electroencephalography bands, their respective frequencies, and most characteristic location in a normal recording

Band	Frequency (Hz)	Characteristic location
β (beta)	>13	Frontal
α (alpha)	8–13	Occipital
θ (theta)	4–7	Central
δ (delta)	<3	Frontal/central

arrangements, several "views" of cortical electrical activity can be established. This improves the likelihood of "seeing" focal abnormalities in cortical activity, such as in a seizure focus, or those associated with a stroke, subdural hematoma, tumor, or other problems.

Making sense of the EEG record

The electrical signal recorded on the scalp is a final summation of a multitude of potentials generated by the area of cortex underlying the recording electrode. Although the brain produces activity at a wide range of frequencies (Hz = cycles/second), clinical electroencephalographers typically divide these frequencies into four major bands (beta, alpha, theta, and delta). Although activity in each band can be seen over the entire cortex, each appears to have an area of cortex over which it is best represented or most characteristically present (Figure 10.2 and Table 10.1).

Without the influence of distantly connected neurons or exogenously administered substances, adjacent neurons (or groups of neurons) tend to fire synchronously. However, the pattern of firing of cortical neurons is influenced by relatively distant structures controlling arousal and sleep, including the reticular formation and the thalamus. When an individual is awake, the reticular formation produces widespread cortical activation, which on EEG is reflected as asynchronous cortical electrical activity – the neurons are not firing together, but are firing independently and at a frequency that roughly reflects the amount of ascending drive that they receive. This means that the waking EEG is characterized by fast (usually high alpha and/or beta) activity, and the individual channels will reflect varying degrees of cortical activity at the frequencies.

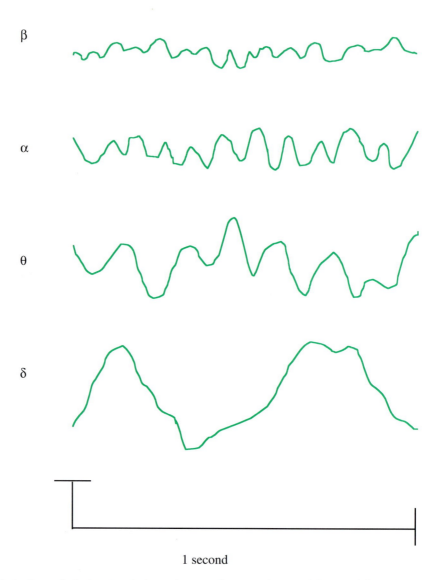

Figure 10.2 Illustrations of electroencephalography waveforms. β, beta activity; α, alpha activity; θ, theta activity; δ, delta activity.

The alpha rhythm may be thought of as the frequency of "idling" cortex. In other words, when a person is awake but has his or her eyes closed, the occipital cortex is not receiving input and will be firing at the alpha frequency. The electrodes over the occipital cortex (O1 and O2) will record predominantly alpha frequencies when the person is in this state. Like a car at a stoplight, the cortex is idling until a signal from the outside provides it with the energy needed to begin firing more quickly. When the person opens the eyes, visual inputs are received and processed, and reticular and thalamic inputs provide the occipital cortex with the "gasoline" needed to begin firing more quickly. To continue with this metaphor, when the gasoline that is the ascending sensory input is withdrawn (as when the eyes close), the alpha rhythm develops again. Although the alpha frequency is most easily recognized on EEG in the visual (occipital) domain, all cortical areas will develop an alpha rhythm when information is not being processed in that domain (for example, when auditory cortex fires at alpha frequency in a silent room).

At sleep onset, there is less reticular activation and consequently the activity of the cortex decreases. Lessened activity produces slower rhythms like theta and eventually delta. As noted above, when an ascending drive is present it desynchronizes cortical activity. Conversely, when the ascending drive is reduced, the EEG becomes more synchronized. It has been suggested that there are brain "pacemakers" that determine the frequency of these slower and more synchronous rhythms, and that the thalamus may be one such pacemaker. Without ascending drive from the reticular formation, the thalamus is prone to fire more slowly. Consequently, at sleep onset thalamocortical rhythms are unmasked (released from the influence of reticular activity). Cortical activity becomes relatively more synchronous as it is driven by deeper, central, and diffusely connected thalamocortical activity, and consequently the EEG shows slower and higher-amplitude waveforms.

When abnormalities are present, the electroencephalographer uses a few basic principles to begin determining the origin of the signals. First, current headed toward an electrode produces a positive EEG deflection and current headed away from an electrode produces a negative EEG deflection. Second, electrical currents from the brain are "spread out" across a relatively wider area of scalp. This means that a strong electrical signal under one electrode (for example, F3) will also be seen by adjacent electrodes (Fp1, Fz, F7), although to a lesser degree. Third, deflections on the EEG tracing occur as a result of differences in the electrical activity between two electrodes; in other words, deflections on EEG tracings reflect differences in electrical potential between the two electrodes being compared (for example, Fp1 vs. A1 in a referential montage).

Using these principles, different recording montages may be used to "view" the area of electrical abnormality. The referential montage (activity at a scalp electrode compared to that at a reference electrode) will demonstrate generalized patterns of cortical activity (as in diffuse intermixed slowing in

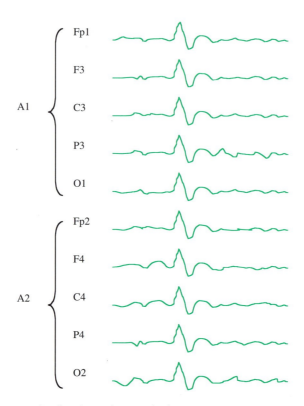

Figure 10.3 Illustration of a generalized spike-and-wave discharge seen on a referential montage.

delirium or generalized spike-and-wave activity in primarily generalized epilepsy) and can also reveal relatively focal abnormalities and asymmetries (as in a spike-and-wave event or focal – asymmetric – slowing in the left frontal lobe). Generalized patterns are especially well seen using the referential montage. Because referential montage EEG tracings reflect differences in the electrical activity between each scalp electrode and a reference electrode, and because a generalized electrical event appears at every electrode except the reference electrodes, when generalized events occur they produce large electrical potential differences between the scalp and reference electrodes. This large potential difference causes a substantial deflection on EEG visible on all channels (Figure 10.3).

Focal events can also be seen on a referential montage, and may suggest an area of abnormal cortical electrical activity. For example, a focal epileptiform discharge occurring under the F3 electrode will appear largest on the EEG channel that includes that electrode, but will also appear on channels created

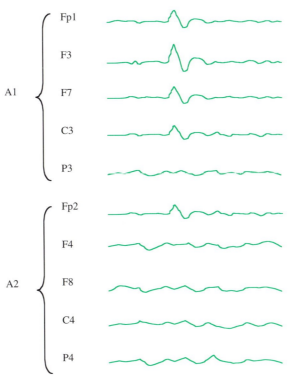

Figure 10.4 Illustration of a spike-and-wave discharge maximal under F3 as seen on a referential montage.

by adjacent electrodes. Remember that current is diffused across the scalp so that activity under one electrode is also detected by neighboring electrodes. This montage is useful for directing attention to an electrically abnormal region of cortex, and suggesting the need for further study of that area using additional montages (e.g., bipolar, transverse, etc.) to better localize the source of the abnormal activity (Figure 10.4).

On a bipolar montage, connecting adjacent electrodes (e.g., Fp1–F3, F3–C3, C3–P3, etc.) creates EEG channels. This montage will demonstrate relatively more subtle potential differences between adjacent electrodes than the referential montage. To illustrate the utility of this sort of montage, we shall consider the EEG signature of a focal epileptiform event. Recall that current moves from the cortex to the scalp and is then diffused across the scalp towards or away from various electrodes. Let's say there is an epileptogenic area of cortex lying underneath C3 (Figure 10.5). The electrical signature of this epileptogenic area is detected by the C3 electrode, but is also seen to a lesser degree on

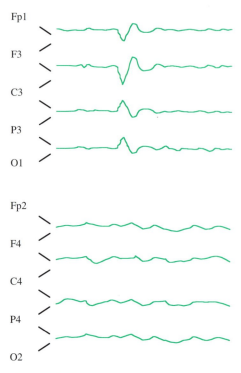

Figure 10.5 Illustration of a spike-and-wave discharge maximal under montage as seen on a bipolar montage. Note phase reversal between channels F3–C3 and C3–P3.

adjacent channels. As is true of many such areas, in this example we will assume that the epileptogenic area is producing a relatively negative electrical potential; this sort of negative (or moving from cortex into the brain) current is that most commonly seen for epileptogenic foci. C3 is seeing a relatively more negative signal than any of its immediate neighbors – in other words, there is a relative potential difference between C3 and the adjacent electrodes. On the EEG tracing, connecting a relatively more positive electrode to a more negative one creates a downward deflection (positive → Negative = dowN), and connecting a relatively more negative electrode to a more positive one creates an upward deflection (negative → Positive = uP). Therefore, connecting F3–C3 produces a negative deflection, and connecting C3–P3 produces a positive deflection. On the EEG record, a positive wave occurs in the C3–P3 channel and a negative wave in the F3–C3 channel. The appearance of a negative wave in one channel and a positive wave in an adjacent channel is referred to as a "phase reversal," and suggests that the area of cortex underlying the electrode common to these channels is relatively near the source of the abnormal signal. By re-arranging the manner in which the electrodes are connected, phase reversals can be localized to a more restricted area of cortex. It is in this manner that abnormal electrical events are typically localized.

Abnormal events and patterns of cortical electrical activity generally fall into two major categories, paroxysmal spikes (and sharp waves) and slow waves. Spikes are relatively high-voltage paroxysmal electrical events with a duration of 70 milliseconds or less, and sharp waves are similar events with a duration of 70–200 milliseconds. In some cases, spikes and sharp waves occur together, forming spike-and-wave complexes. Slow waves are any waveforms in a waking record with a frequency of less than the alpha rhythm (<8 Hz). A pattern of relatively slow (theta or delta) background rhythm with superimposed fast activity is referred to as intermixed slowing. Routine EEG is performed on an awake, resting subject. Several clinical maneuvers, including sleep deprivation, hyperventilation, photic stimulation, and sleep may make some abnormalities more evident.

Clinical use of EEG

Screening EEG may detect apparent abnormalities in 10–20% of general psychiatric patients, but only rarely do such abnormalities alter clinical diagnosis or management. When present, these abnormalities tend to be nonspecific, including rare, non-epileptiform focal (sharp-wave, spike, spike-and-wave) events, low voltage beta, mild diffuse or focal slowing in elderly patients, or "medication effects" (increased beta or slowing). Consequently, using EEG in routine screening of psychiatric patients is unlikely to be clinically useful. However, when there is evidence by history or examination of a neurological condition that may either be primarily responsible for, or significantly worsening, the patient's condition, an EEG may be a useful diagnostic tool. Similarly, when it is unclear whether a neurological condition may be a significant contributor to the patient's psychiatric illness, an EEG may help clarify the diagnosis (for example, in resolving the argument between "psychosis" and delirium). However, even when neuropathology is present, the EEG result is neither perfectly sensitive nor perfectly specific, and must be taken as merely one piece of information in a broader clinical evaluation. An important point to remember is that EEG can be a useful adjunct to clinical diagnosis, but EEG abnormalities without clinical correlates are not necessarily indications of

Table 10.2. Examples of typical electroencephalography (EEG) findings in several neuropsychiatric disorders

Condition	Typical EEG findings
Seizure disorders:	Focal or generalized spikes, sharp waves, and spike-and-wave complexes:
infantile spasms	hypsarrhythmia – nearly continuous high-voltage multifocal spikes or sharp waves and arrhythmic slow waves
absence	generalized, bilaterally synchronous 3 Hz spike-and-waves (ictal)
primary generalized epilepsy	generalized, bilaterally synchronous spike-and-slow waves (ictal), or typical spike-and-wave discharges (2–5 Hz)
complex partial seizures	focal spike or sharp-wave discharges
Tumor or infarction	Focal slowing at the borders of the tumor or infarction and absence of activity overlying necrotic tissue
Anterior brainstem/diencephalic injury	Frontal intermittent rhythmic delta activity (FIRDA), bilateral, reactive to stimuli, and not apparent during sleep; bifrontal theta may be seen with slow growing deep midline tumors
White matter pathology	Continuous polymorphic delta activity that is not reactive to stimuli
Alzheimer's disease (advanced)	Accelerated development of EEG changes of normal aging (some alpha slowing, diffuse theta and delta, decline in low-voltage beta, focal delta in temporal areas)
Creutzfeld–Jakob disease	Generalized, synchronous, periodic (0.5–1 sec) sharp waves lasting 200–400 msec; also known as periodic short-interval diffuse discharges (PSIDDs)
Subacute sclerosing panencephalitis	Typically generalized, synchronous, periodic (4–15 sec) sharp-and-slow wave complexes; also known as periodic long-interval diffuse discharges (PLIDDs)
Herpes encephalitis	Periodic lateralized epileptiform discharges (PLEDS)
Delirium:	Diffuse slowing with irregular high-voltage delta activity:

Table 10.2. (*cont.*)

Condition	Typical EEG findings
acute agitated delirium (AAD)	low-voltage fast activity
acute confusional state (ACS)	diffuse intermixed slowing
uremic or hepatic encephalopathy	triphasic waves

a need for treatment. In other words, it is the patient that needs treatment, not the EEG.

An EEG should be ordered when there is concern regarding a specific problem for which there are likely to be EEG findings and when demonstration of abnormal findings is likely to change clinical management (see Table 10.2). For example, complex partial seizures with intermittent secondary generalization may be diagnosed on clinical grounds alone, and when the history is clear (for example, clear onset of seizures following a traumatic brain injury with no antecedent history of seizures), an EEG may not be necessary. However, when the distinction between seizure types is not clear (as in complex partial vs. absence) based on history, an EEG should be obtained. As another example, an EEG may be used to help determine whether auditory hallucinations, delusions, and thought disorder in a previously delirious patient with schizophrenia represent symptoms of a continued delirium or are better considered as symptoms of the schizophrenia alone. In the case of resolving delirium, mild diffuse intermixed slowing should be present whereas in schizophrenia alone a standard clinical EEG should be relatively normal.

Summary

Electrodiagnostic assessment is an important part of many neuropsychiatric evaluations. To understand the meaning of results obtained from such assessments, it is important to understand the basic principles of clinical neurophysiology, the strengths and limitations of the diagnostic techniques presently available, and the language used in most diagnostic reports. Of the various methods presently available, only clinical (either standard or digital) is widely accepted and available. QEEG, evoked potentials and event-related potentials, and MEG are presently best regarded as research methods with regard to neuropsychiatric conditions. In general, EEG is most usefully applied as a confirmatory test or one to facilitate refinement of the differential diagnosis, and should not be employed as a screening tool for neurological disease in patients for whom there is no clear clinical indication for this testing.

11

Neuroimaging

Introduction

Neuroimaging has become increasingly sophisticated over the last two decades, permitting an understanding of brain–behavior relationships in vivo that previously could only be inferred from post-mortem studies. For example, purely structural neuroimaging techniques such as computed tomography (CT) scanning and magnetic resonance imaging (MRI) have confirmed the association between left temporoparietal stroke and Wernicke's aphasia and between left frontal stroke and Broca's aphasia in living subjects. Functional studies, including functional MRI (fMRI), single photon emission computed tomography (SPECT), and positron emission tomography (PET) imaging, have further improved our understanding of structural–functional relationships in the brain with their ability to demonstrate alterations in regional brain function during experimental tasks or in pathological states. For example, patients with early to moderate Alzheimer's disease often suffer posterior (transcortical sensory or Wernicke's) aphasias and visuospatial impairments. Even in cases where the disease has not yet produced grossly visible atrophy, SPECT or PET scans may demonstrate the bilateral parietotemporal hypometabolism that might be expected to underlie such problems.

In the neuropsychiatric evaluation, structural and/or functional neuroimaging may be extremely useful and provide diagnostically important information. For example, we recently saw a 67-year-old woman with chronic paranoid schizophrenia who had been admitted to the hospital with an "acute psychotic decompensation." She was in her usual state of health, and had been regularly compliant with her antipsychotic medication regimen, until that afternoon, when she began speaking "nonsensically" and appeared quite agitated and confused. In the emergency room, she was described as "psychotic and paranoid" and was admitted to the psychiatry service. Evaluation of the patient was most remarkable for a normal level of arousal, grossly normal attention, mild anxiety, no evidence of responding to internal stimuli and no overt paranoia;

she did demonstrate a complete lack of ability to follow even simple commands, to repeat any phrases, and produced volumes of incoherent speech (a *jargon aphasia*). The patient's history and presentation was less supportive of an acute psychotic decompensation and more suggestive of a new onset fluent aphasia. An MRI of the brain resolved the ensuing debate, demonstrating a left temporoparietal infarction and prompting her transfer to a medical unit for management of her acute stroke. Such studies can facilitate accurate and appropriate diagnosis, and in this case reducing the likelihood of misinterpreting the "nonsensical speech" of aphasic patients as evidence of psychosis, which would not only result in a failure to treat the correct diagnosis but also most likely result in a course of increasing doses of antipsychotic medication that would not only have been unhelpful but also potentially harmful.

Neuroimaging methods that measure physiological changes, such as functional MRI (fMRI), magnetic resonance spectroscopy (MRS), single photon emission computed tomography (SPECT), and positron emission tomography (PET), are capable of providing valuable information about both normal and abnormal brain activity. Although these more high-tech imaging modalities have, at present, few applications in the practice of clinical neuropsychiatry, a growing number of clinical research studies seem to suggest that these technologies (or their successors) will become increasingly useful for both diagnosing neuropsychiatric illness and assessing the effects of treatment (e.g., as has already been done in patients with obsessive–compulsive disorder and major depression using PET imaging).

Even in their present form, both structural and functional imaging studies of the brain are used in clinical neuropsychiatry, particularly in the evaluation of patients with psychiatric symptoms that are suspected to be the result of an underlying neurological or medical problem. Although a detailed review of all of these neuroimaging technologies and their various applications in clinical neuropsychiatry is beyond the scope of this book, a basic familiarity with their strengths and limitations is essential for understanding the clinical indications for their use and the situations in which each may provide particularly useful information.

Neuroimaging Technologies

Computed Tomography (CT) Scanning

CT scanning employs X-radiation to evaluate brain structure. Following the principle of differential absorption of X-rays by tissues of different density, CT

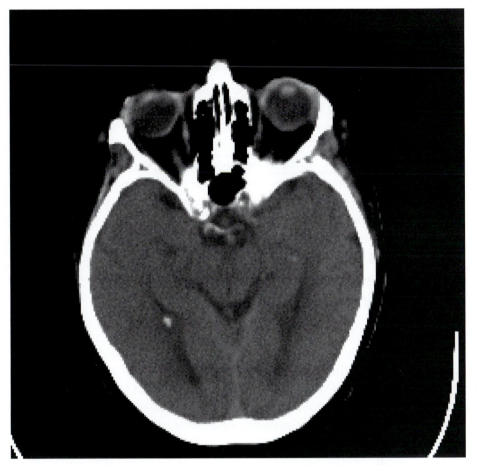

Figure 11.1 Axial computed tomography image of the brain. Courtesy of K. A. Johnson and J. A. Becker, *The Whole Brain Atlas* (http://www.med.harvard.edu/AANLIB/home.html).

applies a mathematical algorithm to create slice-images of the brain from multiple linear X-ray projections through the brain (Figure 11.1). Image enhancement may be obtained using electron-dense iodinated contrast, and is particularly useful for providing greater distinction of lesions involving vascular structures and disruption of the blood–brain barrier (e.g., aneurysmal bleeds, acute epidural or subdural hematomas, and vascularized brain tumors).

Although CT scanning can provide useful information quickly and relatively economically, its principal limitations are its dependence on X-radiation, relatively lower spatial and tissue density resolution in comparison to newer technologies (it is relatively insensitive to subtle changes in gray or white matter), and its susceptibility to artifact. Because it uses X-radiation, CT may not be well suited for use in some patients, particularly in pregnant women. Artifact errors are easily produced when CT images are obtained through a portion of brain containing an admixture of tissue and air, or through tissue and bone (known as partial volume error or partial volume averaging). These are serious limitations on the usefulness of CT scanning in the evaluation of patients with neuropsychiatric disorders. However, CT scanning is probably the best method of evaluating acute neurotrauma that may produce skull fractures or acute bleeding because it is relatively inexpensive, rapidly performed, and widely available. As a result, while the information it can provide may not be as sophisticated as some of the other techniques presented in the following sections, in many emergency settings it may be the most efficient and cost effective method of quickly obtaining information in an agitated, uncooperative, or medically tenuous patient.

Magnetic Resonance Imaging

MRI is a non-radiological (meaning it is not based on X-radiation) imaging technique that was developed for clinical use in an effort to overcome some of the limitations of CT scanning. MRI is based on the measurement of the responses of magnetically active atomic nuclei (mainly protons in water molecules) in brain tissue. When magnetically active nuclei are placed in a sufficiently strong magnetic field, they become aligned along the lines of the direction of the magnetic field. When a short-wave (high frequency) pulse is sent through the field, the magnetically active nuclei will briefly align themselves in the direction of the pulse (or, away from the direction of the standing magnetic field). After the pulse is discontinued, the nuclei will "relax" back to their resting state, thereby realigning themselves in the standing magnetic field. As they relax, they emit the energy absorbed from the radio frequency pulse. Because tissues of different compositions differ in the amount of magnetically active nuclei (protons in water) they contain and in the interaction of those nuclei with the other macromolecules contained in the various tissues in the brain, the protons do not relax back to the plane of the magnetic field at a uniform rate. These differences in the proton relaxation times confer different magnetic "signatures" (also known as relaxation times) to different brain tissues (e.g., gray matter, white matter, cerebrospinal fluid, etc.). These relaxation responses can be recorded, and are used to reconstruct an image based on the differences among the magnetic signatures of different brain tissues.

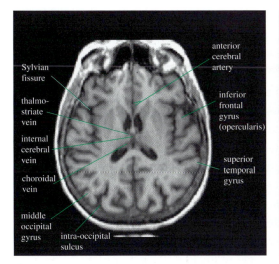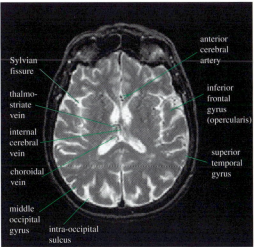

Sylvian
fissure

thalmo-
striate
vein

internal
cerebral
vein

choroidal
vein

middle
occipital
gyrus   intra-occipital
        sulcus

anterior
cerebral
artery

inferior
frontal
gyrus
(opercularis)

superior
temporal
gyrus

Sylvian
fissure

thalmo-
striate
vein

internal
cerebral
vein

choroidal
vein

middle
occipital
gyrus   intra-occipital
        sulcus

anterior
cerebral
artery

inferior
frontal
gyrus
(opercularis)

superior
temporal
gyrus

Figure 11.2 Axial T1 (left) and T2 (right) images of the brain. Courtesy of K. A. Johnson and J. A. Becker, *The Whole Brain Atlas* (http://www.med.harvard.edu/AANLIB/home.html).

The magnetic signatures are typically recorded at two time intervals, designated T1 and T2. The T1 (longitudinal or spin–lattice) relaxation time is the time at which atomic nuclei have lost 63% of the energy produced following their exposure to a radio frequency pulse and are reorienting to the plane of the magnetic field. The T2 (transverse or spin–spin) relaxation time is the time following application of a radio frequency pulse when the atomic nuclei retain 63% of their excitation energy. Accordingly, T1 times are longer than T2 times. Images may also be created based on measurement of the density of protons in tissues (called proton density weighted images), enhanced by variations in the pulse sequences applied, and enhanced by use of suppression techniques to reduce signals from certain physiological tissues (e.g., lipids, water, etc.). Because each type of brain tissue has characteristic T1 and T2 values, reflecting the magnetic response of the protons they contain given the magnetic environment of that tissue, images can be reconstructed that reasonably differentiate between gross tissue types (e.g., gray matter, white matter, CSF, etc.) and also between relatively subtle variations within those tissues (e.g., demyelination, or changes within subcortical gray matter).

On T1 and proton density weighted images, collections of water such as the cerebrospinal fluid (CSF) appear black, gray matter appears gray, and white matter appears white (Figure 11.2). Because the appearance of the anatomy on these images is consistent with intuitive naming conventions (gray is gray, white is white), some refer to T1 images as "anatomic" images. T1 images are better at distinguishing between areas with large differences in the concentration of water, such as the extraparenchymal CSF spaces and the adjacent cortex or the parenchyma and the ventricular spaces.

On T2 images, water and CSF appear white and parenchyma appears gray (Figure 11.2). T2 images are best at revealing subtle differences in tissue density within the brain substance, or areas within the brain parenchyma with significantly different water contents (e.g., lesions in multiple sclerosis). T2-weighting permits relatively sensitive detection of white matter abnormalities; consequently it often reveals so-called white matter "UBOs," or "unidentified bright objects," the clinical significance of which is often uncertain. However, in many neuropsychiatric disorders (e.g., multiple sclerosis, traumatic brain injury) in which there may be particular concern for white matter pathology, T2-weighting and variations of such (e.g., FLAIR imaging) may be very useful.

In addition to providing gross images of brain structure, computer-assisted interpretation is expanding the possible roles for MRI in neuropsychiatric practice and research. Volumetric MRI may be performed on properly acquired image sequences (generally those in which the slice thickness is less than 3 mm, and usually even smaller), and may be used to obtain highly accurate quantification of the intracranial space, total brain volume, and of the volumes of specific brain structures, such as hippocampus, thalamus, amygdala, caudate, and so on. This method of analysis is more sensitive to subtle changes in brain structure than simple visual inspection; however, because it is quite labor intensive and because standard reference databases are yet to be developed and made widely available, this technique is, at present, largely used only as a research method.

Gadolinium DTPA, a paramagnetic agent, is sometimes used as a contrast agent in MRI. A paramagnetic agent changes the local magnetic environment of the tissue through which it passes, and therefore changes the T1 and T2 relaxation times of those tissues (in this case, blood). If the paramagnetic agent leaves the intravascular space (e.g., when there is a disruption of the blood–brain barrier), the contrast agent enters brain tissue and produces an area of enhancement in the brain tissue in which it collects (Figure 11.3). Although the introduction of any foreign substance into the brain and other vascular organs is to be avoided if possible, because paramagnetic agents are non-ionic and non-iodinated they appear to confer a lower risk of adverse

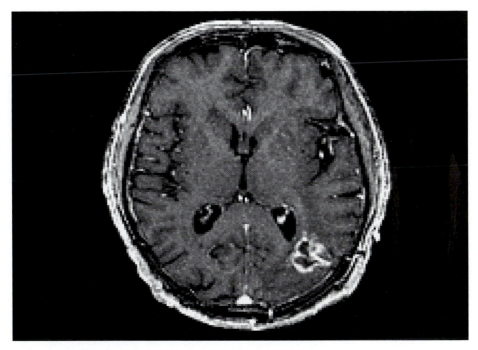

Figure 11.3 T1 image with gadolinium enhancing glioma posterior to the left lateral ventricle. Courtesy of K. A. Johnson and J. A. Becker, *The Whole Brain Atlas* (http://www.med.harvard.edu/AANLIB/home.html).

sequelae (e.g., renal failure) than do the ionic and iodinated contrast agents used with CT scans.

Functional (Echoplanar) MRI

Building on the above principles, fMRI extends the application of MRI to the assessment of brain function. Active neurons use oxygen when they convert hemoglobin to oxyhemoglobin. Because oxyhemoglobin has a longer T2 relaxation time than deoxyhemoglobin, an image that characterizes tissues according to differences in oxyhemoglobin concentrations can be created, by measuring these differences over two or more closely spaced intervals of time. Oxyhemoglobin concentrations are used to infer the metabolic activity of the area in which they are imaged. Therefore, fMRI images may be used to assess not only the structure but also the function of the brain both at rest

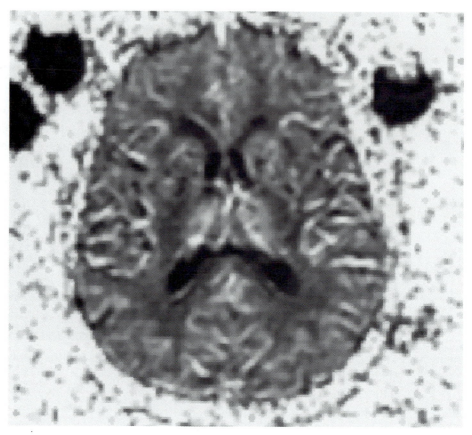

Figure 11.4 Functional magnetic resonance image of patient with Alzheimer's disease. The posterior parietal regions appear relatively less metabolically active bilaterally. Courtesy of K. A. Johnson and J. A. Becker, *The Whole Brain Atlas* (http://www.med.harvard.edu/AANLIB/home.html).

and in response to mental activity. Although fMRI is still largely a research tool, some authors have suggested that it may become clinically useful for the diagnosis of disorders with specific patterns of metabolic abnormality (e.g., temporoparietal hypometabolism in Alzheimer's disease, as seen in Figure 11.4).

Magnetic resonance spectroscopy

Using the principles of nuclear MRS developed for use in the basic sciences, clinical MRS measures the quantities of various cerebral metabolites in brain tissue. From the data acquired using MRS acquisition sequences, determining very specific aspects of both the structural integrity and metabolic activity of the brain using MRI techniques becomes possible. As with fMRI, the ability of MRS to quantify metabolites in brain tissue derives from the fact that each chemical compound has a distinct magnetic resonance signature. In the presence of a magnetic field of sufficient intensity, homogeneity, and stability, the different chemical signatures can be detected. The determination is based on the assumption that the strength of the magnetic resonance signature at a specific frequency is proportional to the amount of the substance that resonates at that frequency. The main types of MR spectroscopy are proton (1H), phosphorus-31 (^{31}P), carbon-13 (^{13}C), or fluorine-19 (^{19}F).

Proton (1H) MRS is the most commonly used form of MRS, and can measure several major metabolic components: N-acetyl aspartate, choline and inositol, lactate, and creatine. N-acetyl aspartate (NAA) is relatively restricted to neuronal cells in the brain (not including glial cells), and the amount of NAA is thought to reflect the number of viable neurons. When neuronal damage or cell loss occurs, as from stroke or traumatic brain injury, decreases in NAA can be detected spectroscopically. Choline is an important constituent of membrane synthesis and breakdown; its spectroscopic peak is increased when membrane integrity is compromised. Inositol is likewise involved in membrane metabolism and increases its spectroscopic peak when there is a breech in membrane integrity. Lactate is a product of anaerobic metabolism; its concentration in the brain increases under conditions of oxidative stress. Creatine and creatine phosphate are relatively stable in most neuropsychiatric disorders, and this peak is often used to establish a reference signal against which to measure other spectroscopic readings. Most other spectroscopic peaks, therefore, are reported as ratios to the creatine/creatine phosphate peak. Finally, proton MRS can also be used to assess other compounds such as glutamate, aspartate, and GABA concentrations. An illustration of a typical proton-MRS spectrum is presented in Figure 11.5.

Phosphorus-31 MRS may be used to obtain information about membrane phospholipids and stability, and is particularly useful for assessing high-energy phosphate metabolism (ATP). Carbon-13 and ^{19}F may be used to radiolabel pharmacologic agents, making ^{13}C and ^{19}F MRS capable of assessing the distribution of pharmacological agents in the brain.

Although MRS is most often used for research, it may have clinical applications in neurodegenerative disorders, tumors, strokes, and traumatic brain injury both diagnostically and therapeutically. MRS may facilitate neurochemical

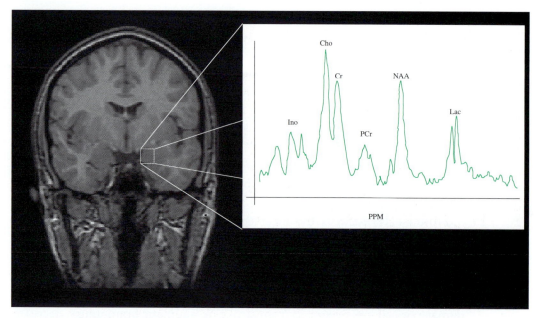

Figure 11.5 Illustration of proton magnetic resonance spectroscopy over the left amygdala. A spectrum of moiety resonances is illustrated in the right window. Abbreviations: Ino, inositol; Cho, choline; Cr, creatine; PCr, phosphocreatine; NAA, *N*-acetyl aspartate; Lac = Lactate.

characterization of neuropsychiatric disorders in living subjects in a manner that is relatively cost effective and more convenient than either PET or SPECT scanning. Additionally, MRS may become useful for assessing both the distribution and metabolic effects of neuropharmacological agents. However, these interesting applications of MRS remain the province of neuropsychiatric research at the present time.

PET

PET scanning is currently the most technologically sophisticated and expensive functional brain imaging technique available. PET images are created by mathematical reconstruction based on the distribution of gamma (photon) emissions produced during the collision of a local electron with a positron emitted from an injected radionuclide. The images produced are of very high spatial resolution, limited only by the distance the positron must travel from the point of emission to collision with an electron in its local environment.

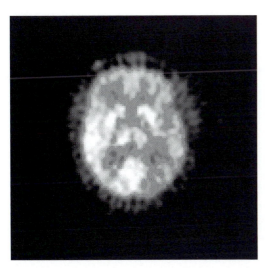 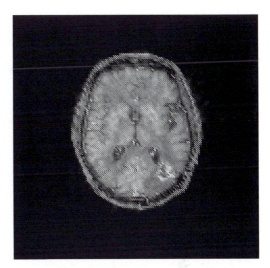

Figure 11.6 Fluorodeoxyglucose (FDG) positron emission computed tomography (PET) image (left) and corresponding T1 image with gadolinium (right) in a patient with a left posterior glioma. Courtesy of K. A. Johnson and J. A. Becker, *The Whole Brain Atlas* (http://www.med.harvard.edu/AANLIB/home.html).

Radiolabeled tracers are available for use in PET to assess regional glucose or dopamine metabolism, blood flow, protein synthesis, monoamine oxidase activity, and neurotransmitter receptor distribution, using either benzodiazepine, serotonin, dopamine, muscarinic, or opioid radioligands. However, the availability of PET scanning is severely limited by its cost and by the need for a local cyclotron to generate the short-lived radionuclide tracers used in this brain imaging technique. Although PET scanning is used clinically in cardiology and in neuro-oncology (Figure 11.6), there are at present no consistently accepted indications for its use in clinical neuropsychiatry. Major barriers to clinical use have included the difficulties in matching imaging physiology data obtained in an individual with the values determined for groups of subjects and in managing the remarkable within-individual variability of the PET data generated.

Nonetheless, some centers do use PET to provide adjunctive information about brain function in neurodegenerative dementias, traumatic brain injury, obsessive–compulsive disorder, and some other neuropsychiatric conditions. PET information may be very useful in correlating functional and structural abnormalities, or in establishing the presence of pathophysiological conditions despite apparently normal brain structure. While these uses are interesting and

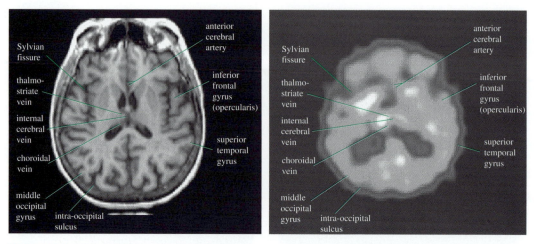

Figure 11.7 Axial T1 (left) and single photon emission computed tomography (right) images of the brain. Courtesy of K. A. Johnson and J. A. Becker, *The Whole Brain Atlas* (http://www.med.harvard.edu/AANLIB/home.html).

potentially very helpful in select cases, the cost and logistical difficulties of PET scanning are likely to limit severely its acceptance and use in clinical neuropsychiatry more generally.

SPECT

SPECT images are obtained by mathematical reconstruction based on the pattern of distribution of direct gamma emissions produced by single photon emitting radionuclide tracers (Figure 11.7). Unlike PET, the gamma emissions come from the injected radionuclide itself, and not from the energy released by the emitted particle's collision with electrons in the local (brain) environment. Radionuclide tracers are available for use in SPECT to assess cerebral blood flow, amino acid concentration (alpha-methyltyrosine), and receptor distribution and activity (acetylcholine, benzodiazepine, serontonin, dopamine, and norepinephrine). SPECT has good spatial resolution; however, although one might think that SPECT offers an advantage over PET by avoiding spatial resolution errors associated with the distance between positron emissions, collision with the local electrons, and the subsequent production and emission of photons, this is not the case and the spatial resolution of

SPECT is indeed relatively inferior to that of PET. Additional advantages over PET include lesser cost, and use of radionuclides with relatively long half-lives permitting use at greater distances from their point of production. A potential disadvantage is that many of the single photon emitting nuclides, such as iodine-123, may interfere with the chemical activity of the molecule to which they are tagged, thereby possibly contributing to misrepresentation of the metabolic activity with which these molecules are involved.

Like PET, SPECT presently has no consistently accepted application in clinical neuropsychiatry. Nonetheless, it is used in some centers in the evaluation of conditions such as the neurodegenerative dementias, stroke and traumatic brain injury (TBI). Because SPECT may provide evidence of decreased metabolic activity, it may be a useful adjunct to structural neuroimaging studies in these cases. For example, clinicians may commonly observe either mildly focal or diffuse cerebral atrophy in dementia cases without knowing whether this finding is meaningful with respect to brain function. Decreased function on SPECT associated with structural neuroimaging findings can enhance interpretation of the latter studies with important information about their relevance to brain activity (e.g., temporoparietal hypoperfusion in Alzheimer's disease). Similarly, many patients with mild TBI report cognitive impairments in the absence of structural imaging abnormalities in the referable areas of the brain. In such cases, SPECT may provide useful information about brain function despite grossly "normal" brain structure. While not routinely used in the evaluation of these or any other neuropsychiatric disorder, SPECT may provide clinically useful information in select cases.

Summary

All of the neuroimaging techniques described in this chapter have been used extensively in neuropsychiatric research. Clinical application of the functional techniques is limited by their respective availability and costs, typically labor-intensive processing requirements, and present uncertainty regarding clinical implications and utility of abnormal findings. However, as noted above some functional studies and most structural imaging studies do have a role in clinical neuropsychiatry. Clinical use of functional neuroimaging methods is probably best reserved for centers with expertise derived from extensive research experience and with sufficiently large databases to permit interpretation of individual findings in the context of a "reference range" for that technique.

Table 11.1. Suggested indications for neuroimaging in clinical neuropsychiatry

Clinical indication	Preferred neuroimaging modality
Acute cognitive deterioration (e.g., trauma, delirium)	CT
Chronic cognitive deterioration (e.g., dementia or delirium)	MRI
New onset movement disorder	MRI
First episode of psychosis regardless of age	MRI
First episode of major disorder over 40 years of age	MRI
Anorexia nervosa	MRI
Any atypical presentation of psychiatric illness	MRI
Failure to respond to standard therapy	MRI
Co-occurring psychiatric symptoms and significant neurologic or neuropsychological deficits	MRI

Notes:

CT: computed tomography; MRI: magnetic resonance imaging.

As a general guideline, structural neuroimaging studies should be under-taken at least once in all cases of neuropsychiatric (including ostensibly primary psychiatric) illnesses in which there is an atypical presentation, a chronic and progressive course, or a failure to respond to standard therapies. Although no primary psychiatric disorder can be diagnosed solely on the basis of neuroimaging, such imaging may reveal neurological or medical conditions that masquerade as primary "psychiatric" conditions. Daniel et al. (1992) suggest indications for structural neuroimaging evaluation of psychiatric syn-dromes, which we have modified and included in Table 11.1. As is clear from the list in Table 11.1, CT scanning is a useful screening procedure in emergency settings when there is an immediate history of cognitive deterioration, partic-ularly following trauma, or in patients unable to cooperate with the relatively longer MRI procedure. For all other indications, MRI is the preferred modal-ity for neuroimaging in clinical neuropsychiatry.

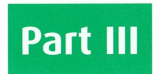

Part III

Applying the approach to neuropsychiatric disorders

12

Delirium

Introduction

Delirium is among the most common neuropsychiatric problems faced by clinicians of all disciplines across all clinical settings. According to the DSM-IV (American Psychiatric Association, 1994), among geriatric patients hospitalized for a general medical/surgical problem, up to 20–25% will become delirious at some point in their hospital course. Although a florid delirium is generally obvious to most clinicians, more subtle forms of this syndrome may initially escape recognition by all but the most astute examiner. Failure to recognize subtle forms of delirium is most likely due, in part, to some widely held misconceptions and oversimplifications about the essential features of this syndrome, and in part because elements of the mental status examination most sensitive to subtle changes in cognition seen in mild deliria are not part of most clinicians' usual or screening mental status examinations.

Most clinicians understand delirium to be a syndrome that can involve disturbance of consciousness, inattention and other cognitive impairments, alteration of perception, altered gait and balance, autonomic nervous dysregulation or a combination of these. It is also well recognized that delirium is most commonly caused by one or more neurological or systemic medical conditions that affect multiple neural systems simultaneously. In the vast majority of cases, delirium is an entirely reversible condition if treatment is directed expeditiously at the underlying cause and is successful. It is also often taught that delirium usually has an acute or subacute onset, and that this feature may be used to distinguish it easily from most dementias, which tend to have a more insidious onset. While both acute (or subacute) onset and fluctuating signs and symptoms are often seen in delirium, neither is necessary for the diagnosis and the absence of either may mislead examiners into believing that the patient is not suffering a delirium.

The fact that the DSM-IV classifies delirium among the cognitive disorders helps to remind us that impaired cognition (specifically, inattention), not onset or course, defines this syndrome. In practice, it is usually true that delirium develops over a short period of time, waxes and wanes with respect both to type and severity of associated features, and is reversible. However, throughout the course of the delirium, inattention nearly always remains an identifiable and important feature of the syndrome. Indeed, some forms of delirium may go unnoticed when the neuropsychiatric practitioner has not assessed attention carefully.

Clinically, both the psychiatric term "delirium" and the neurological term "acute confusional state" may correctly describe the clinical phenomenon under discussion here, and cogent arguments can be made to justify a preference for either term. The neuropsychiatry consultant may use the term that is more familiar to the patient's physician – with a psychiatrist, the patient is delirious, and with a neurologist, the patient is in an acute confusional state. We view the term "delirium" as preferable because of the serious implications associated with it by both psychiatrists and neurologists. Although some clinicians may feel that describing acute but mild inattention and "confusion" as a delirium is an unnecessarily alarmist overstatement of the problem, it is important to remember that the morbidity and mortality associated with delirium is high and that the underlying causes of the condition often constitute grave medical emergencies. Given the high frequency with which patients suffer from deliria during hospitalizations, this term should be used to encourage in the physicians and staff caring for the patient the utmost sense of concern and urgency that this condition warrants. As we consider delirium in this chapter, therefore, we hope to establish that even patients with mild acute confusional states are best served by a thorough consideration of the differential diagnosis of delirium and an approach that regards such conditions as potential medical emergencies. This approach guides accurate diagnostic determination and prompt treatment of the underlying cause.

Diagnostic features

The hallmark feature of delirium is a reduced ability to attend selectively, to sustain attention, to shift attention, and to limit susceptibility to distraction. Alterations in perception (most often visual illusions and/or hallucinations) are also a common feature of this condition, and also represent a disturbance of cognition at its most fundamental levels. Predicated on these disturbances of consciousness are other impairments in memory, language, praxis, recognition, execution, emotion, and behavior. Recalling our view of cognition as relatively hierarchically organized (see Part I), it logically follows that if attention is disturbed then higher cognitive functions will most likely also be disturbed. If a patient cannot attend, they cannot remember, interpret, or respond appropriately to the information presented to them.

In some cases, attentional impairments result from alterations in arousal (or level of consciousness), the lowest functional level in the cognition hierarchy. Impaired arousal results from decreased ascending reticular system activity, and this reduction in reticular driving of the cerebrum produces cognitive impairments at all levels. Even when there is ongoing external stimulation, arousal systems may not be capable of supporting even the most basic cognitive functions of selective and sustained attention. In the opposite case, that of excessive arousal, too much ascending reticular activating drive (or perhaps inadequate ascending inhibition) and or otherwise reduced cerebral inhibition (see *Delirium tremens* in Chapter 17) produces impaired sustained attention due to a tendency to become inappropriately distracted to irrelevant stimuli. This situation has the expected consequences of impairment at higher levels of cognition, including a decreased ability to process information in an organized, efficient, or environmentally relevant fashion. The clinical features of delirium, therefore, may include:

(1) reduced ability to focus, shift, or sustain attention;
(2) hypo-, hyper-, or mixed level of arousal;
(3) other disturbances in cognition (orientation, memory, language, visuospatial, or complex functions);
(4) reduced clarity of awareness of the environment due to fluctuating levels of consciousness;
(5) perceptual disturbances including illusions or hallucinations, and misinterpretations of misperceptions (i.e., delusions);
(6) emotional disturbance and/or lability that may include any combination of any of the following;
   • anxiety or fear,
   • sadness,
   • apathy,
   • anger or irritability,
   • euphoria;
(7) disturbed behavior, including or shifting between
   • restlessness, hyperactivity, and assaultiveness,
   • sluggishness or lethargy;

(8) sleep cycle disturbance;

(9) and course characterized by
  - acute or subacute onset,
  - features tend to fluctuate over the course of a day,
  - reversibility upon correction of the underlying medical condition.

Many patients with delirium will also demonstrate abnormalities on the elemental neurological examination, most commonly primitive reflexes (see Table 8.3). These reflexes emerge when cortical (predominantly prefrontal) inhibition of these reflexes is reduced, as when there is reduced driving of frontal cortices due to decreased function of ascending reticular activating system. These reflexes are not typically present in primary psychiatric disorders, with which delirium is sometimes confused, and therefore may be diagnostically useful. Additionally, as the delirium resolves, these reflexes are again inhibited. Consequently, they can in some cases be a useful accompanying physical examination finding by which to monitor the course and response to treatment of the delirium.

Pathophysiology

Research into the pathophysiological mechanisms causing delirium is surprisingly sparse in light of the frequency of this condition. A variety of biochemical processes are likely to be involved, and the heterogeneity of both the clinical condition and its underlying causes may partially explain the absence of a single compelling explanation for the neurobiological basis of delirium. Whatever the specific mechanisms may be, a simple way of viewing their individual or combined effects is the production of a generalized disturbance of cerebral metabolism (discussed further below). Support for this perspective is supported by the electroencephalography (EEG) findings in delirium.

Delirious patients typically have abnormal EEGs, and the most common finding is a pattern of diffuse, intermixed slowing (see Chapter 10, Table 10.2). This pattern suggests a generalized disruption of cerebral functioning. In the non-delirious state, normal fast activity seen on EEG results from ascending reticular formation activity that facilitates activity of thalamic neurons projecting diffusely to the cortex. This activating "tone" from reticular and thalamic neurons generates activity in the rest of the brain, reflected on the EEG as background activity in the range of 8 Hz or higher. When slower rhythms are seen on EEG, either or both of two processes may contribute.

First, disruption of cortical function by any cause reduces activity in the frontal-subcortical circuits, which secondarily decreases cortical activating influences on the reticular nucleus of the thalamus and the reticular formation, which consequently decreases cerebral activity. Second, primary disruption of the function of the reticular formation and thalamus results in decreased activation of the cerebrum more generally. In both cases, abnormal rhythms on EEG and the clinical signs of globally impaired cerebral function (i.e., delirium) may be observed.

Of note, while EEG changes are generally sensitive to the delirium syndrome, they are often not specific with respect to the underlying disease process, although some EEG changes may be more "characteristic" of some conditions than of others (see Table 10.2). At the same time, EEG changes are generally reversible to the same extent as the delirium. The pattern of EEG changes does follow the clinical presentation of the delirium, with the more commonly observed diffuse intermixed slowing in lethargic, anergic, abulic, inattentive patients (e.g., delirium due to sepsis, post-ictal delirium, etc.), and low-voltage fast activity in hyperactive, hyperaroused, agitated, inattentive patients (e.g., delirium tremens). It has been suggested that the former state is the acute confusional state (ACS), and reflects frontostriatal dysfunction, possibly as a result of inadequate ascending activation. The latter condition of activation is also described as acute agitated delirium (AAD), and is thought to reflect middle temporal gyrus dysfunction. Although these two phenomena have been specifically described, delirium is also seen when function of the high-order association areas of the prefrontal and posterior parietal regions or the inferomedial surface of the occipital lobe is disturbed. The question that arises, given the heterogeneity of areas implicated in the production of delirious states, is whether there may be a common underlying pathophysiology. Is there a final, common pathway that informs the development of the clinical phenomena despite disruption of disparate functional areas of the brain?

Until additional research provides a satisfying answer to this question, it is probably best to adopt a practical view – delirium can be thought of as a pervasive disturbance of cerebral metabolism. Although the constellation of delirium symptoms may develop as a result of many disease processes, impaired cerebral metabolism may result from any of them through one or another pathophysiological mechanism. Common causes of delirium, such as hypoglycemia, hypoxia, hypotension, dehydration, or intoxication, certainly produce cerebral metabolic perturbations. Because the brain has a relatively high metabolic requirement, it has a relatively limited ability to maintain normal function when under metabolic stress. There is also some evidence to suggest that the tolerance for metabolic and cerebrovascular stress may vary among different regions of the brain. It appears that especially vulnerable areas include the reticular formation, the thalamus, the hippocampus, and the frontal (orbital and dorsolateral) lobes. Additionally, the ability to make use of alternate metabolic strategies (glycolytic pathways, ketone metabolism, etc.) seems to differ among brain areas. Further, the activity of neuronal cell bodies and synaptic regions may be differentially affected under such conditions. Clinically, the end result of metabolic stress to the brain is a disruption of function in these metabolically vulnerable brain regions, each of which is critically important to the maintenance of normal attention, memory, and other aspects of cognition, emotion, and behavior.

Differential diagnosis and evaluation

If delirium represents a final common expression of a profound disturbance in cerebral metabolism, it is prudent to regard it as a form of vital organ (brain) failure and as a sign of underlying life-threatening medical illness. Mortality during and following an episode of delirium is very high, by some estimates 14 times greater than that for affective disorders and 5.5 times greater than that seen among hospitalized patients with dementia alone. It has also been reported that up to 35% of patients who develop an episode of delirium die within one year of the occurrence. While this statistic does include patients in the terminal stages of general medical conditions such as cancer, AIDS, and hepatic, renal, cardiac, or pulmonary disease, it suggests that delirium can be a harbinger of life-threatening medical illness. In addition to increased mortality, the cost and morbidity associated with delirium are high, as evidenced by increased lengths of hospitalization and an increased frequency of medical complications among delirious patients.

For all these reasons, the wise clinician will evaluate the delirious patient with the same vigor accorded to the evaluation of any other vital organ failure. Consideration of the differential diagnosis occurs on two levels, beginning with identification of the appropriate clinical syndrome. Delirium as a syndrome must first be distinguished from other syndromes. These include dementia, amnestic disorders, psychotic disorders, mood disorders, substance intoxication, uncomplicated substance withdrawal, factitious disorders, malingering, and isolated cognitive deficits, such as aphasia, apraxia, or agnosia.

Having identified the clinical syndrome as a delirium, its etiology must then be established. Recalling that delirium is always the result of one or more underlying medical (including neurological or substance-related) problems, the evaluation of the delirious patient must involve an assiduous review all available clinical information in an effort to determine both primary and contributing causes. Some conditions increase the likelihood of developing delirium in response to otherwise tolerable metabolic or systemic disturbances. These are the predisposing factors presented in the evaluation section below. Among them are old age, pre-existing central nervous system abnormalities (such as dementia, stroke, or tumor), drug withdrawal, the immediate post-cardiotomy (and probably any post-surgical) period, immunocompromised states (such as AIDS, and possibly chronic immunosuppressive therapy), and severe burns. Additionally, very young age has been suggested to be another predisposing factor, along with sleep and sensory deprivations. With regard to sleep and sensory deprivation, it is not entirely clear that these are specific predisposing factors, and may instead be only contributing factors that lower the threshold for developing a delirium in the face of other predisposing factors or metabolic stresses.

The differential etiology of delirium includes many possible causes. As discussed above, the simplest clinical approach for this differential diagnosis is to consider any and all ongoing problems that may disturb cerebral metabolism. Processes that alter availability of required metabolic fuels (oxygen, glucose, water), delivery of these fuels (hypotension, hypertension), interfere with use of these fuels (toxins, medications and other drugs), or compromise the structural and functional integrity of the brain, all may result in a delirium. These categories can be recalled quickly using the mnemonic A.D.I.I. – Availability, Delivery, Interference, and Integrity. Many conditions may affect more than one of these categories and recognition of this fact can help guide clinical attention to disturbances in each (Table 12.1).

Establishing the diagnosis follows from a thorough assessment of the patient, guided by an integration of clinical findings and consideration of the differential diagnosis. At a minimum, the assessment should include the elements listed below.

(1) *History*, with particular attention given to onset, course, and predisposing factors. All available sources of information should be reviewed, including the medical record (and especially nursing notes), all personnel involved

Table 12.1. Common causes of delirium organized by possible causative mechanisms. The columns list conditions in which there is inadequate availability of metabolic components, inadequate delivery of necessary metabolic components, interference with metabolism, and impairment of the structural or functional integrity of the brain that may disturb cerebral metabolism

Availability	Delivery	Interference	Integrity
Electrolyte disturbance e.g., burns, post-operative, renal disease, dehydration, lithium intoxication	Anemia Hemoglobinopathies	Infectious e.g., intracerebral or extracerebral competition for metabolic fuels, release of toxins from infectious agents	Trauma Hypertension Hydrocephalus
Hypoglycemia	Hypotension e.g., cardiac failure, medication-induced	Acid/base disturbances	Cerebrovascular disorders e.g., stroke, vasculitis, hemorrhage
Hypoxia/anoxia e.g., pulmonary failure, cardiac failure, carbon monoxide poisoning	Cerebrovascular disorders e.g., stroke, vasculitis, hemorrhage	Endocrinopathies	Cerebral infection e.g., encephalitis, meningitis, intracerebral abscess
Deficiency states e.g., B12, Niacin, Thiamine		Toxins e.g., pesticides, heavy metals, solvents	Drug withdrawal e.g., alcohol, barbiturate, benzodiazepine
Endocrinopathies e.g., parathyroid problems, adrenal insufficiency		Medications e.g., anticholinergics, sedatives, illicit drugs, alcohol	Seizure
			Neurogenerative disorders e.g., Lewy body dementia

in the patient's care, the medication record, the family, and (if possible) the patient.

(2) *Physical and neurologic examinations*, and in particular vital signs and any evidence of systemic or neurological abnormalities, and particularly focal deficits or other lateralizing signs. Primitive reflexes may also provide evidence of impaired upper motor neuron (frontal lobe) dysfunction.

(3) *Mental status examination*, including both general and cognitive portions (see Chapter 9). With regard to cognitive examination, a thorough assessment of attention (preferably by digit span, random letter test, or either the verbal or written Trail Making Tests), language (especially naming), memory (including orientation), praxis (particularly construction and writing abilities), and complex cognition should be performed. Difficult behavioral problems should be considered as they relate to problems in perception (e.g., hallucinations or illusions), social intelligence, and motivation and therefore as they relate to the underlying sensory and prefrontal cortices that subserve these functions.

(4) *Laboratory examination*, in cases where there is a question regarding the nature of the syndrome (as in deciding among delirium, dementia, schizophrenia, or depression) the most widely agreed upon single test supporting diagnosis of the delirium is the EEG. As discussed earlier, most delirious patients will demonstrate diffuse intermixed slowing, whereas in most of the other syndromes (advanced dementia being a possible exception) the EEG will be essentially normal. With regard to the etiology of the delirium (see below), basic laboratory examination should include serum chemistries, creatinine and blood urea nitrogen, liver function tests, sedimentation rate, complete blood count, urinalysis and urine toxicology. In cases where these tests do not suggest a specific etiology, lumbar puncture, and CT (computed tomography) or MRI (magnetic resonance imaging) scan of the head may be useful.

Treatment

The first principle in the treatment of delirium is to treat the underlying cause. For patients with otherwise normal brain structure and function, the symptoms and signs of delirium usually resolve quickly with improvement of the primary disorder. Among patients with compromised cerebral function before the delirium (such as dementia, brain injury, advanced age), return to normal brain function may take longer than the time required to resolve the underlying cause. It has been suggested that as many as 40% of these patients may develop chronic signs of impaired cognition, emotion, and behavior, although this statistic may include patients with chronic or progressive illness such as cancer, major organ failure, or AIDS. As a cautionary note, when a return to normal function is delayed the search for as yet untreated underlying problems should be continued.

The second principal in the treatment of delirium is to address the presenting symptoms themselves. This follows from the observation that a specific cause for a delirium may not be identified in as many as 50% of cases. Patient reports suggest that the experience of delirium may be terrifying, and modern medications can substantially reduce the severity of neuropsychiatric symptoms and the distress they produce (in patients, family, and staff) in most cases. Symptomatic management of the delirious patient may also be necessary merely to assure patient safety during periods of agitation and combativeness. There are many approaches to symptomatic management, but we consider those presented herein to be both the most useful and most important. We recommend the following measures:

(1) *Liaison*, raise the level of awareness and concern among the medical and nursing staff about the morbidity and mortality associated with delirium, and encourage expeditious work-up and treatment of the underlying cause. If difficult behavioral problems are discouraging staff from performing duties with their usual level of diligence and care, the physician should educate staff about the neurobiological bases of the delirium, the lack of "volitional" bad behavior on the part of delirious patients, and encourage staff to use their own (usually more) adaptive coping strategies to deliver the care so needed by these patients.

(2) *Environmental interventions*, alter the patient's environment so as to balance sufficient orienting stimulation against over stimulation.
   - The patient should be in a private room if possible to allow sleep and decrease unit disturbance.
   - An attendant should be with the patient at all times. Ideally the attendant should be someone familiar to the patient, but a private nurse or sitter may also suffice.
   - Frequent reorientation and reassurance should be provided by the nurse or attendant, especially during the evening and night, when the effects of sensory deprivation are the greatest.
   - Provide adequate sensory stimulation:

- During the day, leave the curtains open, provide a clock, a clearly visible calendar, familiar pictures or objects, and have a TV or radio on at a reasonable volume.
- If an attendant is not available, placing the patient in a safe chair near the nursing station, where ongoing reorientation and reassurance can be easily provided by staff may be useful.
- At night, keep low-level lighting on in the patient's room. This may facilitate reorientation when the patient awakens during the night.
- Decrease over stimulation:
  - Silence the continuous noise of monitors (e.g., cardiac, ventilators, etc.).
  - Silence monitor alarms quickly.
  - Reduce as much as possible the number of visitors, examiners, or other persons interacting with the patient.

(3) *Medications*, although environmental manipulations alone are sometimes adequate, medications are often also required. Indeed, use of medications may even permit maximal benefit from environmental manipulations.

- Low dose haloperidol is usually our first-choice agent. Starting doses should be in the range of 0.5 mg orally/intramuscularly every 6–8 hours. Intravenous haloperidol is also frequently used, and may be useful when oral or intramuscular administration is impractical. Where the possibility of extrapyramidal side effects of this high potency neuroleptic are a concern, for example in orthopedic or neurosurgical patients who may be in traction or have had a neck brace surgically placed, a relatively lower potency anti-psychotic agent may be preferable. However, the choice of a lower potency agent must be balanced with the possibility of exacerbating the delirium via the anticholinergic, antihistaminic, and antiadrenergic effects of these agents. When absolutely necessary, thioridazine in the range of 10 to 25 mg daily or its parenteral cognate, mesoridazine, at 5 to 15 mg intramuscularly may be useful. At the time of this writing, the newer neuroleptics (e.g., risperidone, olanzapine, etc.) have not been shown to offer an advantage over the standard agents in treating delirium. If increasingly higher doses of either haloperidol (>5 mg daily) or thioridazine (>50 mg daily) are used, it is prudent to reconsider the cause of the problem (including iatrogenic exacerbation of the delirium) and before continuing to increase the dosages of the medication.
- When sedation greater than that provided by haloperidol is required, adjunctive use of lorazepam 0.5–1 mg every 6–8 hours may be useful.

However, lorazepam and other benzodiazepines may cause paradoxical agitation, most commonly in elderly or brain-injured patients. Consequently, when these agents are used, dose and response should be monitored carefully, and a worsening of agitation should prompt reconsideration of this approach rather than increasing the administered doses of these medications. Alternatively, thioridazine 10–25 mg orally every 6–8 hours or chlorpromazine 10–25 mg orally every 6–8 hours may be useful for some patients, as the antihistaminic, anticholinergic, and antiadrenergic properties of these agents may provide the additional sedation needed. However, these agents must also be used with caution, as these mechanisms of effect may themselves worsen delirium in susceptible patients (for example, they should not be used in a patient with an anticholinergic delirium) and may cause significant hypotension. Again, we advise caution when using any of these adjunctive approaches, and generally recommend maximizing the dose of a primary neuroleptic before adding any additional psychoactive agents.

- Benzodiazepines alone are the agent of choice for patients in alcohol or sedative-hypnotic withdrawal. Outside of this use, adjunctive treatment of delirium with benzodiazepines (as noted above) should be avoided whenever possible. The agents predictably impair arousal, memory, and coordination, and carry a nontrivial risk of producing paradoxical agitation in delirious patients. Because paradoxical agitation may be mistaken for the delirium itself, it may prompt additional use of these medications and precipitate a cycle of worsening symptoms and overmedication.
- Chloral hydrate at 500 mg to 1 g can be an effective sedative, particularly at night, and appears to carry less risk of paradoxical agitation than the benzodiazepines.

(4) *Physical restraints*, in general, tend to agitate patients, and should be used only to prevent accidents or disruption of life support apparatus. If used, they should be placed only during periods of agitation, and should be removed promptly during periods of relative calm.

Summary

Delirium is a common neuropsychiatric problem, and a cause of significant morbidity and mortality among hospitalized patients. Although there are many causes, and possibly many pathophysiological mechanisms, of delirium, the condition itself is most usefully regarded as a form of vital organ (brain) failure. Diffuse cerebral dysfunction is often reflected on the EEG, even in relatively mild delirious or confusional states. While not generally specific to the cause of the delirium, an abnormal EEG may be supportive of the diagnosis when there is debate as to the nature of the clinical syndrome observed: schizophrenia vs. depression vs. dementia vs. delirium, with the EEG typically being relatively normal in the first two and markedly abnormal only in the later stages of dementia, in delirium superimposed on dementia (of any severity), or in delirium itself. The differential diagnosis for the causes of delirium is broad, but may be most usefully considered with regard to problems that limit the availability or delivery of essential metabolic requirements, interferes with metabolism, or alters the structural integrity of the brain. Evaluation of delirium follows that suggested in Chapter 8, and focuses in particular on attention, perception, and other aspects of cognition. Treatment is directed at correcting any identified underlying cause expeditiously, and managing the symptoms of delirium with a combination of liaison efforts, environmental manipulations, medications, and (when necessary) physical safety interventions.

13

Dementia

Introduction

Dementia is best defined as an acquired syndrome of persistent impairment in several aspects of basic or complex cognition, without disturbance of level of consciousness. Unlike delirium, dementia often entails a permanent pathological change in brain tissue, rather than a transient metabolic or toxic upset. Dementia is typically a problem of later adulthood and old age (e.g., Alzheimer's disease), although it may be seen in younger adults as well (e.g., patients with Huntington's disease, traumatic brain injury, AIDS, or brain tumors). All causes considered, however, dementia remains most prevalent in older adults. Significant dementia is present in about 5% of individuals in the United States over age 65. By age 80, the prevalence of significant dementia increases to over 20%. It has been estimated that 2–4 million adults in the United States suffer from dementia, and by extension a much larger number of family members, caregivers, and health care professionals experience the impact of dementing illnesses. There are significant economic and emotional costs for patients, their families, and society associated with dementia regardless of the underlying cause. As an example, the National Institute on Aging estimates that the cost of caring for individuals with Alzheimer's disease at about $90 billion per year.

As life expectancies continue to rise, the absolute number of persons with dementia will inevitably increase. Consequently, physicians can expect to encounter greater numbers of patients with dementia proportionate to the increasing age of the population. Although the treatment of dementia is often regarded as the province of neurologists and psychiatrists, all physicians should be familiar with the typical signs and symptoms, differential diagnosis, and available treatments for patients with dementia.

Dementia is a syndrome, or constellation of symptoms. There is no single etiology or pattern that is pathognomonic of the condition, and indeed there is also no universal definition of dementia. The word itself suggests both loss of mind and brain – from Latin, *de-* "down from," or "out of," and *mens-* "mind" or "brain." The term was originally coined to refer to a condition in which a person was "out of brain," reflecting both loss of brain function and (often) brain matter. While this derivation is not nearly specific enough for modern diagnosis, it does capture the fundamental concept behind the clinical syndrome. There are a number of more specific definitions of dementia in the scientific literature, and although there are differences between them, together they may usefully clarify what dementia is and what it is not.

Most authors suggest that prominent disturbance of consciousness is *not* a feature of dementia, which is generally meant to suggest that level of arousal and the basic aspects of attention (e.g., selective and sustained) are relatively normal. Similarly, most definitions require that dementing conditions represent a decline in cognitive functioning from a previously established, stable, and higher functioning baseline. This distinguishes dementia from mental retardation in which there is not a decline in function, but instead a failure to attain age appropriate cognitive abilities. Further, most definitions require that the symptoms of dementia result in a decline in important areas of everyday functioning such as work, interpersonal relationships, and self-care.

Beyond these generalities, there are considerable differences among authors in defining the specific features of impaired cognition that constitute a dementia. This is particularly true when viewed from a discipline specific perspective. For example, the DSM-IV (American Psychiatric Association, 1994) criteria require impairment in memory and in at least one other area of cognitive function such as language, praxis, recognition, or complex cognition. The DSM-IV definition relies on the fact that many, if not most, dementing conditions eventually include memory impairment. This requirement is, however, very conservative. Many patients will experience sometimes not-so-subtle changes in personality, language, and complex cognition prior to developing demonstrable memory impairment (e.g., frontotemporal dementias). In some dementias, and even in some patients with Alzheimer's disease, when memory problems do occur they may not become obvious until well into the course of the illness. For example, some patients with multi-infarct dementia, dementia due to tumors, or dementia due to penetrating brain injuries commonly have extensive cognitive impairment (e.g., aphasia, apraxia, agnosia, complex cognition, and/or motivation) without prominent memory (or at least encoding) impairment. Consequently, some authors do not require memory impairment for the diagnosis of dementia. Instead, they note that impaired memory may simply be one of several areas of impaired cognition supporting the diagnosis.

With that in mind, Cummings & Benson (1992) define dementia by the presence of impairment in any three or more areas of cognition that together result in functional impairment.

For purposes of this discussion, we favor the latter definition in order to include the many patients in whom disabling cognitive impairment warrants clinical concern but whose clinical presentation does not necessarily include impaired memory. This wider definition urges equal clinical attention to all of the major domains of cognition during the evaluation.

Diagnostic features

Since dementia is a syndrome, or a collection of signs and symptoms, its features may vary depending on the specific cause and the areas of the brain affected. Although there may be disagreement over the best method of defining the syndrome, the following summary may be used to guide the evaluation of the patient with dementia. The following are general features of the dementias.

(1) A significant and persistent decline in cognitive functioning from a previously established and stable baseline level of performance.

(2) A relatively normal level of arousal and attention is present (that is, the decline is not due to a delirium).

(3) Multiple cognitive deficits occur in three or more of the following domains:

- perceptual disturbances (illusions, hallucinations);
- memory impairment (amnesia – either in new learning, recall of previously learned information, or both);
- language disturbance (aphasia or dysphasia);
- impaired purposeful execution of tasks on command despite intact comprehension of the task and intact motor skills necessary to perform the task (apraxia or dyspraxia)
- impaired visuospatial skills (most often manifest as constructional apraxia or dyspraxia)
- impaired recognition of objects specific to a single sensory modality despite intact sensory function and language (agnosia);
- impaired complex cognition, which may include:
  - impaired executive functioning (interpretation of perception, reasoning, abstraction, insight, judgment, planning, and/or sequencing);
  - decreased motivation (apathy or abulia);

– social inappropriateness (disinhibition, grossly inappropriate or violent behavior).

(4) The cognitive deficits result in significant impairment in important areas of daily living.

(5) The cognitive impairments are the result of a disruption of normal brain function produced by a neurological disease, a medical condition, or a combination of such factors.

(6) Disturbances of emotion may be present, particularly depressed mood or affective lability.

(7) Disturbances in sleep may be present.

Pathophysiology

The essential pathophysiological feature of dementia is significant and persistent dysfunction of the areas of the brain that mediate cognitive functions or of the connections among these areas. In contrast to delirium, which we presented earlier as a sort of "bottom-up" process (disruption of the most basic aspects of cognition produces disturbances in relatively more complex cognition), most dementias may be thought of as "top–down" processes. Recognizing that there are variations among types of dementia and even within prototypic dementias (e.g., Alzheimer's disease), impairment in relatively higher cognitive functions usually occurs first. Only much later, if at all, do the lower functions of arousal and attention become significantly impaired.

Dementia may result from intrinsic brain disease, from a systemic medical condition (including medications and other substances) that adversely affects the brain, or from a combination of such factors. While a detailed discussion of every potential cause of dementia is beyond the scope of this chapter, the general principles of pathophysiology can be remembered by considering practical classification schemes.

Dementia may be organized by neurological localization, by association with other medical or neurological illnesses, or by its reversibility and the responsiveness of its cause to treatment. Classification by brain localization divides the dementias according to the most affected type of neural structures underlying the clinical presentation:

(1) cortical (e.g., Alzheimer's disease, frontotemporal degeneration);

(2) subcortical (e.g., Huntington's, Parkinson's, and Wilson's diseases);

(3) white matter (e.g., multiple sclerosis, Binswanger's disease);

(4) mixed (e.g., multiple infarct, Creutzfeldt–Jakob disease, neoplasm, trauma).

These distinctions are based on clinically demonstrable differences in the pattern and severity of cognitive impairments associated with dysfunction of each general area. This scheme is particularly helpful in associating the clinical phenomena with the potential etiology of the dementia.

Cortical dementias typically present with normal arousal, attention and speed of processing, suggesting relative preservation of functions mediated by subcortical structures including brainstem, cerebellum, thalamus, basal ganglia, and white matter. The impairments of cortical dementia include those mediated by the neocortex, namely memory, language, praxis, recognition, and complex cognition. When cortex is damaged, the impairment in cognitive function is absolute, meaning that the patient is unable to perform the task subserved by the lost area of cortex (e.g., loss of executive function or frank non-fluent aphasia in a patient with a frontotemporal dementia).

By contrast, subcortical and white matter dementias typically involve relatively more "subcortical" impairments in cognition, including decreased speed of processing, disturbances in the complex aspects of attention, problems with memory retrieval (but not memory encoding), and executive functioning. Hence, the memory problems in subcortical and white matter dementias are usually ones of impaired spontaneous (free) recall, with relatively preserved cued (prompted) or recognition recall. In other words, on memory testing they have difficulty remembering items presented a few minutes earlier, but when given cues or a list of items from which to choose they are more able to recall the correct items. This pattern suggests deficits in retrieval (frontal-subcortical pattern) rather than problems in encoding (cortical pattern).

The subcortical and white matter dementias typically involve relatively less severe impairments of cognitive functions such as language, praxis, or recognition. For example, patients with severe white matter disease may have remarkable impairment of word fluency on formal testing due to slowed language production, but may not demonstrate other word finding problems and agrammatisms associated with the nonfluent aphasias. The character of this language disturbance is rather different than that of the typical nonfluent (cortical) aphasia – the subcortical or white matter dementia patient can produce words and grammatically correct sentences, but the production of such occurs at a remarkably reduced rate. As such, the problem in such cases appears to have less to do with language disturbance due to loss of cortical function *per se*;

instead, this reduced fluency (as opposed to nonfluency) reflects inefficient use of the intact cortex due to disruption of frontal-subcortical circuitry.

Many of the other cognitive deficits in the subcortical and white matter dementias may be similarly understood as reflecting disruption of the activity of frontal-subcortical circuits. By remembering the activity of these circuits (see Chapter 4), one can reasonably predict the pattern of deficits associated with such dementias. These dementias may be further differentiated from one another by the presence of extrapyramidal motor dysfunction suggesting subcortical pathology (e.g., Parkinson's disease) and corticospinal/cerebellar motor dysfunction suggesting white matter pathology (e.g., multiple sclerosis).

Finally, as the term suggests, patients with mixed dementias (e.g., multi-infarct) may present with combinations of deficits referable to cortical, subcortical, and white matter dysfunction. The usefulness of classifying the dementias by the pattern of cognitive impairment with which they present is in its ability to inform the clinician of the most likely areas of dysfunctional brain and thereby to guide the development of the differential diagnosis. Viewed from this perspective, the rationale for our position that impairments on the mental status testing should be regarded as evidence of focal neurological deficits should now be clearer – the examination findings and the patterns of deficit that they establish are referable to relatively focal neural systems, and sometimes even to specific loci.

The second method of classifying dementia is by its association (or lack thereof) with other medical or neurological disease. The three main categories in this classification scheme include:

(1) dementia associated with signs of systemic medical illness (such as hypothyroidism, chronic drug intoxication, or nutritional deficiency);

(2) dementia associated with other neurological signs but without systemic medical illness (as in Huntington's disease, Creutzfeldt–Jakob disease, tumor, normal pressure hydrocephalus, or multiple sclerosis);

(3) dementia itself is the only illness present (Alzheimer's disease, frontotemporal degeneration).

In general, we do not find this classification scheme particularly useful. However, if properly used it may serve to remind one to evaluate the patient for other medical/systemic illnesses causing progressive cognitive impairment and of the potential benefit of obtaining consultation with other medical specialists during both the evaluation and delivery of care to patient with some dementias.

A third method classifies the dementias according to the availability of treatment for their causes, and places special emphasis on identifying potentially reversible causes of cognitive impairment. This scheme divides dementia according to the following characteristics:

(1) *Treatable cause and potentially reversible dementia*, definitive treatment is available for the underlying cause of the dementia and the condition is potentially reversible. This group represents as many as 15–20% of cases of dementia, and etiologies include conditions such as normal pressure hydrocephalus, tumor, subdural hematoma, cerebral vasculitis, metabolic disorders, nutritional deficiency states, chronic meningitis, neurosyphilis, and depression.

(2) *Treatable cause but irreversible dementia*, definitive treatment for the underlying cause of the dementia is available, but the brain damage resulting from that cause and the associated cognitive losses are unlikely to be substantially reversed by treatment. Instances where deterioration can be arrested, but not necessarily reversed, represent as many as 20–25% of cases of dementia, and its causes include conditions such as multiple cerebral infarctions, cerebrovascular disease, hypertension, or alcoholism. For example, preventing stroke recurrence will limit further cognitive decline, but this strategy will not return cognitive functions lost as a result of previous strokes. As another example, achieving abstinence from alcohol may prevent further cognitive decline, but does not reliably result in significant cognitive improvement.

(3) *Untreatable cause and irreversible dementia*, in these cases, the cause of the dementia, even if known, cannot be definitively treated and hence the dementia inevitably progresses. This represents about 55–65% of dementia cases, and includes conditions such as Alzheimer's disease, Huntington's disease, progressive supranuclear palsy, frontotemporal degeneration, and Creutzfeldt–Jakob disease. A word of caution about this category is warranted – the fact that the *cause* of the dementia is untreatable should not be misunderstood as suggesting that the patient with the dementia is untreatable. There are treatment strategies for many aspects of these dementias, including behavioral management, counseling and family work, and neuropsychiatric treatment for symptoms caused by the dementia (as discussed later in this chapter). For example, cholinergic augmentation strategies have been developed for the treatment of dementia due to Alzheimer's disease. While these strategies do not appear to change the underlying progressive neurodegeneration in Alzheimer's disease, they

may at least transiently slow the progression of associated cognitive impairments. While this should not be mistaken for treatment of the disease or for the ability to "reverse" the dementia, it is imperative to remember that there are symptomatic therapies available that may be of significant benefit to some patients.

We find that integrating the first method of dementia classification described above (associating the pattern of cognitive deficits with probable location and hence the related differential diagnosis) with the latter method described here yields the most useful approach to the evaluation and treatment of the dementias.

Differential diagnosis and evaluation

The possibility of a dementia should be considered in any adult in whom there is a persistent loss in cognitive function. As with delirium, the differential diagnosis of dementia should be approached on two levels. The first is that of the clinical syndrome: distinguishing dementia from other syndromes with overlapping clinical features. The most common alternative diagnoses in the differential include delirium, amnestic disorder, substance intoxication or withdrawal, mental retardation, psychotic disorders (e.g., schizophrenia), mood disorder (e.g., major depression), malingering, factitious disorder, benign senescent forgetfulness (in DSM-IV, Age-Related Cognitive Decline), isolated cognitive deficits (aphasia, apraxia, agnosia, etc.), or other mild neurocognitive impairment (in DSM-IV, Cognitive Disorder Not Otherwise Specified, as from mild traumatic brain injury).

The most critical distinction to be made is that between dementia and delirium: it is imperative that delirium be ruled out in order not to overlook a more immediately life-threatening illness. Assessing the levels of arousal and of attention provides the clinical focus for this diagnostic consideration. Beyond this distinction, the most troublesome etiology to exclude is depression. Patients with a relatively rapidly developing dementia characterized by impairment of concentration, recent memory (usually retrieval, not encoding), motivation (which itself may impair apparent cognitive performance), decreased energy and sleep, and depressed mood may simply be experiencing a major depressive episode. This disorder, sometimes referred to as the *pseudodementia of depression* or more simply as the dementia of depression, may be distinguished from its most frequent competitor in the differential diagnosis of dementia, namely Alzheimer's disease, by the patient's often vociferous complaints of impaired cognition (in contrast to the demented patient who attempts to conceal or is unaware of cognitive deficits), poor effort on the mental state examination, and tendency to show substantial improvements in cognitive performance when patiently encouraged to do better. While none of these features, or any combination of them and the many others that have been described, reliably and repeatedly distinguish the dementia of depression from Alzheimer's disease, this profile of symptoms and clinical signs may serve as useful clinical hints at the correct diagnosis.

As a practical matter, most patients presenting with depressed mood and impaired cognition should first receive treatment to correct their depression. A formal diagnosis of dementia should be reserved until the depression has been maximally treated and the patient subsequently re-evaluated. It is important to note, however, that dementia and depression may co-occur. If a patient demonstrates clear and persistent symptoms of cognitive impairments despite treatment of the depression, or if the type and severity of cognitive impairments is simply inconsistent with the mild subcortical pattern of impairment associated with depression (e.g., the patient demonstrates clear aphasia, apraxia, agnosia, or severely impaired complex cognition), a thorough evaluation for other possible causes for the dementia should continue while treatment for depression is ongoing.

The second level of the differential diagnosis of dementia focuses on the underlying etiology. An exhaustive differential diagnosis is well beyond the scope of this work. A simple rule, however, is that almost any category of disease process (i.e., neoplastic, vascular, infectious, metabolic, nutritional, etc.) can be included in the differential diagnosis of dementia. From a practical standpoint, the clinical presentation will guide the development of the differential possibilities. We offer the phrase "VAST DEMENTIA" (Table 13.1) as a mnemonic for important categories of disease with which dementia may be associated.

Establishing the diagnosis follows from a thorough assessment of the patient, guided by an integration of clinical findings and their implications for the differential diagnosis. Although dementia has at times been considered a diagnosis of exclusion, in general such an approach unnecessarily delays treatment for both the patient and the family. When the history and clinical evidence suggest dementia, the diagnosis should be entertained and a thorough evaluation begun. As a minimum, the assessment should include the elements listed below.

Table 13.1. VAST DEMENTIA: a mnemonic to aid in the differential diagnosis of dementia

V	Vascular	stroke (thrombotic, embolic, lacunar), atherosclerotic, arteriosclerotic, hypertensive
A	Anoxic	prolonged hypotension, carotid stenosis, near-drowning, respiratory arrest
S	Sensory	impaired vision, impaired hearing
T	Toxic	alcohol, substances of abuse (toluene), toxins (lead), medications (anticholinergics)
D	Degenerative	Alzheimer's, Huntington's, Parkinson's, and Pick's diseases, Creutzfeld–Jakob
E	Endocrine	hypothyroidism, hypoparathyroidism, hypo/hyperpituitarism, diabetes
M	Mass lesion	neoplasm (meningioma, glioma, metastatic), chronic subdural hematoma
E	Emotional	depression, conversion disorder, factitious disorder, malingering
N	Nutritional	niacin, B12, thiamine, folate, cobalamin, iron, copper (Wilson's disease)
T	Traumatic	traumatic brain injury, normal pressure hydrocephalus
I	Infectious	tuberculosis, syphilis, AIDS, abscess, encephalitis/meningitis (late effect)
A	Autoimmune	multiple sclerosis, vasculitis, lupus cerebritis, rheumatoid cerebritis

(*1*) *History*, particularly onset and predisposing factors. A slowly progressive course may suggest an insidious process (often but not necessarily neuro-degenerative), whereas a step-wise development of multiple discrete deficits (including motor signs) might suggest a cerebrovascular cause (e.g., thrombotic, embolic, or lacunar stroke). With regard to predisposing factors, both personal and family medical histories deserve investigation. Any evidence suggesting co-morbid medical conditions requires particular attention, especially when the history suggests the presence of cardiovascular disease, hypertension, diabetes, inflammatory diseases, endocrine, or other illness that may directly or indirectly, as secondary complications of such illnesses or their treatments, compromise brain function. A number of illnesses producing dementia are the result of genetic disorders, including some types of Alzheimer's disease, some frontotemporal dementias, some cases of Parkinson's disease, and of course Huntington's disease. The presence or absence of such problems in the family history should be determined to help guide formulation of the differential diagnosis. In determining the history, all available sources of information should be reviewed, including the medical record, personnel involved in the patient's care, the medication record, the family, and (if possible) the patient.

(2) *Physical and neurological examinations*, particularly vital signs and any evidence of systemic or neurological abnormalities. In the general physical examination, vital signs are of importance both for ruling out delirium and in the evaluation for disorders involving autonomic instability (e.g., Parkinson's plus syndromes). On the elemental neurological examination, cranial nerve abnormalities (including visual fields), motor (voluntary or extrapyramidal) or sensory signs, impairments of gait or coordination, and abnormal or asymmetric reflexes invaluably guide the development of the differential diagnosis. Even in the absence of such findings, the presence of abnormal primitive reflexes (see Chapter 8) alone may provide evidence of impaired upper motor neuron (frontal lobe) dysfunction.

(3) *Mental status examination*, including both general and cognitive portions (see Chapter 9). On the general mental status examination, assessment of emotion should be a high priority, and the suspicion for depressed mood should be great. With regard to cognition, at a minimum a short standardized cognitive screening test (e.g., Mini-Mental State Examination (MMSE), Blessed Information-Memory-Concentration Test, Blessed Orientation-Memory-Concentration Test, and the Short Test of Mental Status) should be administered and compared to normative data (usually based on age and education). When these measures reveal deficits, more detailed cognitive testing is usually needed to determine more carefully the type and severity of cognitive impairments.

It is important to note that a normal screening examination with the MMSE does not necessarily preclude a diagnosis of dementia. For example, many patients with subcortical and white matter dementias will score normally on such tests; however, if the cognitive examination is expanded to include assessments that rely on speed of processing and executive functioning these patients predictably do less well. In such cases, we sometimes refer to the use of the MMSE in the evaluation of subcortical and white matter dementias as comparable to the use of a stethoscope in the evaluation of an arthritic joint – it is just not the best tool for the task at hand. Therefore, where the history suggests the possibility of either subcortical or white matter pathology, more detailed (and time-dependent) assessments of cognitive performance should be performed.

(4) *Laboratory examination*, as noted in Chapter 12, most mildly demented patients will have a relatively normal appearing standard clinical electroencephalography EEG, although slowing on the electroencephalography (EEG) does tend to increase in proportion to the degree of cognitive

impairment. In cases where there is initial uncertainty regarding the presence of delirium, dementia, or both after the clinical examination, an EEG may sometimes be a useful diagnostic tool. Quantitative EEG (QEEG) may also be a useful diagnostic tool in some cases. However, interpretation of QEEG should be made only by an experienced clinical electroencephalographer with additional expertise in QEEG. Since there are relatively few such experts in the world, routine use of diagnostic QEEG is impractical in most centers.

Specific laboratory tests should be ordered to confirm the presence of a suspected underlying etiology. When ordering tests, the guiding principle is selecting those that may reveal reversible causes of dementia. After the history and physical examination are completed, it is customary to undertake a battery of standard tests, including serum chemistries, creatinine and blood urea nitrogen, liver function tests, vitamin B12, folate, thyroid stimulating hormone (TSH), and serum syphilis serology. Although different centers may differ with respect to the specific tests included in such "screening" batteries, the set presented herein reflects both our own practice and the recommendations of most review texts in this area. Second, specific histories or physical findings may indicate second line tests such as human immunodeficiency virus (HIV) antibody, antinuclear antibody, erythrocyte sedimentation rate, ceruloplasmin, complete blood count, and urinalysis/urine toxicology. Although disagreement about the utility and scope of laboratory screening tests has been very controversial, most experts agree that the majority of conditions causing reversible dementia will be detected by a combination of neuroimaging (computed tomography, CT, or magnetic resonance imaging, MRI), a urine or serum toxicology screen, thyroid function tests including TSH, vitamin B12 and folate, and a syphilis serology test (FTA-ABS). In other cases, lumbar puncture may also be needed (e.g., central nervous system infection, multiple sclerosis), and in the case of normal pressure hydrocephalus this procedure may not only be diagnostic but also therapeutic.

The question of whether a neuroimaging study, and if so which type of study (CT, MRI, single photon emission computed tomography or SPECT, positron emission tomography or PET), should be performed has been a subject of much debate. Unfortunately, most of this debate is focused on the cost of such procedures, rather than on the potential value of the information that neuroimaging provides. Based on the foregoing discussions of the localization of cognitive functions to specific neural networks in the brain, we believe that clinicians should regard an abnormal mental status finding as equivalent to a focal deficit on the elemental neurological examination. Hence, the laboratory work-up of such findings should proceed with the same vigor as that of any other focal neurological deficit. We therefore suggest that patients with dementia should have a structural neuroimaging study (CT or MRI) at least once during their evaluation. This is equivalent to saying that a chest X-ray should be performed in every patient with pulmonary disease at least once (and sometimes more than once) during the evaluation and treatment of their illness. The results of such studies can provide definitive information on the cause of a patient's dementia (e.g., the presence of tumor, chronic subdural hematoma, multiple sclerosis lesions, lacunar infarctions, or diffuse white matter disease, or the absence of such), and such information invariably affects both diagnosis and management of the dementia and its cause. For most, economy of diagnosis will lead to economy of successful, appropriate treatment, and is in the best sense of the word "economy."

(5) *Neuropsychological evaluation*, particularly when additional information on the pattern and the extent of cognitive impairments is needed to clarify the diagnosis and guide treatment planning. A neuropsychological assessment directed at specific aspects of cognition and psychological functioning may help refine the differential diagnosis (e.g., more clearly distinguishing between subcortical and cortical patterns, or assessing the potential contribution of depression or anxiety to the clinically observed deficits). Further, the results of testing help identify areas of relative strength that can be supported when developing a treatment plan for both patient and family (e.g., medication regimens, compensatory behavioral strategies). Finally, repeating the testing after a year or two may provide information about the type and rate of progression of illness (e.g., Alzheimer's disease, frontotemporal dementia) and/or progress and degree of recovery (i.e., alcohol dementia, traumatic brain injury). Such information may be extremely valuable not only for treatment planning, but also for counseling patients and their families as to prognosis and the timing of additional psychosocial needs and interventions (see below).

Treatment

A comprehensive review of treatment options for dementia is also beyond the scope of this book, but a number of general principles and a few specific suggestions may be more easily made. Foremost among all approaches is aggressive treatment of the underlying cause of the dementia, particularly when a potentially reversible or arrestable cause is identified. Additionally, and certainly in the case of the irreversible dementias, symptomatic management should be undertaken and directed at minimizing the adverse effects of the illness on the daily life of the patient and caregivers. Finally, all treatment approaches should also include discussion and planning for future with both patient and family. Given this framework, we usually suggest the following elements of treatment.

(1) *Supportive/educational*, many demented patients have difficulty accepting their diagnosis and limitations. They and their families need support in dealing with the diagnosis and their reactions to it. Education, especially when a specific diagnosis can be given, is helpful in preparing patients and families for the course of their illness and the psychological and social adaptations they will need to make.

The patient and family should be encouraged to make use of community resources, including day programs, caregiver support groups, and the patient's usual social supports. Important social supports include friends, local social and religious organizations, and national resources such as the Alzheimer's Association and the National Institutes of Health/National Institute on Aging Alzheimer's Disease Education and Referral Center. Resources of this kind can be an invaluable part of any treatment plan, and may help the patient and family receive assistance that is beyond that available from their professional caregivers.

(2) *Behavioral/compensatory*, these measures attempt to compensate for cognitive and functional impairments. For example, when memory is the primary deficit, notes or signs in the home, pill boxes and timers for medications, and frequent reminders from family or caregivers about important information may be helpful to patients. When language is affected, optimizing verbal communication and developing effective nonverbal communication skills (e.g., picture boards with common items to which the patient can point and thereby communicate needs or problems) may be helpful. When praxis is affected, the patient may need more structured care in order to attend adequately to activities of daily living. Finally, maintaining the patient in a familiar environment often lessens the adverse effects of cognitive impairment by limiting the need for new learning or alterations in routines. A major environmental change, such as hospitalization, can be very disorienting for the moderately to severely demented patient. With the lack of the normal environmental cues on

which the patient has depended, there may be a relatively abrupt decline in function. Limiting such changes in environment or attempting to include old cues and routines in the new environment may lessen the impact of such changes.

(3) *Medication:* medication use in dementia has traditionally been directed toward symptomatic relief of abnormal mood states, perceptual disturbances, and troublesome behaviors such as agitation and aggression. In recent years, cholinesterase inhibitors as tacrine, donepezil, rivastigmine, and galantamine have become available for the symptomatic treatment of impaired cognition in some patients with dementia, particularly those with Alzheimer's disease. Careful use of these medications in appropriate patients may lessen the short-term impact of an otherwise relentlessly progressive dementia by temporarily slowing cognitive decline. These medications may also beneficially affect other aspects of cognition, emotion, and behavior (e.g., mood regulation, motivation, aggression) although such suggestions are at this writing only speculative.

Although most patients tolerate judicious use of medications for symptomatic treatment, in general all medications should be used with caution in this population due to their relatively high risk for developing a medication-induced confusional state or frank delirium. In general, a "start low, go slow" approach to initiating and adjusting medication doses is advisable.

When medications are necessary, a symptom-targeted approach is suggested. The following guidelines may be useful in this regard.

• *Sleep disturbance* is a common problem. Although traditionally used sedative hypnotic agents such as benzodiazepines may be of occasional use in non-demented patients, they should be avoided wherever possible in patients with dementia. The benzodiazepines and similar agents may be excessively sedating in these patients, and such effects can be particularly long-lasting due to the combined effects of accumulation of their active metabolites in lipid tissues and decreased efficiency of metabolism, excretion, or both, in elderly or chronically medically-ill patients. These medications may consequently have the unintended but potentially serious effects of causing excessive sedation and of exacerbating cognitive impairment during waking hours. Because the benzodiazepines increase gamma-aminobutyric acid (GABA) function, they predictably impair cognitive speed, efficiency, and flexibility, and may interfere both with memory encoding and retrieval, and in a small number of patients this adverse effect extends beyond the cognitive impairment attributable to sedation alone. It goes almost without saying that iatrogenic memory impairment is to be avoided in dementia patients whenever possible. Benzodiazepines also impair coordination, thereby placing patients with dementia at increased risk for falls. Finally, dependence on these agents can occur, and withdrawal may be particularly dangerous for patients with dementia. Finally, benzodiazepines may cause paradoxical agitation in the demented patient.

Given the various potential problems with benzodiazepines in patients with dementia, we suggest using one of the following alternatives for treatment of insomnia in demented patients: trazodone 25–50 mg by mouth at bedtime, chloral hydrate 500 mg, or diphenhydramine 25–50 mg. Wherever possible, use of such agents should be terminated as quickly as possible. In patients requiring ongoing treatment, we favor using trazodone among the medications listed here.

- *Psychosis, agitation and aggression* are also common problems in demented patients. Although agitation and aggression may occur as behavioral disturbances in their own right, these problems are often the result of underlying psychotic symptoms (particularly visual or auditory hallucinations and/or paranoid delusions). A number of approaches have been suggested, each of which may be of use in some patients.
  - Haloperidol, 0.5–1 mg orally at bedtime, may be useful for the nightly agitation (or sundowning) or in those whose agitation is related to the presence of perceptual disturbances (hallucinations) or misinterpretations (illusions). Atypical antipsychotics (e.g., risperidone 0.5–1 mg, olanzapine 2.5–5 mg) are also be useful for demented patients. In both cases, very small starting doses may be increased to the point of improvement of symptoms or the development of side effects. Most, however, will receive beneficial effect from relatively small doses.
  - Valproate, 125–250 mg orally at night or twice daily, may also be useful for treatment of agitation that is not obviously related to perceptual disorders or psychotic symptoms. Low doses may occasion improvement without the development of untoward side effects. Of course, doses can be increased until either symptomatic improvement or untoward side effects occur, but again low doses seem helpful for most patients.
  - Buspirone, 5–15 mg per day (usually in divided doses of 5 mg), has been reported to be of use in some agitated demented patients.

    – Propranolol may be useful for some patients, although its hypotensive and cardiac effects may preclude its use in many elderly, demented patients. When used, starting doses may be in the range of 10 mg by mouth twice daily, with gradual increases in dose titrated to effect and cardiovascular tolerance.

- *Depression*, either depressed mood or major depressive disorder, is also commonly seen in patients with dementia and should be treated aggressively. Even among patients who do not fulfill diagnostic criteria for major depressive disorder, mild depression may adversely affect both cognition and everyday functioning. While antidepressants are generally safe, the side effect profile of the chosen agent should be carefully considered. In general, medications with significant anticholinergic properties, such as amitriptyline and imipramine should be avoided. Similarly, use of monoamine oxidase inhibitors offers high clinical risk due to the difficulty of monitoring compliance with the medication, the potential for coadministration of agents with serious drug–drug interaction effects, and the patient's limitations in voluntary compliance with dietary restrictions, all of which are compounded by the dementia. When indicated, the following medications appear to have reasonably benign side effect profiles when begun at low doses, with the dosage increased as necessary (beyond the starting doses listed here) and as tolerated:

    – Sertraline 25–50 mg orally once daily;
    – Fluoxetine 5–20 mg orally once daily;
    – Buproprion 50–75 mg orally twice daily;
    – Nortriptyline 25–50 mg orally at bedtime;
    – Trazodone 25–50 mg orally at bedtime.

- *Impaired cognition* may improve in response to treatment with cholinesterase inhibitors in some patients with dementia. Presently, these treatments are only approved for use in patients with Alzheimer's disease, although they may also be of benefit in patients with other forms of dementia, such as traumatic brain injury. At the time of this writing, tacrine, donepezil, rivastigmine, and galantamine are available for this treatment. Donepezil appears to have a relatively more benign side effect profile than that of either tacrine or rivastigmine and appears to lack the hepatoxicity encountered with tacrine. Additionally, administration of donepezil is substantially less complicated than that of either tacrine or rivastigmine, both in the dose titration (starting and maintenance dose are often the same with donepezil) and schedule for daily administration (once per day with donepezil). *Ginko biloba* has also been suggested to be helpful for some patients with impaired cognition.

Given these limited options, donepezil is, in our opinion, the simplest choice presently for the treatment of impaired cognition. In appropriate patients it may be given as 5–10 mg by mouth daily. Because some patients may experience nausea and vomiting and because these effects appear related to the rate of dose increase, it is best to begin with 5 mg by mouth daily. If tolerated, the dose may be gradually increased to 10 mg to see if any additional benefit is achieved with the higher dose. While it is not entirely clear that there is any consistent advantage of 10 mg over 5 mg daily, some patients who fail to respond adequately at the lower dose may do so with the higher dose.

(4) *Social and medicolegal issues* should also be addressed early in the treatment, and revisited in an ongoing fashion throughout treatment. The effect of cognitive impairment on the patient's work and social life, especially family relationships, should be determined. This includes assessing the patient's ability to work, to manage finances and legal affairs (wills, advance directives), and to perform personal ADLs (activities of daily living). The assessment should also include evaluation of the family's ability to provide necessary support, or willingness to assume responsibility for areas in which the patient is no longer competent to make decisions. Choosing the individual in the patient's life who will be responsible for decision making, including obtaining power of attorney or guardianship when it becomes necessary, is a difficult task but should not be delayed until the time when the patient is no longer able to participate in such decisions.

If the family or other supports are not able to provide adequately for the care and safety of the patient, or if there has been evidence of neglect or abuse, the appropriate local authorities should be involved (for example, in the United States this authority is the local Department of Social Services, Adult Protective Services team). In many states in the United States, physicians are mandated to report suspected cases of neglect or abuse of the elderly. If the family needs additional assistance, home health care aides or visiting nurses can provide invaluable help to the patient and family. Their assistance to the family may allow the patient to remain in a familiar environment for a longer period of time.

Similarly, caregivers can burn out, and respite hospitalizations for the patient (depending on the available resources) may be an option that allows caregivers much needed breaks. Physicians should regularly inquire as to the caregiver's emotional and physical status, and encourage them to obtain assistance and respite for their own and the patient's welfare.

Summary

Dementia is best defined as an acquired syndrome of persistent impairments in several aspects of basic or complex cognition, without disturbance of level of consciousness. Dementia is typically a problem of later adulthood and old age (e.g., Alzheimer's disease), although it may be seen in younger adults as well (e.g., patients with Huntington's disease, traumatic brain injury, AIDS, or brain tumors). There are significant economic and emotional costs for patients, their families, and society associated with dementia regardless of the underlying cause. Dementia is a syndrome, or constellation of symptoms. There is no single etiology or pattern that is pathognomonic of the condition, and indeed there is also no universal definition of dementia. However, we find the most useful definition of dementia as the development of impairment in three or more areas of cognition that represents a change from a higher functioning baseline and that causes significant functional impairment.

When evaluating a patient with dementia, the history should seek to reveal the course and progression of the dementia and to ascertain whether it is associated with other medical problems. The physical and neurological examinations should aim to reveal any focal or lateralizing neurological problems, movement disorders, or other medical conditions the presence of which might usefully guide the formulation of the differential diagnosis. The mental status examination should be designed to reveal the pattern of the patient's cognitive deficits (e.g., cortical, subcortical, white matter, or mixed). Standard laboratory evaluation should include tests for reversible causes of dementia, and should in every case include at least one structural neuroimaging examination (CT or MRI). Neuropsychological testing should be considered when bedside examination leaves substantial doubt as to the diagnosis and when seeking to help the patient and family to develop strategies to compensate for the patient's cognitive impairments.

When possible, aggressive medical interventions to fully treat or at least arrest any identified medical cause or contributor to the dementia should be undertaken. Treatment of the dementia should follow a symptom-targeted approach, and should include identification and treatment of cognitive, emotional, and behavioral problems. In general, treatment will consist of a combination of educational, behavioral/compensatory, medication, and social/medicolegal interventions.

14

Obsessive–compulsive disorder

Introduction

Obsessive–compulsive disorder (OCD) is a disabling illness characterized by the presence of recurrent obsessions, compulsions, or both. Obsessions are experienced as intrusive, inappropriate, and persistent ideas, thoughts, impulses, or images that cause marked anxiety or distress. Compulsions are repetitive behaviors or mental acts, the ostensible goal of which is to prevent or reduce anxiety or distress related to obsessions. The performance of compulsive acts may reduce anxiety but does not provide pleasure or gratification. The obsessions and compulsions of OCD are excessive, ego-dystonic, unlikely to be related to a real-life problem, and do not effectively neutralize or prevent the problem against which the patient believes they are directed.

During most of the twentieth century, OCD was believed to be the result of deep-seated neurotic conflict, with the obsessions and compulsions symbolically representing intolerable intrapsychic conflicts. Unfortunately, treatments focused on bringing these unconscious conflicts to light in the service of treating the illness met with no predictable effect or success. Indeed, it may be argued that apparent remissions produced by such treatments may have merely reflected the natural course of OCD, in which spontaneously occurring periods of relief are both predictable and at best inconsistently related to environmental influences.

In recent years, our understanding of OCD has improved, and it is now generally believed that OCD is fundamentally a neurobiological disorder with a significant genetic component. In this context, obsessions and compulsions may be usefully understood to represent the cognitive and behavioral products of inappropriately reverberating frontal-subcortical circuits. While the etiology of the overactivity in these circuits remains uncertain, intrapsychic conflict does not appear to be either a necessary or a sufficient explanation for this activity or the development of OCD.

We feel strongly that OCD is a paradigmatic neuropsychiatric disorder, and that an understanding of the neurocircuitry involved not only provides a firm foundation for understanding and treating patients with OCD but also offers an opportunity for understanding the neurobiology of cognition, emotion, and behavior more generally. To that end, we have included this chapter in the book, and offer a brief review of OCD from the perspectives described previously in Parts I and II. It is our hope that by offering an understanding of the structural and functional neuroanatomy of OCD will provide both an intellectual framework within which to understand symptoms and treatment and a clear illustration of the value of the approach we have described. It is our further hope that understanding OCD in these terms will also facilitate the development of empathy for the experience of helplessness OCD patients face as a consequence of a neurobiology gone terribly awry.

General considerations

Although estimates of the prevalence of OCD have varied over the last several decades, the most recent estimates (included in DSM-IV) suggest a one-year prevalence of 1.5–2.1% and a lifetime prevalence of about 2.5%. OCD typically has its onset in late adolescence or early adulthood, with modal age of onset between ages 6 and 15 years in males and 20 and 29 years in females, and is equally common in both sexes. There does appear to be a genetic component to OCD, with higher rates of concordant diagnosis in monozygotic twins than dizygotic twins, and higher rates of OCD among first degree relatives with OCD or Tourette's Disorder. The disorder generally has a gradual onset followed by a waxing and waning course, although in a small number of cases symptoms are both progressive and inexorable.

OCD is often associated with other major psychiatric disorders, including major depressive disorder, other anxiety disorders, eating disorders, obsessive–compulsive personality disorder, and alcohol abuse/dependence. However, the highest psychiatric comorbidity of OCD is in individuals with Tourette's Disorder, in whom 35–50% also meet criteria for OCD. Interestingly, among individuals with OCD, only 5–7% have comorbid Tourette's Disorder but 20–30% of people with OCD report current or past tics.

Current diagnostic criteria for OCD

The DSM-IV offers a clear set of criteria for the diagnosis of OCD, and interested readers are referred to this text for additional details. In brief, OCD requires the occurrence of either obsessions or compulsions that cause marked subjective distress, occupy a significant portion of the patient's time (more than one hour per day), and/or significantly interfere with the patient's functioning, including social activities or relationships. *Obsessions* are defined as recurrent and persistent thoughts, impulses, or images that the patient experiences as intrusive, inappropriate, and anxiety provoking or distressing. The thoughts, impulses, or images are not simply excessive worries about real-life problems, and in general the patient recognizes that they are a product of his or her own mind; when they do not recognize this, the OCD is qualified as "with poor insight." The patient's attempts to ignore or suppress the obsessions are not consistently successful (although some patients may be able to do so for brief periods of time). One attempt at suppression, or neutralization, of the obsession is the development of related compulsions.

Compulsions are defined as repetitive behaviors or mental acts that the person feels driven to perform in response to an obsession, or according to rules that must be applied rigidly. Compulsions appear to be aimed at preventing or reducing distress of the obsessions to which they are related. However, the compulsions are not connected to the obsessions in a realistic way and/or they are clearly excessive. Hence, they do not tend to neutralize immediately the obsessions, and therefore take up an inordinate amount of the patient's time and energy to perform.

As with all of the major psychiatric disorders, if obsessions and compulsions occur in the context of another Axis I disorder, the OCD diagnosis can only be made if the content of the obsessions or compulsions is not restricted to the other disorder. For example, if the obsessions occur in the context of an eating disorder, their context must extend beyond preoccupation with food (e.g., also fears of contamination, or excessive safety or symmetry concerns). Additionally, to diagnose idiopathic OCD, the obsessions and compulsions must not be due to the direct physiological effects of a substance (e.g., a drug of abuse, or a medication) or a general medical condition (e.g., Parkinson's disease). As we will discuss at the end of this chapter, this is a particularly important issue in neuropsychiatry, as there are a host of neurological disorders that can produce obsessive and compulsive symptoms.

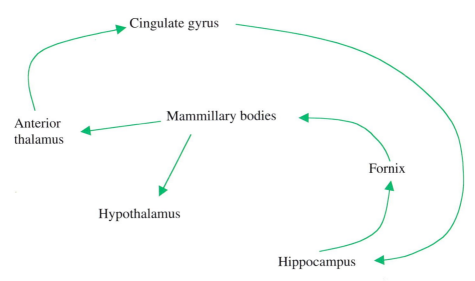

Figure 14.1 The Circuit of Papez. Although now somewhat outdated both conceptually and anatomically, this circuit remains a useful starting point for considering the neurobiology of obsessive–compulsive disorder.

Neurobiology of OCD

Though much has yet to be learned about the neurocircuitry of OCD, it is clear that the illness is neurologically based. Though obsessions and compulsions may come to have psychological meaning for the patient with OCD, it is fairly well accepted at this time that the etiology of OCD does not lie in unresolved intrapsychic conflict and its cure is not to be found in psychodynamic therapy. Instead, the cause of OCD appears to be aberrant functioning of frontal-subcortical and limbic-subcortical circuits, disrupted either by idiopathic (likely genetic and epigenetic) factors, or by various traumas. Post-surgical, post-infectious, and post-traumatic OCD have all been described, and the presentations of these post-traumatic OCDs may be phenomenologically indistinguishable from the primary disorder. Early descriptions of the involved brain areas focused on the Papez Circuit (Figure 14.1; see also Chapters 2 and 5). This area was felt to hold promise since it was believed to contain brain elements relevant to thought, memory, emotion, and behavior.

More recent investigations have refined our understanding of brain dysfunction in OCD using computed tomography, magnetic resonance imaging, regional cerebral blood flow scans, positron emission tomography, and single photon emission computed tomography. These technologies have been used to document differences between normal control subjects and patients with OCD. These investigations have variously demonstrated both unilateral and bilateral hemispheric abnormalities, but have consistently pointed to abnormalities in the basal ganglia (particularly the caudate nucleus), in the orbital regions of the frontal lobe, and in the thalamus. Other studies, including postmortem investigations, have demonstrated gliosis of the caudate nucleus, necrosis of the globus pallidus, lentiform nucleus lesions, and increased ventricular size and patients previously diagnosed with OCD.

It is now felt that the neurocircuitry of OCD principally involves the frontal lobes (orbitofrontal cortex and dorsolateral prefrontal cortex), the basal ganglia (and particularly the caudate nucleus), and the thalamus. The dysfunctional circuits appear to involve the direct and the indirect basal ganglia pathways to the thalamus and the connection of the thalamus to the cortex (Figure 14.2).

Let us briefly review the normal functioning of the circuit diagrammed in Figure 14.2. The elements of the circuit include the limbic cortex and neocortex, the striatum (caudate and putamen), the globus pallidus (including direct and indirect pathways) and the thalamus. The pathway begins with the cortices activating the striatum, which in turn inhibits the direct basal ganglia pathway. Inhibition of the direct basal ganglia pathway (striatum to globus pallidus interna) results in decreased inhibitory signal to the thalamus, resulting in thalamic disinhibition. Thalamic disinhibition results in further cortical activation, which then begins the circuit again.

Simultaneously, activation of the striatum sends an inhibitory signal to the indirect basal ganglia pathway. In this pathway, this inhibitory signal is received by the globus pallidus externa. The globus pallidus externa ordinarily inhibits the subthalamic nucleus; therefore, inhibition of the globus pallidus externa results in disinhibition of the subthalamic nucleus. Once disinhibited, the subthalamic nucleus then sends an excitatory signal to the globus pallidus interna, which sends an inhibitory signal to the thalamus. Thalamic inhibition relatively decreases cortical activation, which attenuates the "drive" of this circuit.

The actual workings of the direct and indirect pathways are somewhat more complex than illustrated above. A more detailed view would likely include the structures included in Figure 14.3, which makes clearer that the pathways illustrated in Figure 14.2 are really a distillation of the essential elements of a much more complex network of multiple frontal-subcortical and limbic-subcortical circuits. Both diagrams illustrate the parallel and reciprocally modulating

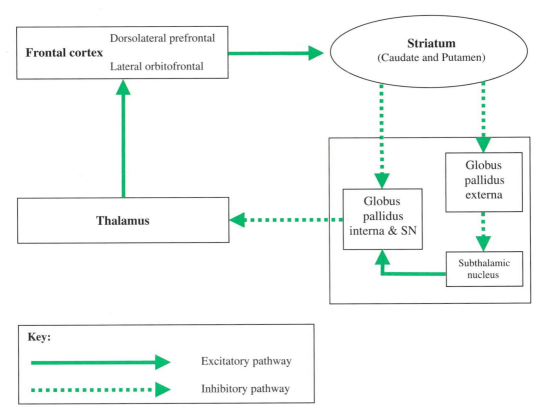

Figure 14.2 A simple schematic of the frontal-subcortical circuitry most relevant to obsessive–compulsive disorder. SN: substantia nigra.

nature of these two circuits, as they flow through the same fundamental elements of the circuits, and to other multiple circuits and structures. To make this complex neurocircuitry more understandable and immediately relevant to our current discussion of OCD, several points deserve further highlighting.

Under normal circumstances the direct basal ganglia pathway in the orbitofrontal-subcortical circuit disinhibits the thalamus, which subsequently further activates the orbitofrontal cortex. In a sense, this circuit establishes a positive feedback loop, and each reverberation of the circuit could, in theory, further infuse the circuit with increasing energy. Without some other modulating input, this circuit would continue to engage in recycling the same information over and over again.

It can be reasonably argued that the purpose of the orbitofrontal circuit under normal circumstances is to permit one to hold information of

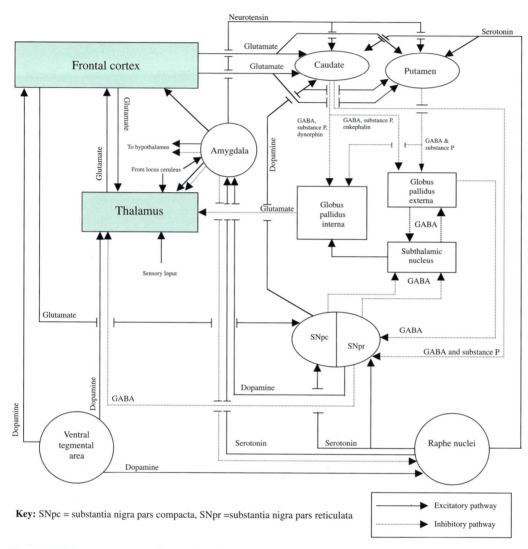

Figure 14.3 A more complex illustration of the neurocircuitry most relevant to obsessive–compulsive disorder. While many of the major pathways are illustrated here, space does not permit a delineation of orbitofrontal and dorsolateral prefrontal pathways, nor are all other afferents and efferents from parallel modulating circuits illustrated. Where neurotransmitters and neuroactive substances are known, they are indicated adjacent to their respective pathways

emotional or survival (i.e., limbic) significance (i.e., safety, grooming, mating, eating, gathering, etc.). Remember from our discussion of the orbitofrontal-subcortical circuit in Chapter 4 (Complex cognition) that the orbitofrontal cortex may be metaphorically thought of as the "limbic police," and viewed as the area that participates in keeping limbic impulses in check, suggesting a possible neurobiological basis for obsession. This is the condition we referred to earlier (in a somewhat tongue-in-cheek but still illustrative manner) as a state of "limbic martial law," where the activity of the orbitofrontal-subcortical circuit continuously "holds and controls" information about such limbic impulses. As discussed in Chapter 4, the several frontal-subcortical circuits subserving cognition, emotion, and behavior are reciprocally connected at multiple levels. Hence, excessive drive in the orbitofrontal circuit may secondarily influence (and perhaps increase) the dorsolateral prefrontal (executive function and behavioral planning) and anterior cingulate (motivation) circuits. Since these circuits are involved in the development of ideas, plans, sequences, responses, and strategies, and in motivation (respectively), increased activity in these circuits would be expected to bring these limbic concerns into conscious awareness and perhaps also therefore facilitate the development of compulsions. Again, without some modulating input to these circuits, the excessive recycling of limbic information, excessive motivation, and related behaviors will persist, and the continuously obsessing patient will be literally "driven" to perform compulsions again and again.

Under normal circumstances, modulating circuits are present and do attenuate the activity of the orbitofrontal circuit. The principal modifying circuit appears to be that driven by the dorsolateral prefrontal cortex. This area frontal-subcortical circuit subserves executive function, and is capable of exerting its effects on cognition and behavior in a manner related to, but not inexorably bound by, activity in the orbitofrontal circuit. The dorsolateral prefrontal circuit may be usefully thought of as responding to the information held in the orbitofrontal circuit, permitting the individual to regulate the type and duration of response to this information. In other words, it allows the conscious brain to recognize the issue of concern (e.g., cleanliness), and make a decision to act on it (e.g., wash hands) and then stop both the concern and the reaction (e.g., only wash hands once). Clearly, if this circuit is not functioning or communicating with the orbitofrontal circuit properly, the person will not be able to cease responding to the concerns in an appropriate and expeditious manner.

In addition to these ideas about the neurocircuitry of OCD, a few additional review comments on the neurochemistry of these circuits are warranted. Without question, multiple neurotransmitter systems are at work here. However, a simplified view places: (1) glutamatergic and dopaminergic influence at the level of the striatum; (2) serotonergic influence at the level of the striatum; and (3) GABA-ergic (gamma-aminobutyric acid) influence at the globus pallidus interna and at the thalamus. The benefit of understanding this circuitry as it relates to OCD is that it begins to provide a rational foundation for therapy. Interventions that take advantage of the known circuitry and/or the predominant neurotransmitter systems at each level may be expected to alter the activity of the circuits in predictable ways and therefore to alter patient symptoms.

Serotonin modulates activity of these circuits in a complicated fashion, but increases in serotonin within the system (as provided by selective serotonin reuptake inhibitors, or SSRIs) appear to attenuate activity at the level of the striatum and to facilitate behavioral inhibition. Decreased inhibitory outflow from the striatum should result in increased globus pallidus interna activity, and therefore increased thalamic inhibition. This should have the effect of attenuating the "drive" of this circuit, and should therefore decrease OCD symptoms. Indeed, SSRIs (including the serotonergically active tricyclic agent, clomipramine) have been shown to be effective pharmacological agents for treatment of OCD, an observation that follows logically from the known circuitry.

Similarly, activation of the dorsal prefrontal cortex, as happens with the techniques employed by cognitive therapy, appears to attenuate "drive" in the orbitofrontal circuit. The exact mechanism by which this occurs is not entirely known, but in simple terms it may be that increasing the "inhibitory" circuitry in the dorsolateral circuit either overrides the "excitatory" activity in the orbitofrontal circuit, or perhaps inhibitory activity in one produces complementary inhibition in the other. In either case, increased activity of the dorsolateral prefrontal circuit is produced by cognitive therapy and is the most likely explanation for the effectiveness of this therapy for OCD.

Neurosurgical interventions continue to be available as treatment in the most severe and refractory cases of OCD. Generally, these procedures include bilateral capsulotomy, cingulotomy, subcaudate tractotomy, or limbic leukotomy. In bilateral gamma-knife capsulotomy, lesions are placed in the internal capsule between the caudate nucleus and the globus pallidus. Decreased inhibitory outflow from the caudate to the globus pallidus decreases inhibition of the globus pallidus, permitting the globus pallidus to increase inhibitory outflow to the thalamus and decrease the "drive" in the circuit. Though the beneficial effects of such procedures often take several months to develop fully, and necessarily entail the potential complications of any neurosurgical procedure, the logic of a surgical approach to treatment of the patient with refractory OCD appears to be very similar to that of the pharmacological or psychotherapeutic methods.

The functional neurocircuitry of OCD may also help explain the high rate of alcohol abuse and dependence among individuals with OCD. Such patients often report that their use of alcohol began as an attempt to control their symptoms. Although alcohol has effects on many neurotransmitter systems (see Chapter 17) one of its principal effects is facilitation of the activity of GABA receptors. In the above diagram, a GABA-ergic agent would simulate the action of an activated globus pallidus interna by increasing inhibition of the thalamus. As with the above mentioned agents, increased thalamic inhibition decreases the "drive" in the circuit and might decrease OCD symptoms. Clearly, development of tolerance, withdrawal, and the multiple other complications of alcohol abuse and dependence eventually make this an ineffective and otherwise harmful pharmacological "treatment." Nonetheless, understanding the neurocircuitry may help explain both the appeal of alcohol for many OCD patients and the difficulty these patients have achieving alcohol abstinence.

Evaluation

In most cases, the etiology of OCD will represent the idiopathic illness described earlier in this chapter. However, the differential diagnosis must first consider whether the clinical presentation is most consistent with OCD or with another neuropsychiatric disorder. In cases where there is no overt suggestion of comorbid or predisposing neurological disorder, the differential will reasonably include psychotic disorders (which may include obsessions, perseveration, or both), mood disorders (obsessions vs. preoccupation and excessive guilt), other anxiety disorders (e.g., post-traumatic stress disorder, generalized anxiety disorder), eating disorders (e.g., anorexia nervosa), obsessive compulsive personality disorder, somatoform disorders, factitious disorders, malingering, and substance disorders. Importantly, these conditions are not mutually exclusive, and patients may suffer from more than one such problem simultaneously. The important consideration is whether during periods of relative remission of one or the other set of symptoms (e.g., depression and obsessions) the other set persists nonetheless; a history that suggests two independent illnesses with related but at least somewhat separate courses may be very useful in deciding whether obsessions and compulsions represent an independent disorder or are instead merely symptoms of another condition (e.g., schizophrenia, major depressive disorder). When the history or examination is at all atypical (see below), the possibility of a secondary obsessive– compulsive syndrome must be considered and an additional neurological differential diagnosis constructed. The evaluation of OCD should include the following items:

(1) *History*, with attention to age of onset and course, family history, and any suggestion of comorbid psychiatric, substance, neurological, and medical disorders.

(2) *Physical/neurological examination*, although a standard part of the evaluation of any patient with OCD, is particularly important when the history or presentation are atypical because of the increased likelihood of another significant and causative neurological condition.

(3) *Mental status examination*, including both a thorough clinical cognitive examination and the use of a scale to quantify the severity of OCD symptoms (e.g., the Yale–Brown Obsessive Compulsive Scale (Y-BOCS) that can be repeated as an objective measure of response to treatment. As discussed below, particular attention should be given to the evaluation of executive function, as significant neuropsychological impairment may suggest the presence of an underlying neurological disorder and may influence the potential benefits of treatment, and particularly cognitive–behavioral treatment.

(4) *Laboratory evaluation* where indicated (see below), and especially when tricyclics or lithium are likely to be employed. The inclusion of neuroimaging in the initial evaluation is arguable, but is certainly indicated for any patient with atypical history, presentation, or treatment response (see below).

(5) *Neuropsychological evaluation* may be very useful when the bedside examination suggests significant cognitive impairment or where the diagnosis is unclear or confounded by comorbid psychiatric problems.

If in the course of this standard evaluation any of the following atypical features are observed, a more intensive neurological evaluation (including neuroimaging, laboratory tests, and neurological consultation) is indicated:

• Late or abrupt onset.
• Absent family history.
• Chronic refractory illness.
• Neurological abnormalities (parkinsonism, chorea).
• Significant or unexpected neuropsychological deficits (executive dysfunction).

These atypical features will occur in only a small percentage of all cases of OCD. When any of these is present, particularly in the refractory, neurologically abnormal, or neuropsychologically impaired patient, the differential diagnosis should include the neurological conditions listed in Table 14.1. If the history and clinical evaluation suggest that one of these problems is present, a

Table 14.1. Differential diagnosis of other neurological disorders associated with obsessive–compulsive disorder

Frontal lobe disorders	Striatal disorders	Globus pallidus disorders	White matter disorders
Frontotemporal dementia	Parkinson's disease	Postencephalitic disorder	Multiple sclerosis
Epilepsy	Basal ganglia calcification	Parkinsonism	Right frontal white matter lesions
Tumor	Huntington's disease	Progressive supranuclear palsy	
Traumatic brain injury	Sydenham's chorea (post-	Manganese intoxication	
Stroke	Streptococcal chorea)	Pallidal anoxia and ischemia	
Anoxia or ischemia	Caudate anoxia, ischemia		
	Tourette's Disorder		
	Neuroacanthocytosis		
	Lesch-Nyhan syndrome		
	Rett syndrome		

detailed neuropsychiatric evaluation should be performed and may include one or more of the following elements:
- neurological examination and consultation;
- neuropsychological evaluation;
- neuroimaging, usually MRI;
- antineuronal antibodies, erythrocyte sedimentation rate (ESR), antinuclear antibody (ANA), anti-DNase B assay, pregnancy test.

Treatment

The most common treatment modality for OCD is an 8–12 week trial of pharmacotherapy with one of the SSRIs or the strongly serotonergic tricyclic antidepressant, clomipramine. As a general rule, most patients with OCD require doses at the higher end of ranges listed in Table 14.2. In some cases lower doses may suffice, but this is true only in a minority of patients with OCD. Since there is no definitive evidence suggesting that one medication is clearly more effective than the others, the clinician's recommendation will depend largely on the side-effect profile that the patient is willing to accept and also considerations about the patient's compliance. This latter issue is particularly important for patients who may, by virtue of neuropsychological impairments, ambivalence regarding treatment, or habit, have a tendency to miss or "forget" doses, and for whom a medication with a relatively longer half-life may be most useful. By contrast, patients with underlying neurological disease, including and especially movement disorders, may be better treated by selection of an agent with a relatively shorter half-life, as rare but potentially serious adverse effects of these medications (i.e., akathisia, restless leg syndrome, dystonia) may abate more quickly once they have been discontinued.

When effective, treatment should continue for a minimum of 6–12 months. Because this is a chronic, relapsing disorder, and because there is no evidence to suggest that extended treatment is associated with adverse consequences, it is probably prudent to maintain the patient on an effective medication indefinitely if this is the only treatment modality employed.

When a single agent does not provide sufficient benefit, augmentation with agents such as buspirone, lithium, clonazepam, methylphenidate, or other antidepressants may be useful. Additionally, some patients will respond to a combination of the commonly prescribed anti-OCD medications. Neuroleptics may be of benefit to patients with poor insight (which may be almost delusional) or with tics (as in Tourette's Disorder), but should be used judiciously and are not recommended for use without concurrent administration

Table 14.2. Commonly prescribed medications for obsessive–compulsive disorder

Generic name	Trade name	Dosage (mg/day)
Clomipramine	Anafranil®	≤250
Fluoxetine	Prozac®	≤80
Sertaline	Zoloft®	≤200
Paroxetine	Paxil®	≤60
Citalopram	Celexa®	≤60
Fluvoxamine	Luvox®	≤300

of an anti-OCD agent. In general, neuroleptics should not be used at all in cases of OCD where insight is relatively preserved. The basis for this may be that the relatively strong dopamine blockade by typical neuroleptics predictably worsens prefrontal cortex function, and more obviously dorsolateral prefrontal function. The apparent effect of typical neuroleptics among patients with typical OCD is a trivial reduction in symptoms, a weakening of the ability to use cognitive strategies as part of the treatment plan, and the emergence of unacceptable acute or chronic (and sometimes permanent) medication side effects including tardive dyskinesea.

As discussed earlier, recent studies suggest that cognitive–behavioral therapy for OCD may be just as effective as pharmacological therapy, and that concurrent pharmacotherapy and cognitive–behavioral therapy may afford the best long-term control of symptoms. While the scientific efficacy literature is encouraging, there is concern that the implementation of cognitive–behavioral therapy is not standardized between individual therapists in the community. As such, the effectiveness of cognitive–behavioral therapy in clinical practice may produce somewhat more variable results than those reported in the literature. With this concern in mind, a combined medication and therapy approach for all patients seems most prudent.

Neurosurgical treatment is a legitimate and potentially effective treatment option for patients who have failed to respond to all other treatments. Failure is generally defined as persistent and severe symptoms (Y-BOCS of at least 26), and persistent disability (Global Assessment of Function score of 50 or lower) despite systematic treatment with all currently accepted pharmacological and behavioral therapy treatments alone or in combination for at least five years. In some cases, pharmacological treatment will have been legitimately discontinued due to intolerable side effects. More pragmatically, failure may be defined as persistent symptoms after two SSRI trials, three trials of medication combinations, a trial of electroconvulsive therapy (ECT), and a trial of behavioral treatment, *plus* incapacitation and active suicidal thoughts. In most centers, such failure is a prerequisite for neurosurgical referral and the treatments listed in the preceding section. Among them, recent literature seems to suggest that gamma-knife capsulotomy may be of most benefit.

ECT may also provide some relief from OCD symptoms when pharmacotherapy and psychotherapy have failed. Though it is generally not as effective as neurosurgical interventions, some authors advocate a trial of ECT prior to neurosurgery for OCD. In cases where ECT or neurosurgery are considered, it is important to have completely evaluated the possibility of other etiologies for the patient's presentation with appropriate vigor. In similar fashion, transcranial magnetic stimulation may emerge as a potential alternative treatment for not only treatment-resistant patients with OCD, but perhaps also as an adjunctive or alternative treatment to pharmacotherapy.

Summary

OCD is a disabling condition characterized by intrusive and distressing ideas, images, or impulses (obsessions) and repetitive, ritualized behaviors (compulsions) that at least appear to be designed to neutralize the anxiety associated with obsessions. Recent neuroimaging studies suggest that OCD is fundamentally a disorder affecting the function of and interaction between several frontal-subcortical circuits, including the lateral orbitofrontal-subcortical circuit and the dorsolateral prefrontal-subcortical circuit. The symptoms appear to be related to overactivity of the orbitofrontal-subcortical circuit and to be reduced by either reduction in this circuit or increased activity in the dorsolateral prefrontal-subcortical circuit. The effect of increased activity in the latter circuit seems to be a relatively increased ability to inhibit, or more effectively modulate, activity in the former circuit.

The neuropsychiatric evaluation of OCD should attempt to distinguish between the idiopathic (or primary) illness and secondary OCD-like conditions produced by underlying neurological disorders. In general, atypical of onset, family history, neuropsychological or neurological status, or response to treatment all suggest the possibility of a secondary OCD-like syndrome. Treatment involves using relatively high doses of strongly serotonergic medications, cognitive behavioral therapy, or both. In refractory cases, electroconvulsive therapy or even neurosurgical interventions may be needed to provide relief from this potentially disabling neuropsychiatric illness.

15

Diminished motivation and apathy

Introduction

Motivation is best described as an individual's direction, intensity, and persistence toward achieving specific goals, and is the process by which the behavior, emotion, and thought associated with achieving those goals is started, directed and sustained. Apathy is a state of diminished motivation – a reduction in goal-directed motor, emotional, and cognitive activity – due to central nervous system disturbance.

Apathy may be a symptom or a syndrome in a variety of neuropsychiatric disorders (e.g., depression, dementia, delirium) or may be an independent syndrome due to neurological or medical causes. Whether present as symptom or syndrome, apathy may be a significant contributor to clinical disability due to the lack of motivation needed to comply with prescribed treatment, to function socially or occupationally, or to care for oneself properly. For this reason, an understanding of the causes, neurobiology, and treatment of apathy may meaningfully assist in the management of patients with this problem, and improve outcome. Marin, Duffy, Campbell and colleagues offer an excellent review of this literature in *Psychiatric Annals* (Volume 27, Number 1, 1997), from which much of this chapter is derived and to which readers are referred for a more extensive but entirely practical overview. In this chapter, we will review in a more limited fashion the clinical characteristics, neurobiology, differential diagnosis, and treatment of apathy.

Clinical characteristic of diminished motivation and apathy

Most people are familiar with diminished motivation as a dimension of everyday behavior, whether in regard to some part of work, recreation, relationships, or personal growth. The "senioritis" commonly experienced by high school students in the spring of their senior year may be used to illustrate "normal" apathy. The student with "senioritis" is not bothered by his or her diminished motivation towards completing school assignments, although many teachers and parents find this marked decrease in motivation towards schoolwork both concerning and aggravating. However, unless the diminished motivation develops to the point of endangering the student's chances of graduation or jeopardizes their entrance into college, most parents and teachers simply ascribe this circumscribed area of progressively decreasing motivation to "normal behavior." Individuation and passive–aggressive issues notwithstanding (though clearly in the differential diagnosis for this behavior), this common example of *forme fruste* apathy illustrates that there exists a continuum of normal motivational states. Our concern manifests when movement along this continuum extends into the pathological range, with diminished motivation compromising function in areas such as school or occupational performance, relationships, or even more fundamental functions like eating, clothing oneself, obtaining shelter, or maintaining health.

Apathy may be a feature of neuropsychiatric, neurological, and medical disorders, including schizophrenia, depression, dementia, stroke, multiple sclerosis, and traumatic brain injury, among many others. The essential features are a lack of overt behavior, a lack of emotional reaction to circumstances, and an apparent lack of thought or concern about these (or any other) issues. For example, recent descriptions of the deficit syndrome (or "negative symptoms") of schizophrenia – which include prominent avolition (lack of will or motivation), alogia (lack of thought reflected as a lack of words or speech), and affective flattening – are essentially synonymous with the present definition of apathy. Importantly, apathetic symptoms contribute significantly to the morbidity associated with the schizophrenias, given their impact on self-care and adherence to prescribed treatments.

Marin (1991) has proposed working criteria for the syndrome of apathy (adapted here as Figure 15.1) that usefully frame the concept of apathy and the issues requiring consideration in the evaluation of this problem. Based on this concept of apathy, Marin et al. (1991) developed and validated a tool for the assessment of apathy, the Apathy Evaluation Scale (AES). The AES appears to accurately characterize apathy, and to distinguish it from depression, with reasonable validity and reliability. We will return to a discussion of the use of the AES later in this chapter.

The Apathy Syndrome

The Apathy Syndrome is present when there is a clinically significant decrease in goal-directed behavior resulting from diminished motivation, and when diminished motivation is the dominant feature of the syndrome (in other words, the diminished motivation is not better accounted for by depression, dementia, delirium, schizophrenia, etc.).

To meet criteria for the Syndrome of Apathy, the patient must demonstrate a clinically significant decrease in motivation, relative to his or her previous functioning or the patient's cultural standards. Diminished motivation must be present in each of these areas:

    a. Goal-directed behavior (e.g., lack of initiative, perseverance, productivity, effort, time spent in activities of interest, socialization) resulting in dependence on others to structure and support activity

    b. Goal-directed cognition (e.g., lack of intellectual interest, curiosity, initiative, concern, or perseverance regarding personal, social, occupational, or other functional issues)

    c. Emotional experience and responsiveness (e.g., flat affect, lack of emotional responses to either positive or negative events and experiences)

Figure 15.1 Apathy, a neuropsychiatric syndrome. (Adapted from Marin, 1991.)

Neurobiology of motivation and apathy

In addition to improving clinical recognition of apathy, defining apathy in terms of its motoric, cognitive, and affective components is consistent with our present understanding of the neurocircuitry of motivation and its disorders. Kalivas et al. (1994) and Duffy (1997) offer outlines of this circuitry based on a review of a combination of animal and human lesion analyses, neurocircuitry analyses in primates, and discussions of neuropsychological and neuroanatomic correlates in humans. A comprehensive illustration of both the macroscopic selectively distributed network subserving motivation and the microcellular (i.e., receptor) level interactions that sustain the activity of this network in the human brain is well beyond the scope of this book. With this in mind, it is our intent that our readers regard the model presented only as a basic conceptual framework that may be used when pursuing additional reading and learning about this topic elsewhere.

Neurocircuitry

In our earlier discussion of complex cognition (Chapter 4), we outlined a very basic structure of the major frontal-subcortical circuits (presented again in

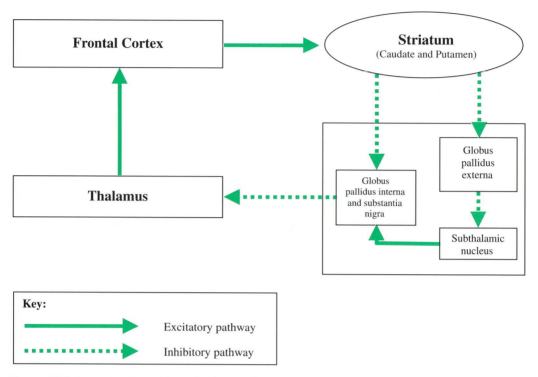

Figure 15.2 General outline of frontal-subcortical circuitry.

Figure 15.2), including that of the anterior cingulate circuit. In our earlier presentation, we referred to the anterior cingulate circuit as the frontal-subcortical circuit most involved in the development and maintenance of motivation. As we will discuss in this section, the neural substrates of motivation are substantially more complex than that illustrated by this very simple framework. However, we will use this framework as a starting point from which to move on to a more complex presentation of the neurocircuitry of motivation. This presentation requires the description of two additional neural networks subserving motivation, the extended amygdala and the ventral striatopallidum, and their interconnections and interactions with the frontal-subcortical circuitry described previously.

Extended amygdala

The extended amygdala, as used in this discussion, includes the centromedial portion of the amygdala, the ventral portion of the substantia innominata, the stria terminalis, and the caudomedial portion of the "shell" of the nucleus accumbens. The extended amygdala is the gateway through which information enters the motivation circuit. Highly processed multimodal sensory information is projected to the extended amygdala from the secondary and hetermodal association areas, the hippocampus/dorsolateral prefrontal limbic division (see Chapter 5, Emotion), the frontal-subcortical circuits (including the anterior cingulate, or motivation, circuit) via the thalamus, and visceral afferents via the hypothalamus, parabrachial nucleus and the sensory thalamus. These various types of information conveyed to the thalamus from these sources are integrated in the extended amygdala and establish an automatic, ongoing, and unconscious "awareness" of the internal and external environment that (as we describe below) is used in establishing the motivational "tone" of the organism.

The information contained in this rudimentary awareness appears to be subjected to a form of "filtering" (or assignment of emotional and motivational valence) before being fed-back into to the various circuits from whence it came. The methods by which this information is filtered are subjects of ongoing scientific investigations, but the basic processes appear to be based on a combination of "hard-wired", or evolutionarily preserved, responses to specific classes of visual, auditory, and visceral stimuli and also learned responses (including modifications of hard-wired responses) to these sorts of stimuli based on prior experience of and response to such stimuli. Once this filtering and assignment of emotional and motivational valence is accomplished, the extended amygdala also effects automatic behavioral responses. Output of the extended amygdala is communicated (in parallel) to:
- the locus ceruleus (which produces norepinephrine and facilitates arousal);
- the medial portion of the hypothalamus (which activates the hypothalamic–pituitary axis);
- the lateral hypothalamus (which activates the sympathetic nervous system);
- the periaqueductal gray region of the midbrain (which facilitates automatic motor responses and "freezing");
- the parabrachial nucleus (which influences respiration);
- the thalamus and the ventral striatopallidum (from whence information is fed-back into the frontal-subcortical circuits).

In this fashion, the extended amygdala facilitates associative (or conditioned) learning, develops a schema for automatic (e.g., pre- or unconscious) assignment of relative "survival values," or emotional and motivational valences, to incoming sensory information. Hence, the extended amygdala participates in the entry of motivationally relevant information into the complex of frontal-subcortical and limbic-subcortical networks involved in motivation, and is capable of generating automatic behavioral responses to information in cases where it is subjected to information of sufficiently strong motivational valence.

Ventral striatopallidum

The ventral striatopallidum is an extended region of the ventral striatum (caudate and putamen) that also includes the ventral pallidum (ventral portion of the globus pallidus), the olfactory tubercle, and the nucleus accumbens. The ventral striatopallidum appears to be involved in communicating information between the extended amygdala (which is nearly equivalent to the ventral compartment referred to in Mayberg's model of emotional experience – see Chapter 5) and the dorsal striatopallidum (which refers to the dorsal portions of the subcortical structures – those that are involved in the frontal-subcortical circuits described in Chapter 4). The ventral striatopallidum appears to be a conduit through which the information processed by the extended amygdala is relayed back into the frontal-subcortical circuits. The activity of the ventral striatopallidum is heavily influenced by dopaminergic projections from the ventral tegmental area (to the nucleus accumbens) and the substantia nigra (to the pallidum), and it appears to play a critical role in binding information from the extended amygdala into a number of selectively distributed neuronal networks and for sustaining of the motivational state of the organism.

The extended amygdala and the ventral striatopallidum overlap anatomically and functionally, and the activity of both areas involves the nucleus accumbens. The nucleus accumbens is a complex structure that is most simply regarded as playing a major role in stimulus reward and hence the development of motivational valence. The nucleus accumbens is significantly influenced by dopamine received from the ventral tegmental area and substantia nigra pars compacta. Dopaminergic neurons project from these brainstem areas into the nucleus accumbens, extended amygdala, and ventral striatopallidum, are largely excitatory, and tend to increase the activity of their target areas. It is likely that the high-reward and behaviorally reinforcing properties of pro-dopaminergic agents (e.g., cocaine, amphetamine) are related to their influence on these structures of the motivation circuitry. Additionally, the extended amygdala and ventral striatopallidum also have descending influences on the brainstem dopaminergic nuclei, thereby effecting a mechanism by which increased motivational states can be perpetuated.

The smaller networks that define the extended amygdala and the ventral striatopallidum appear to be essential elements of the much larger networks subserving motivation in all three major domains: cognition, emotion, and behavior. Although the exact nature and operation of these smaller networks is not yet fully understood, they appear to provide much of the fundamental motivational valence and reward properties attached to stimuli, whether internal or external. Given this additional background, we will follow Duffy's (1997) description of the four subcircuits that appear most relevant to the development and maintenance of motivation.

Motivational working memory circuit

This circuit includes the ventral tegmental area, nucleus accumbens, and ventral pallidum. This highly reciprocal circuit receives information from the sources described above, including the prefrontal cortex and hippocampus. In simple terms, this circuit can be thought of as momentarily "holding" the information from these sources and comparing the motivational valence of the "held" information with that of previously presented stimuli. This activity is ongoing and continuous, and is the basis by which the overall motivational "readiness" of the organism is maintained, thereby serving the role of a motivational rheostat. In other words, this circuit defines the motivational state of the system and promotes or inhibits behavioral responses to the various incoming stimuli in a continuous fashion.

Importantly, this circuit includes two subcircuits within it that subserve different behavioral responses to motivationally charged stimuli, a "limbic" circuit and a "motor" circuit. The limbic portion of the motivational working memory circuit appears to have a relatively lower threshold for responding to stimuli than does the motor portion of this circuit. Upon receipt of stimuli with modest emotional or motivational valence (a moderate stressor), the limbic portion of the circuit is activated. Via this circuit's connections to the hypothalamus and ventral tegmental areas in particular, increased autonomic activity and arousal are generated, and a readiness for behavioral responding is established. If the intensity of the stressor increases (in other words, it becomes a noxious stressor), the motor portion of this circuit is automatically engaged and, by way of its additional connections to hypothalamic, basal ganglia, and brainstem areas, automatic and stereotypic motor responses are generated.

As noted earlier, there are substantial dopaminergic inputs to the nucleus accumbens and related areas from the ventral tegmental area and the substantia nigra. Dopamine appears to have differential effects on the limbic and motor portions of the motivational working memory as a result of differences in their threshold for dopamine-mediated activation – the limbic circuit responds to relatively lower levels of dopamine than does the motor circuit.

One consequence of this differential sensitivity to dopamine is that relatively lower level stimulation simultaneously activates the limbic motivational working memory circuit and the other frontal-subcortical circuits, thereby driving thinking about (dorsolateral circuit) the stimuli, its limbic/survival/social significance (lateral orbitofrontal circuit), and motivational responding (anterior cingulate and related circuits). However, in the face of stronger ascending input, the motor circuit is activated and much of the input from the other frontal-subcortical circuits may be supervened by automatic motor reactions (e.g., pulling one's hand away from a hot object, jumping out of the way of an oncoming truck).

Dorsolateral prefrontal circuit

In this context, the elements of the dorsolateral prefrontal circuit includes the previously described dorsolateral prefrontal-subcortical circuit (see Chapter 4) and its connections to the ventral pallidum, medial dorsal nucleus of the thalamus, other prefrontal cortices, nucleus accumbens, and ventral tegmental area. This circuit subserves executive function, and is instrumental in integrating motivationally relevant information into cognitive and behavioral responses. The dorsolateral prefrontal cortex appears to exert a predominantly inhibitory influence on the motivational circuits via its action on the nucleus accumbens, thereby offering a mechanism by which to modulate or attenuate the automatic limbic and motor responses that might otherwise be generated by the subcircuits described above. The interaction between the ventral compartment (extended amygdala) and dorsal compartment (dorsolateral prefrontal circuitry) is linked by the ventral striatopallidum, as described above, and perhaps also by the rostral (infracallosal) cingulate as described by Mayberg (1997; see Chapter 5). Simply put, this circuit permits one to put the brakes on automatic responding and to think about both a stimulus and potential responses to it before moving into action – the dorsolateral prefrontal cortex facilitates developing a rational and appropriate behavioral response to motivationally charged stimuli.

Arousal circuit

This system involves the ventral pallidum, ventral tegmental area, and the pedunculopontine nucleus. The function of this circuit is to integrate arousal into motivation. The reciprocal connections between the pedunculopontine region, the ventral pallidum, and ventral tegmental area serve to integrate cognition, autonomic status, and arousal status with regions subserving motor responses. Information leaving the pedunculopontine nucleus is directed both to the motor system and back to the ventral tegmental area that (mediated by this area's dopaminergic projections throughout the motivation circuitry) infuses the circuits with the individual's arousal status. Activation of the pedunculopontine nucleus itself produces spontaneous fight or flight reactions, appetitive behavior, and stereotypic rhythmic displays.

Reward memory circuit

This circuit involves the ventral tegmental area, the amygdala, and the nucleus accumbens. Connections among these areas are strengthened or weakened based on the outcome of the motor behaviors resulting from the activity of the circuit. Since two of these three areas are also intimately involved in the working memory circuit described above, the additional input of information processed by the amygdala would be predicted to permit the reward memory circuit to influence the state of the motivational working memory circuit in such a way that rewarding (or reinforcing) stimuli drive the overall system in the direction of repeating the experience of such stimuli, and decrease the drive towards re-experiencing aversive stimuli. Since this area reciprocally receives input from the motivational working memory circuit, the elements of the reward memory circuit are also influenced in turn by other elements of the motivational circuitry. Through some more specific mechanisms of this sort, the connections between the elements of the reward memory circuit, and also between this circuit to the other motivational circuits, is modulated. Given that these areas are important in the gatekeeping functions of the motivation circuits, and that they serve to drive the organism as a whole toward increased reward (and also away from continued experience of aversive stimuli), this circuit helps determine the sorts of stimuli that will pass through the gates and drive future behavior. In other words, these elements help form the reward memory that develops from experience.

Neurochemistry

Since a comprehensive review of the neurochemistry involved in the motivational circuits is both beyond the scope of this presentation and also not fully established, we will restrict our discussion here to only a few of the major elements.

The ventral tegmental area is the principal source of mesolimbic and mesocortical dopamine and the substantia nigra is the major source of striatal dopamine. Since we have already reviewed the role of these areas in the motivation circuitry, noting that dopamine is substantially needed to maintain normal motivation is at this point sufficient restatement of our previous comments. Modulation of dopamine activity produces concomitant changes in arousal, autonomic activity, sensorimotor integration, motivation, and the resulting behavior.

As stated in the previous section on the motivational working memory circuit, the ventral and dorsal striatopallidum differ in their responsiveness to dopamine. The ventral system tends to respond to lower levels of dopamine, consistent with its essential role in facilitating communication between the ventral (extended amygdala) and dorsal (including dorsolateral prefrontal and motor) systems. The dorsal system is somewhat less sensitive to dopamine, but responds autonomously to relatively large amounts of dopamine (e.g., those from a large amount of cocaine or amphetamine). Consequently, progressively increasing cerebral dopamine availability produces increases in arousal and autonomic activity, motivation, goal-directed behavior, and eventually automatic and stereotyped behavior.

The prefrontal cortex, as discussed in the previous section, appears to have a predominantly inhibitory role on activity of the motivational circuits. This inhibition appears to be the result of modulation of subcortical dopamine activity (including that in the nucleus accumbens and the activity of the ventral tegmental area) by the prefrontal cortex and probably also via the activity of the amygdala and hippocampus. The prefrontal cortex appears to be able to increase the threshold for activation of limbic and subcortical structures by dopamine. In other words, the prefrontal cortex decreases the ability of environmental stress to elicit excessive arousal, autonomic activity, or automatic behaviors.

The motivational circuitry is also influenced by the action of other neurotransmitters and excitatory amino acids throughout the relevant circuitry. A simplified (albeit still quite complex) illustration of this neurochemical circuitry is provided in Figure 15.3. In this Figure, the dopaminergic projections

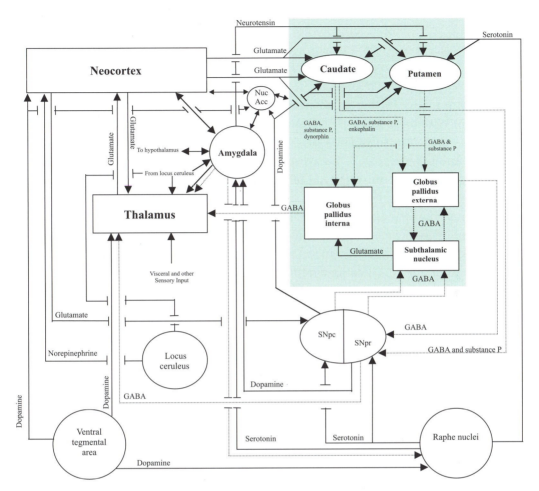

Figure 15.3 A partial illustration of the neurocircuitry of motivation. Note that this circuitry is a modified version of that used to illustrate the neurocircuitry of complex cognition. In this figure, network connections between the structures are not complete, but instead highlight those connections most important to the motivation circuitry. Excitatory neurochemical connections are illustrated with solid lines and inhibitory connections with dashed lines. This convention is generally intuitive with the exception of the serotonergic projections from the raphe nuclei that, though neurochemically excitatory, are behaviorally inhibitory at the connections illustrated here (amygdala and striatum). The striatopallidum (both ventral and dorsal portions) is encompassed in the gray box, and the reciprocal connections of the elements of this circuit to the nucleus accumbens (Nuc. Acc.) are roughly illustrated by the bi-directional arrow between them. The relevant connections between the ventral tegmental area and both mesocortical and mesolimbic areas are shown, as are the important connections between the substantial nigra (SNpc, pars compacta; SNpr, pars reticulata) and the striatopallidum.

to the nucleus accumbens are grossly illustrated, without distinction regarding projections to the nucleus accumbens shell region or core region. These distinctions are relevant for a fuller understanding of the neurocircuitry of motivation, but are beyond the scope of this book. Readers interested in pursuing this matter further are referred to the excellent review by Heimer et al. (1997).

Within the nucleus accumbens, the actions of neurotransmitters and other neuroactive substances at NMDA (N-methyl-D-aspartate), AMPA (alpha-amino-3-hydroxy-5-methylisoxazole-4-propionic acid), mu- and delta-opioid receptors are most relevant to modulating the level of activity within the motivational circuit. In general, the activity of such neurochemicals within the nucleus accumbens increases the activity of the circuit. For example, the action of nicotine at cholinergic nicotinic receptors eventually leads to increased dopaminergic activity in the nucleus accumbens. This "downstream" dopaminergic effect of nicotine on the motivational circuitry may possibly explain the nature of the highly-reinforcing properties of this agent and the mechanisms by which this reinforcement occurs (as discussed in the reward subcircuit, above). Additionally, this view of motivation may also contribute to understanding the mechanisms underlying the experience of increased motivation and clarity of focus described by many people who use nicotine. The effects of other neurotransmitters and neuroactive substances (e.g., neurotensin, cholecystokinin, tachykinin, substance P) are also presently under investigation.

Before concluding this section, the role of serotonin in this system also deserves comment. The interaction between serotonergic neurons, cholinergic neurons, and dopaminergic neurons is extremely complex. It is now clear that the serotonin receptor subclasses vary significantly with respect to their effects on promoting or inhibiting cholinergic activity, and that their secondary effects on dopamine are also varied. For the present discussion, serotonin is regarded as a modulator of frontal-subcortical circuit activity (illustrated in Figure 15.3). Given the behaviorally inhibitory effect of serotonin at the level of the striatum, increasing serotonin levels (e.g., as done with serotonin reuptake inhibitors) is not only unlikely to improve significantly impaired motivation, it may instead decrease frontal-subcortical circuit activity and thereby diminish motivation.

If this view is correct, it may offer some insight into the phenomena of emotional "numbing," diminished motivation, and perhaps even diminished libido (frank sexual dysfunction notwithstanding) experienced by some patients while taking selective serotonin reuptake inhibitors. It is possible, however, that as more receptor-specific serotonin agonists and antagonists (particularly those with downstream pro-dopaminergic and pro-cholinergic effects) are developed, rather different effects of serotonin modulation of motivation may be observed.

Differential diagnosis of diminished motivation and apathy

As stated previously, apathy may present as symptom of a more extensive neuropsychiatric syndrome or may be the presenting feature of an underlying medical or neurological problem that disrupts the structure or function of the neurocircuitry presented in the preceding section. Hence, the differential diagnosis of apathy is approached on two levels. First, it must be determined whether the patient's presentation is most consistent with the Apathy Syndrome or instead with another neuropsychiatric, medical, medication-related, or socio-environmental problem of which diminished motivation is a feature (see Table 15.1). Although much ado is made of the difficulty of distinguishing depression from apathy, if the concept of apathy is understood and the evaluation uses valid and reliable methods (discussed in the next section) then this distinction may be made with relative ease and clarity. In most other cases, distinguishing the Apathy Syndrome from apathy as a symptom of the other clinical conditions in the differential diagnosis should be relatively straightforward. For example, patients with schizophrenia may have apathetic symptoms, but they most often have a number of other prominent and functionally significant problems (hallucinations, delusions, disorganized thought and behavior) that clearly distinguish them from patients with apathy alone (i.e., the Apathy Syndrome).

If apathy is the dominant (or only) feature of the patient's presentation, then characterizing the scope and severity of the problem and determining its etiology are the next step in developing the differential diagnosis. By definition (see Figure 15.1), the Apathy Syndrome requires a simultaneous diminution in goal-related action, emotion, and cognition, and that diminished motivation is the dominant feature of the clinical presentation. If diminished motivation in all three of these domains is present, then the Apathy Syndrome is the correct diagnosis. Patients with the most profound and severe forms of the apathy syndrome may be described as suffering from abulia (loss of will, or the inability to initiate action despite some goal-directed planning) or, in the most severe form of apathy, akinetic mutism. If criteria for the apathy syndrome are not fulfilled, but diminished motivation in one or more specific functional

Table 15.1. The differential diagnosis of diminished motivation, including some of the more common neuropsychiatric, medical, medication- and toxin-related, and socio-environmental conditions with which diminished motivation and apathy may be associated

Neuropsychiatric disorders	Medical disorders	Medications and toxins	Socio-environmental
Frontotemporal dementia	HIV encephalopathy	Typical antipsychotics, particularly those with potent dopamine receptor type-2 blockade, including:	Bereavement, or grief
Late-stage Alzheimer's disease	Hypothyroidism	• haloperidol	Adjustment disorder with depressed mood
Motor aprosodia	Apathetic hyperthyroidism	• fluphenazine	Other significant life stresses, including:
Parkinson's disease	Pseudohypoparathyroidism	• thiothixene	• role change
Huntington's disease	Testosterone deficiency	Selective serotonin reuptake inhibitors	• significant object loss or separation
Fahr's disease (idiopathic basal ganglia calcification)	Chronic fatigue syndrome	Excessive doses of anti-adrenergic agents (e.g., propranolol)	• institutionalism
Progressive supranuclear palsy	Lyme disease	Felbamate	• incarceration
Wilson's disease (hepatolenticular degeneration)	Congestive heart failure	Chronic alcohol abuse	Passive-aggressive coping style
Catatonia (neurological or psychogenic)	End-stage pulmonary disease causing chronic cerebral hypoxia	Chronic marijuana abuse	Efforts towards separation and/or individuation, which may be developmentally appropriate (adolescents) or inappropriate (adults)
Multiple sclerosis	Hepatic failure	Second ("dusted") phase of phencyclidine intoxication	
Normal pressure hydrocephalus	Renal failure	Stimulant withdrawal, including:	
Binswanger's disease	Neoplasms, including:	• cocaine	
Central and extrapontine myelinolysis	• primary CNS tumors	• amphetamine	
Anoxia	• systemic effects of tumors of non-CNS origin	• methamphetamine	
Radiation leukoencephalopathy	Severe malnutrition, including B12 deficiency	Reserpine	
Wernicke's encephalopathy		Manganese intoxication	
Stroke		Carbon monoxide poisoning	
Postconcussional syndrome		Toluene intoxication or abuse	
Klüver–Bucy syndrome		Lead intoxication	
Herpes encephalitis			
Delirium			
Schizophrenia			
Major depression			
Schizoid personality disorder			
Severe anorexia nervosa			

domains is present (e.g., diminished goal-related motor behavior, emotion, or cognition) and if such problem(s) are the dominant (or only) clinical feature, it may nonetheless be correct to describe the patient as suffering from diminished motivation or apathy with respect to a specific functional domain. Whether present as the full Apathy Syndrome or as functionally significant diminished motivation in a specific domain, determining the etiology of the problem is the next major task in developing the differential diagnosis.

Problems with motivation may result from focal lesions to one or more elements of the neurocircuitry presented in the preceding section. For example, lesions of the mesial frontal cortex, the anterior cingulate gyrus, or the connections between these areas may result in dramatic decreases in motivation and are the classic lesions responsible for the apathy syndrome. Such lesions may be the result of rupture of anterior communicating artery aneurysms, meningiomas of the falx cerebri, multiple sclerosis, trauma, or normal pressure hydrocephalus, among many such causes. Again, conditions capable of producing apathetic states will in some cases be obvious (e.g., as in anterior communicating artery aneurysm rupture). Regardless of whether the underlying cause is obvious or more subtle, the important point here is to consider all such causes of the apathy syndrome in the differential diagnosis whenever patients present with this problem.

Less commonly, but still consistent with our review of the relevant neurocircuitry, diminished motivation may also result from thalamic lesions, such as those produced by thrombosis of the great cerebral vein and/or straight sinus, and particularly those lesions affecting the anterior thalamus and/or the mediodorsal nucleus of the thalamus. Lesions to other elements of the frontal-subcortical circuits (e.g., striatum, globus pallidus, white matter and especially the posterior limb of the internal capsule) may also result in diminished motivation. Importantly, most such causes of diminished motivation are associated with other features of frontal-subcortical circuit dysfunction, including movement disorders (as with Parkinson's disease, Huntington's disease, Fahr's disease, and Wilson's disease), eye movement disorders (as with Parkinson's disease, progressive supranuclear palsy, and schizophrenia), and cognitive (executive) dysfunction. Consequently, apathy in the context of these conditions may be understood in terms of the affected neurocircuitry, but in practice the clinical presentation will generally include problems in addition to diminished motivation.

Cortical injury to areas other than the mesial frontal lobes may also result in clinical conditions that phenomenologically overlap with apathy. For example, lesions of the amygdala (as in the Klüver–Bucy syndrome) may produce diminished goal-related behavior (placidity) and goal-related emotion (reduced attachment of appropriate emotional valence). Disturbances of dorsolateral prefrontal dysfunction (particularly on the left) may produce problems initiating, maintaining, sequencing, and persisting with cognitive tasks. Although patients with this presentation are often described as having a "dysexecutive syndrome," Duffy (1997) suggests that it may also be reasonable to conceptualize such patients as suffering from diminished motivation in the cognitive domain.

Additionally, structural and/or functional disturbances of the brainstem nuclei (e.g., ventral tegmental area, locus ceruleus, cholinergic nuclei) involved in the motivation circuitry may also produce apathetic states. Although vascular insult is the most likely cause of dysfunction of these areas, trauma and central pontine myelinolysis may also produce similar problems.

In summary, apathy may be a symptom of a number of neuropsychiatric syndromes or an independent clinical syndrome. Some authors suggest that when criteria are met for the syndrome of apathy in the context of another neuropsychiatric disorder, the specific diagnosis of the Apathy Syndrome should be made (for example, (1) Schizophrenia, undifferentiated type, residual phase and (2) Apathy Syndrome). Whether explicitly stating this additional diagnosis significantly contributes to understanding the patient's condition is debatable, but doing so may be useful where it promotes more careful clinical attention to apathetic features and facilitates the integration of specific treatment of this problem into the patient's overall treatment plan.

Evaluation and treatment of diminished motivation and apathy

Identification and treatment of apathy may significantly decrease the morbidity of the illnesses that produce it. Clinically significant diminished motivation not only affects the patient's ability to participate in treatment making decisions, comply with treatment, and meet the basic demands of everyday life, it frequently results in significant problems for the patient's caregivers and family. Just as parents and teachers may become aggravated with the "senioritis" of the graduating high school student, families and careproviders that misunderstand apathy due to neurological, neuropsychiatric, or medical problems as "volitional" often become frustrated and angry at these patients. In the worst cases, when apathy is not considered in the differential diagnosis of treatment non-compliance, the patient may simply be written off by all involved in his or her care as passive–aggressive or (worse) "not yet ready for treatment."

Evaluation

Recognizing apathy, either the syndrome or symptoms, is important because there are relatively specific pharmacological and behavioral interventions that might not be considered if this diagnosis is missed (e.g., pro-dopaminergic or pro-cholinergic medications). The optimal treatment of apathy and diminished motivation requires an interdisciplinary treatment team including neuropsychiatrists, neuropsychologists, physical and occupational therapists, social workers, case managers, the family, and the patient. Establishing the diagnosis follows from a thorough assessment of the patient, guided by an integration of clinical findings and their implications for the differential diagnosis. When the history and clinical evidence suggest the presence of clinically significant diminished motivation, a thorough evaluation should be undertaken. At a minimum, the assessment should include the elements listed below.

(1) *History*, particularly onset and predisposing factors. A slowly progressive course may suggest an insidious process (often but not necessarily neurodegenerative), whereas a step-wise development of multiple discrete deficits (including motor signs) might suggest a cerebrovascular cause (e.g., thrombotic, embolic, or lacunar stroke). Any evidence suggesting co-morbid medical conditions requires particular attention, especially if it includes cardiovascular disease, hypertension, diabetes, inflammatory diseases, or other illness that may directly or indirectly, as through secondary complications or through treatment, compromise brain function. A number of illnesses associated with diminished motivation are the result of genetic disorders, including familial types of Alzheimer's disease, frontotemporal dementia, Parkinson's disease, and Huntington's disease, among others. The presence or absence of such problems in the family history should be determined to help guide formulation of the differential diagnosis. In determining the history, all available sources of information should be reviewed, including the medical record, personnel involved in the patient's care, the medication record, the family, and (if possible) the patient.

(2) *Physical and neurological examinations*, particularly vital signs and any evidence of systemic or neurologic abnormalities. In the general physical

examination, vital signs are of importance both for ruling out delirium and for ruling in disorders involving autonomic instability (e.g., Parkinson's plus syndromes). On the elemental neurological examination, cranial nerve abnormalities (including visual fields), motor (voluntary or extrapyramidal) or sensory signs, impairments of gait or coordination, and abnormal reflexes invaluably guide the development of the differential diagnosis; injury to the areas subserving these functions may affect the neurocircuitry of motivation directly or may involve circuits that are proximate to those subserving motivation. Even in the absence of such findings, the presence of abnormal primitive reflexes (see Chapter 8) alone may provide evidence of impaired upper motor neuron (frontal lobe) function consistent with that expected in patients with diminished motivation or apathy.

(3) *Mental status examination*, including both general and cognitive portions (see Chapter 9). On the general mental status examination, assessment of emotion should be a high priority, and the suspicion for depressed mood should be great. Additionally, affective variability in response to humor, sentimental or sad topics, or even mild provocation should be observed. When bedside screening examinations reveal cognitive deficits, more detailed cognitive testing is usually needed to determine more carefully the type and severity of such.

If diminished motivation is present, either the Apathy Evaluation Scale (Marin et al., 1991) and/or the Neuropsychiatric Inventory (Cummings et al., 1994) should be used to quantify the severity of the problem, and to establish a clear baseline from which to measure the patient's subsequent responses to treatment.

(4) *Laboratory examination* should be undertaken to confirm the presence of a condition suspected on the basis of the history and physical, neurological, and mental status examinations. Although there is no consensus regarding screening laboratory tests for patients with diminished motivation, several standard tests such as serum chemistries, creatinine and blood urea nitrogen, liver function tests, complete blood count, vitamin B12, folate, thyroid stimulating hormone (TSH), and urinalysis/urine toxicology comprise a relatively inexpensive test battery that will reveal or confirm the presence of the majority of common medical causes of apathy (particularly apathy associated with reversible dementia).

As stated in previous chapters, we believe that every patient with a major neuropsychiatric syndrome deserves at least one structural neuroimaging study (computed tomography or CT, magnetic resonance imaging or MRI) during their evaluation, and patients with apathetic syndromes are no exception. This is particularly true for patients with only the Apathy Syndrome, as this syndrome is most often the result of structural insult to the circuits discussed earlier. Because tumors, aneurysms, stroke, and multiple sclerosis are treatable (or at least somewhat arrestable) causes of diminished motivation, a neuroimaging study, and preferably an MRI, to evaluate the patient for these problems is appropriate. Even where irreversible causes of apathy are revealed, such neuroimaging studies may usefully inform treatment expectations and prognosis for recovery and rehabilitation. Although the cost of such studies is often used to argue against undertaking them, we again reiterate here that for most, economy of diagnosis means economy of successful, appropriate treatment, and is the best sense of the word "economy."

(5) *Neuropsychological evaluation* is also very important to include in the evaluation, and may help with the assessment of not only apathy but also the pattern, extent, and severity of associated cognitive impairments. A neuropsychological assessment directed toward defining the pattern of cognition and psychological impairment may help refine the differential diagnosis. Further, the results of testing help identify areas of relative strength that can be supported when developing a treatment plan for both patient and family (e.g., medication regimens, compensatory behavioral strategies) and information that may be useful for counseling families struggling with adapting to the patient's motivational impairments.

Treatment

Where a reversible cause of diminished motivation is identified, treatment should be directed at reversing or arresting that underlying problem. In some cases, identification and treatment of the pathophysiological state producing apathy (e.g., severe hypothyroidism, high-potency typical antipsychotic medications) may prove sufficient to either eliminate or at least significantly reduce the apathetic state.

When the condition causing diminished motivation cannot be fully reversed (e.g., trauma, ruptured anterior communicating artery aneurysm), pharmacotherapy is appropriate. Medications with pro-dopaminergic properties have been the most useful agents in treating apathy. While some antidepressants (e.g., buproprion, protriptyline, venlafaxine, fluoxetine) have been suggested to be stimulating or activating, there is less evidence for their efficacy in the treatment of apathy than there is for more specifically dopaminergic agents. Table 15.2 lists medications for which there are reasonable reports (mostly case reports) from which to infer efficacy for the treatment of diminished motivation and apathy.

While the treatments listed in Table 15.2 are often quite effective, Campbell & Duffy (1997) suggest that several issues should be considered when dopaminergic agonists are used to treat diminished motivation and apathy. First, given the anecdotal nature of the treatment literature in this area, obtaining informed consent from the patient and family/caregivers before undertaking any empiric trial of these medications is very important. Once such consent is obtained, a start-low go-slow approach is most appropriate and will often mitigate the treatment-emergent adverse events associated with these medications. Although some patients (including children) may respond to relatively low doses, high doses may be required to treat apathy effectively. Surprisingly, patients with diminished motivation and apathy do not generally develop tolerance to the therapeutic effects of these agents, and may be maintained at stable doses for extended periods of time.

Although many clinicians may be concerned about producing an iatrogenic psychosis through use of these medications, this adverse event is relatively rare among patients without a pre-existing psychotic disorder. However, use of these agents in patients with psychotic disorders does pose a risk of worsening their psychotic symptoms, and should be undertaken with great caution. In these patients, use of an atypical antipsychotic may lessen the likelihood of iatrogenic diminished motivation due to typical antipsychotics and may even improve apathy (among other negative symptoms). At present there is no literature to suggest a similar effect of atypical antipsychotics on diminished motivation due to neuropsychiatric disorders other than schizophrenia. Additionally, cholinergic augmentation with medications like tacrine, donepezil, and rivastigmine may also improve motivation, although this suggestion is at best highly speculative at present.

The non-pharmacological interventions for the treatment of apathy are similar to those for other patients with impaired executive or functional capacity. A structured environment, one in which the team of caregivers, including both professionals and the patient's family, can function as an "auxiliary ego" or a "peripheral brain" (terms used by some of our patients and families), and help engage the apathetic patient in activities of daily living and encourage some degree of socialization and reward. Since the severity of apathy occurs on

Table 15.2. Medications used to treat diminished motivation and apathy. Recommended starting and maximal daily doses of these medications are described in the middle column, and the neurotransmitter effects relevant to their therapeutic effect on motivation are listed in right hand column

Medication	Dose range	Relevant neurotransmitter effect
Bromocriptine	2.5 mg TID – 20 mg TID	(+) dopamine
Levodopa/carbidopa	10/100 mg BID – 50/250 mg QID	(+) dopamine
Pergolide	0.05 – 1.5 mg TID	(+) dopamine
Amantadine	50 mg BID – 100 mg TID	(+) dopamine
Methylphenidate	2.5 mg BID – 20 mg TID	(+) dopamine/norepinephrine
Dextroamphetamine	2.5 mg BID – 20 mg TID	(+) dopamine/norepinephrine
Buproprion	75 mg BID – 150 mg TID	(+) dopamine/norepinephrine
Selegiline	5 – 10 mg QD	(+) dopamine/phemylethylamine
Protriptyline	15 – 60 mg QD	(+) norepinephrine, (–) acetylcholine/histamine
Tacrine	40 mg QD – 40 mg QID	(+) acetylcholine
Donepezil	5 – 10 mg QD	(+) acetylcholine

Notes:

BID, twice daily; TID, three times daily; QID, four times daily; QD, once daily.

a continuum, if there is some capacity for reward memory and stimulus driven motivation, such strategies may facilitate recovery of some spontaneous behavior.

However, when apathy is entrenched, it is often the environment (especially the family) that will be the principal focus of treatment. Education about the nature of apathy, explanation about the neurobiological basis of apathy, and attempts to decrease blaming the patient for passivity or laziness are crucial to the patient and family's mutual well being. Reassignment of the patient's premorbid roles to other family members will likely be necessary, and the family's reaction to such role reassignment should be monitored and addressed carefully. Families with limited problem solving skills and inflexible coping strategies may need intensive assistance. Finally, as apathetic patients are easily manipulated, care must be taken to watch for signs of exploitation or abuse.

Summary

Apathy refers to a reduction in goal-directed thought, emotion, and behavior, and may be a symptom of a number of neuropsychiatric syndromes or an independent clinical syndrome produced by injury to the motivation neurocircuitry. Diminished motivation and apathy contribute to significant morbidity in affected patients and distress in persons caring for them. The neurocircuitry of motivation is complex, but appears to involve an extensive network of frontal-subcortical and limbic-subcortical networks, and their connections to several important brainstem nuclei. The most important brainstem nuclei relevant to motivation include the ventral tegmental area and substantia nigra (which produce dopamine).

The differential diagnosis of apathy occurs on several levels: determination of the correct syndromal diagnosis (apathy vs. depression vs. schizophrenia vs. dementia, and so on), and consideration of the various etiologies for apathy both in isolation and in the context of other comorbid neuropsychiatric conditions. In cases where the degree of apathy is out of proportion to that expected in the context of another neuropsychiatric disorder, it may be prudent to make an independent diagnosis of apathy in order to call attention to and direct treatment considerations toward improvement of this condition.

The evaluation of apathy should include a detailed history, physical, neurological, and mental status examination, laboratory evaluation for reversible causes of apathy, neuroimaging, and possibly neuropsychological evaluation.

In all cases, the character and severity of apathy should be evaluated using a validated and reliable scale (e.g., the Apathy Evaluation Scale) before treatment is instituted and this sort of assessment should be repeated during treatment in order to accurately gauge the effectiveness of any and all interventions. Treatment is multimodal, but generally includes pharmacotherapy (usually with dopaminergically active medications), behavioral modification and compensatory strategy building, family education, caregiver counseling (if needed), and attention to social and medicolegal issues and vulnerabilities.

16

Parkinson's disease

Introduction

Parkinson's disease (PD) is a movement disorder caused by degeneration of the extrapyramidal motor system. It was first described by James Parkinson in 1817 as "paralysis agitans," which he characterized as the combination of tremor, muscle rigidity, bradykinesia, and postural instability. The tremor of PD is classically a coarse, high amplitude, low frequency (3–5 Hz) that is present at rest when awake and absent during action or sleep. Although the tremor may affect the head, tongue, lips, trunk, hands, or legs, it is most commonly seen in the hands as a "pill-rolling" tremor. The muscle rigidity of PD varies somewhat between the upper and lower extremities, having a more consistently "cogwheel" quality (stiffness with multiple "catches" on passive flexion-extension manipulation by an examiner) in the upper extremities and a more "plastic" quality (uniformly increased resistance) in the lower extremities. Bradykinesia means "slowness of movement," and refers to problems starting or repeating volitional movement, reduce motor fluidity, motoric "freezing," diminished arm swing, and flat and expressionless ("masked") facies. The postural instability may result from a combination of reductions in motor fluency needed to make the postural compensations used for balancing, postural hypotension (part of the autonomic instability of PD), and perhaps the gaze disturbances (impaired convergence, limited up-gaze, lid retraction) caused by PD.

These motor symptoms are the hallmark features of idiopathic PD, but may also be produced by related neurological disorders and some drugs and medications. In such contexts, they are referred to collectively as "parkinsonism" or "parkinsonian syndrome." Although the core symptom complex that defines PD has changed little since Parkinson first described it, cognitive impairment, depressed mood, anxiety, and psychosis are now more clearly recognized as frequent comorbid problems that significantly complicate the course of PD. Since we understand that the frontal-subcortical circuits subserving motor function, eye movement, executive function, social behavior, motivation and emotional regulation operate in parallel through the same subcortical structures (Figure 16.1; see Chapter 4 for review), it seems intuitively obvious that PD should include an extended constellation of symptoms and signs of problems in these areas. However, such ideas are relatively new additions to our understanding of PD, and ones that merit particular attention here as an example of an illness with predominantly subcortical pathology capable of producing a range of neuropsychiatric symptoms consistent with the concepts presented in Part I of this book. With this in mind, in this chapter we review Parkinson's disease and offer a method of understanding the most common neuropsychiatric problems attendant to this illness based on the concepts presented in previous chapters.

General considerations

The worldwide prevalence of PD is approximately 150/100 000, and increases after age 65 to nearly 1110/100 000. Although the typical age of onset is between 50 and 65 years, idiopathic PD may develop at a much younger age as well. At any given time, nearly one million Americans are affected by this disease, and many experience significant neuropsychiatric morbidity, especially dementia, depression, and anxiety. Dementia occurs in 10–40% of patients, and increases with increasing age. Depression is equally common, affecting 15–50% of patients, and anxiety (either symptoms or full anxiety syndromes) presents a significant problem in up to 40% of patients with PD. The average duration of illness is about eight years, although there is significant variability in illness duration: some patients' illnesses progress very rapidly (1–2 years) or very slowly (up to 30 years).

Although the cause of PD is not known, both environmental and genetic factors have been suggested. Living in a rural environment has been implicated as a risk factor in some cases of PD, a finding that has led some authors to conclude that in sporadic (non-genetic) cases environmental neurotoxins may be etiologically involved. The nature *versus* nurture (or genetic *vs.* environment) dichotomy is challenged by the increased risk for PD conferred by the presence of gene variants that regulate the metabolism of some neurotoxins and pharmacological agents, certain mitochondrial DNA producing dysfunction of this organelle, and a family history of PD demonstrated in some PD patients. Such findings suggest that it is more likely to be the case that idiopathic PD arises

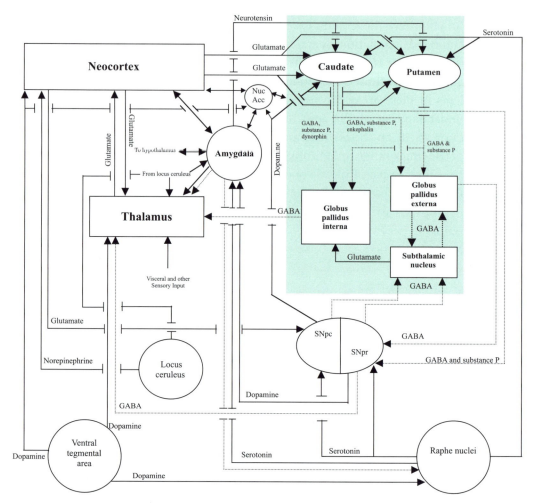

Figure 16.1 A partial illustration of the neurocircuitry of Parkinson's disease. Note that this circuitry is a modified version of that used to illustrate the neurocircuitry of complex cognition. In this figure, network connections between the structures are not complete, but instead highlight those connections most important to Parkinson's disease. Excitatory neurochemical connections are illustrated with solid lines and inhibitory connections with dashed lines. This convention is generally intuitive with the exception of the serotonergic projections from the raphe nuclei which, though neurochemically excitatory, are behaviorally inhibitory at the connections illustrated here (amygdala and striatum). The striatopallidum (both ventral and dorsal portions) is encompassed in the green box, and the reciprocal connections of the elements of this circuit to the nucleus accumbens (Nuc. Acc.) are roughly illustrated by the bi-directional arrow between them. The relevant connections between the ventral tegmental area and both mesocortical and mesolimbic areas are shown, as are the important connections between the substantia nigra (SNpc, pars compacta; SNpr, pars reticulata) and the striatopallidum. Dashed arrows indicate inhibitory pathways and solid arrows indicated excitatory pathways.

from the adverse consequences of an interaction between genetic susceptibility and environmental factors.

Among patients with a family history of PD (about one-third of cases), a small number demonstrate an autosomal dominant inheritance mapping to either chromosome 2 or 4. Again, it is likely that other genetic factors are involved in PD more generally, and additional research into the interaction between genetic susceptibility and environmental factors will undoubtedly shed additional light on the etiology of this disease.

Traditionally, PD has been thought of as a disease producing a loss of nigrostriatal dopaminergic neurons. In fact, patients with PD have been found at autopsy to have loss of dopaminergic cells in the substantia nigra, loss of cholinergic neurons in the nucleus basalis of Meynert (nbM) and the formation of Lewy bodies (hyaline inclusions) in the dorsal vagus nucleus, nbM, locus ceruleus, dorsal and median raphe nuclei, and in the ventral tegmental area. Cortical cell loss also occurs, and cortical interneurons producing somatostatin and corticotropin-releasing factor (CRF) may also be affected in some patients. Although many areas of the brain are affected by PD, those mentioned here are of particular interest for understanding the neuropsychiatric aspects of PD, as they involve dopaminergic, cholinergic, serotonergic, and noradrenergic systems. As has been discussed elsewhere in this work, these neurotransmitter systems play important roles in a wide range of cognitive, emotional, and behavioral functions. From a clinical perspective, this information is useful as it may guide the selection of treatment for neuropsychiatric problems that develop during the course of PD.

Neuropsychiatric aspects of PD

Impaired cognition

Impaired cognition is a significant problem for many patients with PD, with a prevalence of about 10–30%. By comparison, the prevalence of significant cognitive impairment (i.e., dementia) is approximately 2–4% among all persons age 65, with an increasing prevalence of about 1–2% per year thereafter. Cognitive impairment is more common with late-onset PD, being nearly twice as high in patients with onset after age 70 than in those with onset before age 60. The observation that impaired cognition is more frequent among patients with PD than is impaired cognition in comparably aged cohorts suggests that PD itself confers an increased risk for this problem.

Not surprisingly, the cognitive impairment of Parkinson's disease typically follows the pattern of a subcortical dementia. Impaired cognition in PD predominantly involves decreased speed of thought, inefficiency of information processing (bradyphrenia), and impaired complex attention, although language, visuospatial processing, and executive functions may be impaired in some patients as well. Clinically, impaired cognition appears to come in two forms, one being fairly mild and the other more severe. The milder (and more obviously subcortical) type is most characterized by cognitive deficits such as executive dysfunction and impairment of the more complex aspects of attention, both of which are most referable to disruption of frontal-subcortical circuits that parallel the motor circuits affected by the disease.

The more severe type of cognitive impairment involves not only these deficits, but also memory and more global impairment referable to cortical dysfunction. This latter group, identified primarily by the presence of prominent memory impairment, is best described as having a dementia due to PD. Although the severity of motor symptoms does not apparently differ significantly between PD patients with mild cognitive impairment and dementia, those with more severe (cortical) dementia appear to respond less robustly to dopaminergic treatments.

The mechanisms that underlie cognitive impairment in PD may be understandable from the perspective of our discussions in previous chapters. Recall from our discussion of complex cognition (Chapter 4) that adequate function of the frontal-subcortical circuits requires relatively intact function of brainstem and lower diencephalic nuclei, including the substantia nigra, ventral tegmental area, locus ceruleus, cholinergic nuclei, and raphe nuclei, as they project into the basal ganglia. Although the effect of dysfunction of these circuits is most often thought of in terms of their effect on subcortically-mediated motor function (e.g., extrapyramidal motor function), such dysfunction also affects the circuits subserving complex cognition from the "bottom-up" by interfering with the delivery of activating and modulating neurotransmitters to their subcortical components.

Decreased delivery of activating neurotransmitters (particularly dopamine) to the basal ganglia should, at a minimum, impair sustained and complex attention and executive function, diminish motivation, and decrease the ability of the orbitofrontal lobes to regulate limbic activity, and decrease the efficiency and coordination of information processing between these various circuits. While the causes of cognitive impairment in PD are possibly multifactorial, they certainly involve disturbances of frontal-subcortical circuitry resulting from decreases in ascending nigrostriatal dopamine. When decreased dopaminergic tone is the primary etiology of the motor and cognitive impairments, both may be improved pharmacologically by the administration of pro-dopaminergic agents.

It has been suggested that more severe cognitive impairments may indicate additional losses of cortical neurons, including perhaps also loss of cholinergic neurons in the nbM, dysfunction of noradrenergic projections from the brainstem, and disruption of serotonergic function. When dopaminergic and noradrenergic agents are used to treat PD in the setting of predominantly subcortical dysfunction, they not only act by increasing subcortical activity, but also most likely by activating frontal cortices. When the frontal cortices are activated, the circuitry we outlined (see Chapter 4) suggests that they are better able to further increase subcortical activity. Therefore, administration of dopaminergic and noradrenergic agents most likely facilitates restoring the activity of frontal-subcortical and frontal-association area cortices (and hence cognition) to a relatively more normal state by increasing both subcortical and cortical activity; this activity is to some degree self-perpetuating, as increased activity in and between these circuits may facilitate additional activity. Although increasing dopaminergic and noradrenergic activity does not typically restore cognitive functions entirely, many patients with mild cognitive impairment due to PD will report modest benefits in speed of information processing, motivation, attention, and executive functioning.

However, when prefrontal and other cortical areas are affected by PD, relatively more irreparable damage to the frontal-subcortical circuits has occurred. In such cases, one would predict that the cognitive functions subserved by these circuits should be more severely impaired and less responsive to dopaminergic (or other neurochemical) augmentation. In essence, these patients simply have less remaining cortex upon which these agents can act. This relative lack of functionally useful cortex places a ceiling on the possible cognitive benefits that augmentation of subcortical (striatal) activity alone can accomplish. In our relatively hierarchical model of neuroanatomy and cognition, these more severely demented PD patients have not only "bottom–up" (subcortical) pathology but also "top–down" (cortical) pathology driving their clinical presentation.

Psychosis

Psychotic symptoms (e.g., hallucinations and delusions) may develop in PD as a result of treatment with dopaminergic agents or as a relatively late feature of dementia due to PD. The major risk factors for the development of these symptoms are related to the chronicity of treatment with and dose of dopaminergic agents, the severity of the dementia, and chronic sleep disturbance. Estimates of medication-related psychosis in PD range from 20% to 60%, and appear to result more often from treatment with dopaminergic agents (and particularly L-dopa, bromocriptine, and pergolide) than with anticholinergic drugs or monoamine oxidase inhibitors. When patients with PD develop psychotic symptoms, the most common symptoms include unusually vivid dreams with a hallucinatory quality, visual hallucinations, and less commonly paranoid delusions. The dopaminergic agents used to treat PD reduce the motor symptoms of PD by augmenting dopaminergic transmission from the substantia nigra and ventral tegmental area to the striatum and cortex respectively. However, an unintended consequence of this dopaminergic augmentation is the development of dopaminergic receptor hypersensitivity (particularly in the mesolimbic cortex) which appears to facilitate the development of medication-related psychotic symptoms. Interactions between dopamine and serotonin, and subsequent effects on serotonin-modulated GABA (gamma-aminobutyric acid)-ergic neurons (most likely leading to reduced neuronal inhibition) may also play a role in the development of medication-related psychotic symptoms among patients with PD.

Psychosis (usually visual hallucinations and paranoid delusions) also appears to develop more frequently among patients with dementia due to PD. In one study (Naimark et al., 1996), almost 36% of patients with PD and dementia developed psychotic symptoms, including hallucinations, delusions, or both. The patients with PD, dementia, and psychosis experienced greater problems with insomnia, agitation, personality disturbance, cognition, and confusion than their non-psychotic counterparts. Additionally, these patients were less able to maintain their own care and experienced significantly greater challenges to continued home-management.

Although neuropathological studies have revealed associations between cortical neuron loss and dementia, no consistent additional neuropathological features have been identified that distinguish patients with and without psychosis among patients with PD and dementia. The more recent description of diffuse Lewy body dementia, which often presents with psychosis and may overlap neuropathologically with PD, suggests that an increased presence of cortical (and perhaps mesocortical) Lewy bodies may be related to the development of psychosis in PD. However, this suggestion is merely speculation at this point and requires further investigation.

Emotion dysregulation, anxiety, and apathy

Depression occurs frequently in PD, having a prevalence of about 15–30% among all patients with PD. By comparison, the prevalence of major depression in comparably aged cohorts is about 5–9% for women and 2–3% for men. The magnitude of this difference suggests, at a minimum, that patients with PD are at significantly increased risk for depression and further suggests the possibility that the neurobiology of PD itself predisposes patients to depression. Depression significantly complicates management of the motor symptoms of PD, and is often a source of distress and embarrassment for affected patients. Careful distinction must be made, however, between symptoms of depression, affective instability, anxiety, apathy or diminished motivation, and psychological distress due to the progression of PD motor symptoms.

Affective instability in PD and parkinsonian syndromes is characterized by episodic crying, irritability, and sometimes laughing, with an inter-episodic return to euthymic mood, and should not be mistaken for depression. Indeed, some patients with PD develop classic pathological crying and laughing. As discussed in Chapter 5 (Emotion), in such cases there is dissociation between the motor expression of affect and the conscious appreciation or experience of affect. In other words, although the patient is crying and appears to be sad, he or she in fact feels nothing consistent with his or her expression. Although prototypical pathological laughing and crying is relatively uncommon, affective dysregulation that does produce episodes of both expression and experience of brief but intense sadness or irritability is a relatively common feature of PD. As discussed below, distinguishing between affective instability and depression in PD is important because there are different treatment implications for each.

Anxiety symptoms are relatively common in patients with PD, having been reported in up to 40% of these patients. Anxiety symptoms may occur with or without affective or mood disturbance, although comorbidity with depression is relatively common. Anxiety may produce tearfulness and agitation, and distinguishing this problem from depression and affective lability is quite challenging. In some patients, the temporal relationship between motor episodes of freezing and anxiety may usefully guide the evaluation of this problem – motor freezing due to PD may either abort or precipitate panic. If either pattern is clearly observed, and if the episodes of anxiety do not occur in other contexts, an anxiety disorder due to PD may be more easily diagnosed. More mild anxiety states due to the progressive loss of motor, cognitive, and general functions are also very common. Whether anxiety states arise out of the intrinsic disease (e.g., loss of noradrenergic or serotonergic projections), are products of "psychological reactions" to the disease, or result from some combination of these factors is not yet clear. However, the identification and distinction between anxiety and depression is important because each entails somewhat different treatment considerations.

Apathy or diminished motivation is a condition in which the person has lost the drive necessary for normal cognition, emotion, and/or behavior. As discussed in the chapter on apathy and diminished motivation, the anterior cingulate-subcortical circuit and the larger neuronal networks in which it participates have been strongly implicated in the development of diminished motivation. This circuit is highly dependent on ascending dopaminergic input. When dopamine is less available to this circuit, as is intrinsic to PD, its activity and influence on other cognitive, affective, and motor centers decreases, and a state of apathy or diminished motivation may be produced.

Clinically, patients with apathetic states may appear depressed: their expressions may be flat, their cognitive and motor behavior slow, they may respond little and appear to have no real interest or derive no pleasure from their usual activities. The overlap between the intrinsic features of PD, diminished motivation, and depression is therefore understandably murky, as diminished motivation may be an intrinsic and progressive feature of PD itself. However, diminished motivation is not equivalent to depression: apathetic patients lack many of the other usual features of depression such as hopelessness, helplessness, worthlessness, excessive inappropriate guilt and preoccupation, and suicidality. Consequently, a meaningful distinction can be made between apathy and depression clinically, and presumably also neurobiologically (discussed more below). Not surprisingly, the treatment implications of apathy in PD are different from those for depression, with the former being relatively responsive to dopamine and the latter remarkably less responsive to dopamine and more responsive to serotonergically active medications.

Although emotional factors related to loss of physical function and progressive disability should not be discounted in the differential diagnosis of depressed mood in PD, they are not sufficient to produce the sustained and significant depression that is so often encountered in these patients. Grief and adjustment problems often develop in the context of chronic illness, but are typically of relatively shorter duration (weeks to a few months) and of lesser severity than is depression. Indeed, many patients with such illness cope well and do not develop persistent depressive states. However, it may be reasonably argued that the task of adjusting to continually worsening disability and loss of function is never fully completed. Consequently, while grief and adjustment difficulties are understandable and usually relatively short-lived events for most patients with PD, their occurrence should not be minimized, trivialized, or otherwise dismissed and patients struggling with these issues (either acutely or chronically) should be offered the opportunity for counseling and/or psychotherapy. If adjustment and grief issues become increasingly severe, depression should be suspected. This severity issue is particularly important for the distinction between grief and depression: the presence of diffusely generalized hopelessness, helplessness, guilt and worthlessness, and particularly suicidality are not consistent with grief, and should prompt immediate evaluation of and treatment for depression.

Depression in PD may be a function of the neurobiology of PD itself. The observation that predominantly right-sided symptoms (or left frontal-subcortical pathology) may be more strongly associated with depression in PD is highly suggestive of a pathophysiological relationship between these conditions. Such an association is understandable and predictable based on the review of the laterality of emotion presented in Chapter 5. Onset of depression in PD is highly variable, and is without any clear association to patient age, age of onset, severity or duration of parkinsonian symptoms. One possible interpretation of these observations is that the patient's subjective perceptions of illness severity, progressive disability, or loss associated with PD are not sufficient explanations for the development of depression. Additionally, the course of depression in PD does not follow the typical natural course of major depression. Without treatment, an idiopathic major depressive episode lasts between six and twelve months. By contrast, major depression due to PD has a very low remission rate in the first year, and may extend beyond even two years from the onset of depressive symptoms despite ongoing treatment. This pattern of chronic and treatment-resistant depression is much more consistent with a hypothesis of depression resulting from fundamental and persistent disturbance in the neurobiology itself rather than from simple adjustment difficulties or "psychological reactions" to the disease.

While dopamine does appear to be related to affective instability in PD (e.g., crying, irritability, or pathological laughing and crying), there is little evidence to support a direct relationship between dopamine depletion or replacement and depression in PD. Instead, noradrenergic, serotonergic, and possibly cholinergic dysfunction appears to be more strongly related to the development of depression in PD. The intrinsic and interrelated activity of the brainstem nuclei producing these neurotransmitters, the secondary role of dopamine in regulating the activity of these nuclei, and the predictable dysfunction of all of these nuclei and the systems they subserve during the course of PD suggest that depression would be expected to be a predictable and common problem in PD.

By inference from pharmacological studies of depression in PD, norepinephrine and serotonin appear to be more clearly related to depressive symptoms in PD than does dopamine. Where dopaminergic agents may transiently improve mood among PD patients without overt depression, neither the dopaminergic agents nor strongly dopaminergic antidepressants effectively relieve depression in PD. By contrast, strongly noradrenergic tricyclic antidepressants are of benefit in such cases, suggesting that noradrenergic dysfunction is a more likely contributor to the development of depression in PD.

Serotonin has been strongly implicated in the development of primary depressive disorders, and this line of inquiry has been applied to the study of depression due to PD. Patients with PD and depression demonstrate lower cerebrospinal fluid (CSF) levels of 5-HIAA (5-hydroxyindoleacetic acid, a metabolite of serotonin) than comparable patients with PD and no depression, and with healthy comparison subjects. This finding is not unique to PD with depression, as similar findings have been observed among patients with idiopathic depression. Interestingly, patients with PD alone demonstrate CSF 5-HIAA levels between those of healthy comparison subjects and patients with PD and depression. This suggests that moderate serotonin depletion may be a feature of PD, and may therefore confer some increased risk for developing depression during the natural course of PD. Whether the additional depletion of serotonin observed in depressed PD patients represents an intrinsic biological difference between these patients and other patients with PD, the product of an interaction between PD and other biological or environmental factors that facilitate the development of depression in these patients, or both is not yet clear.

Differential diagnosis

Parkinsonism may develop as a result of a number of conditions, including other neurodegenerative diseases (e.g., the Parkinson-plus syndromes), neurological trauma, vascular disease, infections, metabolic disorders, and medications. Levy & Cummings (1999, 2000) have summarized the elements of the differential diagnosis of PD elsewhere. The most common conditions in this differential are included in Table 16.1.

Sorting through the differential diagnosis of parkinsonism presents a complex clinical challenge, but a few general principles may be helpful to

Table 16.1. Conditions in the differential diagnosis of parkinsonism

Neurodegenerative disorders	Trauma	Vascular	Infection	Metabolic	Medications
Idiopathic Parkinson's disease	Traumatic brain injury	Lacunar infarction of elements of the frontal-subcortical circuitry	Post-encephalitic parkinsonism, or encephalitis lethargica	Wilson's disease	Typical antipsychotics
Progressive supranuclear palsy	Brain tumors	Binswanger's disease	AIDS	Hypothyroidism	Lithium
Striatonigral degeneration	Hydrocephalus, including normal pressure hydrocephalus		Neurosyphilis	Hypoparathyroidism	High-dose diazepam
Idiopathic basal ganglia calcification			Creutzfeldt–Jakob disease		Selective serotonin reuptake inhibitors
Shy–Drager syndrome	Subdural hematomas				Carbon monoxide
Olivopontine cerebellar atrophy					Manganese
Huntington's disease (rigid variant)					MPTP (1-methyl-4-phenyl-1,2,3,6-tetrahydropyridine

reduce the level of complexity to some degree. First, idiopathic PD typically presents with at least modest degrees of asymmetry – in the early stages, either predominantly right-sided or left-sided symptoms may be observed. In contrast, parkinsonism developing from medications and toxins is typically more symmetric (assuming the patient does not have underlying but otherwise asymptomatic PD that is "unmasked" by such agents). This distinction is particularly useful when trying to distinguish between idiopathic and medication-related parkinsonism in patients with a condition that requires treatment with antidopaminergic medications (e.g., schizophrenia).

Second, an atypical history (e.g., sudden onset, clear temporal relationship to relevant medications or environmental toxins, recent or chronic infectious disease) tends to suggest a more unusual cause of parkinsonism. In many of these cases, parkinsonism will be but one feature in a much larger array of new-onset neurological symptoms. In cases where previously occult infection (e.g., neurosyphilis) is the etiology of the parkinsonism, this distinction may be less meaningful and the challenge of accurate diagnosis may remain significant.

Third, the Parkinson-plus syndromes usually present with either atypical or additional motoric, cognitive, emotional, or behavioral problems. For example, progressive supranuclear palsy typically involves axial rigidity, a hyper-erect posture, marked paralysis of volitional vertical gaze or frank ophthalmoplegia, and a true bulbar palsy, all of which are not usual features of PD. Diffuse Lewy body disease (or diffuse Lewy body dementia) may initially present with psychosis (hallucinations and delusions), agitation, and depression; parkinsonian symptoms may only become obvious after the disease has progressed for some time. As we previously discussed, psychotic symptoms in idiopathic PD are most often related to treatment with dopaminergic agents or to a significantly progressed dementia in a setting of known PD. Consequently, an initial presentation with psychotic features should be regarded as extremely unusual for idiopathic PD and should instead suggest diffuse Lewy body disease. The course of cognitive symptoms may also facilitate making the distinction between PD and Lewy body dementia. In PD, cognitive impairments are typically mild and consistent, whereas in Lewy body dementia cognitive impairments may fluctuate. This difference may facilitate distinguishing between these conditions, although it entails the further complication of distinguishing between Lewy body dementia and a chronic confusional state (or, delirium). Additionally, prominent early autonomic dysfunction is more suggestive of Shy–Drager syndrome than PD, and the additional presence of marked cerebellar or pyramidal symptoms suggests olivopontine cerebellar atrophy.

Finally, when the distinction between idiopathic PD and the parkinson-plus syndromes cannot be clarified from the outset, treatment response may be used to direct further consideration of the differential diagnosis. Early idiopathic PD generally responds reasonably well to dopaminergic therapy, whereas the response of the parkinson-plus syndromes may be markedly less robust. When the differential diagnosis cannot be easily clarified using these insights, where the patient has a clinical presentation more complex than that outlined here, and/or where the patient has not responded (or has responded poorly or adversely) to standard treatments, consultation with a movement disorder specialist should be pursued.

Evaluation

Establishing the diagnosis follows from a thorough assessment of the patient, guided by an integration of clinical findings and their implications for the differential diagnosis. When the history and clinical evidence suggest parkinsonism due to a cause other than medications (usually typical antipsychotics), a thorough evaluation should be undertaken. At a minimum, the assessment should include these elements.

(1) *History*, particularly onset and predisposing factors. A slowly progressive course usually suggests an insidious process that will most often be one of the neurodegenerative disorders in the Parkinson's disease spectrum. Acute onset more often suggests an atypical cause such as stroke, trauma, infection, or medications. With regard to predisposing factors, both personal and family medical history should be obtained. Although the discovery of a strong positive family history is not essential, and may not impart specific implications for the treatment of the patient, discovery of an autosomal dominant pattern should prompt discussion of risk and early monitoring with the patient's family. Any evidence suggesting co-morbid medical conditions requires particular attention, especially if it includes cardiovascular disease, hypertension, diabetes, inflammatory diseases, or other illness that may directly or indirectly further compromise brain function. In determining the history, all available sources of information should be reviewed, including the medical record, personnel involved in the patient's care, the medication record, the family, and the patient.

(2) *Physical and neurological examinations* are essential, and particular attention should be given to the assessment of vital signs and any systemic or neurological abnormalities. In the general physical examination, vital signs are of importance for the evaluation of disorders involving autonomic

instability (e.g., Parkinson's plus syndromes). On the elemental neurological examination, cranial nerve abnormalities (especially eye movements), motor (voluntary or extrapyramidal) or sensory signs, impairments of gait or coordination, and abnormal or asymmetric reflexes may invaluably guide the development of the differential diagnosis. Even in the absence of such findings, the presence of abnormal primitive reflexes (see Chapter 8, Neuropsychiatric evaluation) alone may provide evidence of upper motor neuron (frontal lobe) dysfunction.

(3) *Mental status examination* (MSE), including both general and cognitive portions (see Chapter 9). On the general MSE assessment of emotion should be thorough and the suspicion for emotional dysregulation (either depression or affective dysregulation) should be high. With regard to cognition, at a minimum a short standardized cognitive screening test should be administered and compared to normative data usually based on age and education. When these measures reveal deficits, more detailed cognitive testing is usually needed to determine more carefully the type and severity of cognitive impairments.

Since Parkinson's disease typically produces a pattern of subcortical cognitive impairment, a "normal" score on screening examination with the mini-MSE (MMSE) does not necessarily contradict the patient's or family's reports of cognitive impairment. Therefore, where the history suggests the possibility of either subcortical or white matter pathology, more detailed (and time-dependent) assessments of cognitive performance should be performed as described in the Chapter 9. Tasks of complex attention (Trail Making Test A and B), word list generation, alternating sequences, visual constructional tasks, and memory tasks focused on the manner and quality of information retrieval are particularly useful in the examination of these patients.

(4) *Laboratory examination*, there are no specific laboratory tests to confirm the diagnosis of idiopathic Parkinson's disease, but some may be useful to determine whether another etiology should be suspected. This is particularly true when dementia is a prominent feature of the presentation, and in such cases, tests that may reveal reversible causes of dementia should be performed (see Chapter 13, Dementia). Typically these include serum chemistries, creatinine and blood urea nitrogen, liver function tests, vitamin B12, folate, thyroid stimulating hormone (TSH), and serum syphilis serology. If the history or physical examination suggest the presence of other causative factors, tests such as human immunodeficiency virus (HIV) antibody, anti-

nuclear antibody, erythrocyte sedimentation rate, ceruloplasmin, complete blood count, and urinalysis/urine toxicology may be useful.

As suggested in the chapters on neuroimaging (Chapter 11) and dementia (Chapter 13), we suggest that every patient with new onset movement disorder should have a structural neuroimaging study (CT or MRI) at least once during their evaluation. It is true that anatomical neuroimaging will often fail to reveal any abnormal findings in patients with idiopathic PD. However, the results of such studies provide important information with regard to the likelihood of other possible causes for the patient's movement disorder (e.g., the presence of tumor, chronic subdural hematoma, multiple sclerosis lesions, lacunar infarctions, or diffuse white matter disease). The results of such studies invariably affect both diagnosis and management of the disorder, even if only to further support the clinical suspicion of idiopathic PD based on the absence of other significant findings.

(5) *Neuropsychological evaluation* is often helpful when the patient experiences cognitive impairment. Determining whether the pattern is most consistent with a subcortical dementia, a cortical dementia in PD, or with other problems (e.g., Alzheimer's disease, depression, anxiety) is often aided by neuropsychological evaluation. When cognitive deficits are demonstrated, knowing their extent and severity is diagnostically helpful and important for treatment planning. The results of testing may help identify areas of relative strength that can be supported when developing a treatment plan for both patient and family (e.g., medication regimens, compensatory behavioral strategies).

Treatment

Motor symptoms

Dopaminergic agents, including dopamine precursors (e.g., L-dopa) or dopamine agonists (e.g., bromocriptine, pergolide, ropinirole, and pramipexole) are the mainstay treatments for the motor symptoms of PD. The majority of patients with idiopathic PD treated with these agents experience significant symptomatic improvement of the movement disorder, with akinesia responding better than tremor or rigidity. Newer agents such as pramipexole and ropinirole appear to be more specific to dopamine type-2 receptors than the other dopaminergic therapies, and as such they may be more effective and less likely to produce unwanted side effects, with the possible exception of psychosis. It has become increasingly clear that L-dopa, though very effective, becomes less effective and associated with fluctuating response (e.g., on–off phenomena) as the duration of treatment lengthens. Consequently, newer agents and other classes of medications are now emerging as first line therapies for the motor symptoms of PD.

The motor symptoms of PD may also respond to selective monoamine oxidase (MAO-B) inhibitors (e.g., selegiline, also known as L-deprenyl), catechol-O-methyltransferase (COMT) inhibitors (e.g., tolcapone), anticholinergic agents (e.g., trihexyphenidyl, benztropine), or mixed dopamine/anticholinergic agents (e.g., amantadine). Selegiline appears to increase the average time that elapses before patients need L-dopa, and may therefore be a prudent choice for the initial therapy for the motor symptoms of PD. COMT inhibitors slow the peripheral metabolism of L-dopa, and may reduce the on–off phenomena associated with L-dopa therapy and the dose of L-dopa required for effective symptomatic control. Anticholinergic agents and amantadine are best regarded as adjunctive therapies, as they may improve the tremor and rigidity not addressed by the dopaminergic agents. However, the anticholinergics may, among their many side effects, exacerbate cognitive impairment or produce frank delirium in some patients. Therefore, caution is warranted when using these agents in patients with cognitive impairment, dementia, or psychosis due to PD.

Electroconvulsive therapy (ECT) is generally regarded as a treatment for depression or psychosis, with or without PD. However, ECT performed for the treatment of psychiatric problems due to PD has also demonstrated reductions in motor symptoms in up to half of patients undergoing this procedure, independent of the effect of this treatment on psychiatric symptoms (Faber & Trimble, 1991; Moellentine et al., 1998). Similar benefit may be possible using transcranial magnetic stimulation, and at least one report suggests that this therapy may be both safe and effective for the treatment of motor symptoms caused by PD (Mally & Stone, 1999).

Pallidal fetal tissue transplants, deep brain (pallidal) stimulation, pallidotomy, thalamic stimulation, and thalamotomy are surgical procedures for the treatment of motor symptoms caused by PD. Early reports suggest that these treatments may effectively treat the motor symptoms of PD in carefully selected patients. However, these procedures present small but not trivial risks of surgical complications, and will require further investigation before entering into the mainstay of treatments for PD. Importantly, several studies have carefully evaluated the cognitive effects of these procedures, and have failed to find significant or consistent effects on cognition, although there is some suggestion that they may reduce anxiety and perhaps depression. While these procedures are, at present, not expected to offer much promise for the treatment of impaired cognition in PD, these early reports do suggest that when performed correctly in carefully selected patients they may offer improvement in motor function without necessarily further compromising cognitive function.

Cognition

At present, there is little information to guide the treatment of cognitive deficits caused by PD, with the few published studies offering variable promise of effective therapy. Cognitive impairment modestly improves with L-dopa treatment, including memory, visuospatial ability, perceptual organization, and sequencing. However, as the disease progresses, these gains are not maintained and cognitive impairment becomes increasingly difficult to treat effectively. Selegiline may modestly improve attention and episodic memory in non-demented Parkinson's disease patients (Lees, 1991), or in subtle ways not easily demonstrated on standard neuropsychological tests (Dalrymple-Alford et al., 1995). One might predict that selegiline would be beneficial for the full dementia of Parkinson's disease, but only one long-term open-label and small sample (8–10 year) trial has been conducted to test this hypothesis; this study failed to show any benefit of selegiline on the cognition of patients with PD and progressive dementia (Portin & Rinne, 1983). Tolcapone, in combination with L-dopa, has been observed to significantly improve attention, auditory verbal short-term memory, visuospatial recall, constructional praxis, and motor symptoms in one group of patients with PD (Gasparini et al., 1997). The pro-cholinergic cognitive enhancers such as donepezil or tacrine are tempting treatments to try in these patients, but one would intuitively worry about the effect of these medications on the motor function of PD. At present, there are no studies available to specifically address the benefits and complications of using these agents to treat impaired cognition in patients with PD.

Given the paucity of useful pharmacological treatments for impaired cognition in PD, neuropsychological (including cognitive remediation) therapies should be strongly considered. Such therapies may help patients develop compensatory strategies that permit them to improve function despite their deficits, and may help both patients and families adapt to troubling consequences of progressive cognitive impairment.

Psychosis

Reducing or withdrawing the offending antiparkinsonian agent(s) is generally held to be the first-line approach to alleviating treatment-emergent psychosis in PD, but this approach is often limited by the re-emergence of unacceptable motor symptoms. Typical antipsychotic agents may effectively reduce psychotic symptoms, but since these agents act via blockade of dopamine type-2 receptors they predictably exacerbate parkinsonian symptoms. When reduction of dopaminergic agents is not practical, use of atypical antipsychotics (e.g., clozapine, olanzapine, quetiapine, etc.) may produce better results. These agents antagonize 5HT-2A receptors (among others) and appear to more selectively bind to mesolimbic dopamine receptors. As a result of this relatively more selective action, they appear somewhat less likely to worsen parkinsonism when used at relatively lower doses.

Reviews of the treatment of psychosis in PD suggest that clozapine is the most consistently effective and well-tolerated antipsychotic agent in this population. In the treatment of medication-related psychosis in PD, as many as 90% of these patients will experience benefit from clozapine without worsening of extrapyramidal symptoms. Some patients may even experience improvement of their motor symptoms during treatment with clozapine. The doses of clozapine needed to effect such benefits may be surprisingly small, with substantial improvement occurring with doses as small as 6.25 mg per day. However, even with small doses, the standard protocol for monitoring white blood cell count weekly is nonetheless required in the United States. Some patients will not tolerate the doses of clozapine required to effectively treat their psychotic symptoms, and others may not be good candidates for this treatment for a variety of other reasons (e.g., medication intolerance, refusal of blood monitoring, or lack of response); in such cases, treatment with another atypical antipsychotic should be attempted.

Low-doses of risperidone may effectively treat psychosis due to PD without worsening the motor symptoms of the disease (Workman et al., 1997), although there is significant debate about using this agent with this population. Although risperidone may antagonize dopamine type-2 receptors to a lesser degree than the typical antipsychotic agents, even relatively small degrees of this antagonism may result in treatment-emergent akinesia in patients with advanced PD. Olanzapine has also been demonstrated to be effective in the treatment of psychosis due to PD (Aarsland, 1999), although it may be somewhat less well tolerated in this population than clozapine (largely due to over-sedation).

Quetiapine may be an effective alternative to all of these agents, though additional research is needed to ascertain how useful an alternative it may be. Regardless of the specific agent used, a start-low go-slow approach is always appropriate and continual re-evaluation of psychotic and motor symptoms as treatment continues is inarguably essential. Where possible, standardized scales that facilitate rigorous and repeatable assessments of both motor function (e.g., the Abnormal Involuntary Movement Scale, or AIMS) and psychosis (e.g., Brief Psychiatric Rating Scale, or BPRS) should be used to establish a pre-treatment baseline and to permit accurate assessment of the effects of treatment.

Emotion dysregulation, anxiety, and apathy

Both tricyclic antidepressants and selective serotonin reuptake inhibitors are commonly used to treat depression in PD, but there are as yet no double-blind placebo-controlled studies establishing the effectiveness of these agents in this population. The selective serotonin reuptake inhibitors decrease dopamine turnover, which may have the unintended consequence of exacerbating PD symptoms or producing akathisia and dyskinesias in some patients. However, this risk may be reduced by the ongoing administration of antiparkinsonian agents. In practice, improvement of depression in PD following treatment with selective serotonin reuptake inhibitors is relatively common and often well tolerated. An alternative strategy is to use buproprion, given the possible actions of this agent on dopamine, norepinephrine, serotonin reuptake.

If the evaluation suggests that apathy is a significant contributor to the patient's presentation (or is the primary problem), use of a more dopaminergically active medication is warranted. The treatment approach may include cautiously increasing the patient's antiparkinsonian medication (including amantadine), using a dopaminergically active antidepressant like buproprion or perhaps venlafaxine, or perhaps prescribing modest doses of psychostimulants such as methylphenidate or dextroamphetamine. The primary concern with these approaches is the need to avoid the development of treatment-emergent psychosis, but with careful monitoring and cautious dosing such treatments can often be quite effective.

If the evaluation suggests that anxiety is a significant contributor to the patient's presentation (or is the primary problem), we advocate combined use of psychotherapy and an antidepressant with anxiolytic properties, and in particular selective serotonin reuptake inhibitor. If these medications are ineffective, buspirone may be a useful alternative. Although benzodiazepines may ultimately be necessary, these medications predictably impair gait, coordination, memory, and arousal in a non-trivial number of patients, and may put patients at increased risk of physical injury from falls or from functional disability from over-sedation.

At the present time, the best evidence suggests that for the treatment of depression due to PD in the setting of ongoing treatment with dopaminergic antiparkinsonian agents, a serotonergically active antidepressant is probably the best choice for treatment, although noradrenergically active agents may also be reasonable choices. Again, a start-low go-slow approach is indicated, although some patients will eventually require standard antidepressant doses to achieve a clinical benefit. As suggested earlier, scales to assess the type and severity of mood or anxiety symptoms (e.g., Beck Depression Scale, Beck Anxiety Scale, Hamilton Rating Scale for Depression or Hamilton Rating Scale for Anxiety) should be used to establish a pretreatment baseline and to assess the effects of treatment.

Summary

Parkinson's disease is a highly prevalent neuropsychiatric disorder caused by structural and functional disturbances affecting (at least) frontal-subcortical circuits. The types of neuropsychiatric symptoms that frequently accompany motor disturbances in PD, namely cognitive impairment or dementia, psychosis, depression, affective lability, anxiety, diminished motivation, and problems in psychological adaptation, are predictable consequences of the known neuropathology of PD and its effects on neuronal networks that subserve cognition, emotion, and behavior.

Alterations in dopamine availability appear to produce not only motor disturbances but also cognitive impairments and apathy, all of which are referable to dysfunction of frontal-subcortical circuits. More severe cognitive impairments are often predicated on additional losses of cortical neurons; although patients with such losses may exhibit some responsiveness to dopaminergic therapy, the effect of such treatments appear to be less robust in this group. This observation follows from our present understanding that prefrontal cortical areas are required for the development and perpetuation of signals in the frontal-subcortical circuits. Diminished motivation and apathy are also common problems in PD; again, such problems are predictable consequences of reduced dopamine availability in the frontal-subcortical networks involved in motivation. In general, all of these problems are best treated with dopaminergic agents.

One unfortunate consequence of dopaminergic therapies is the production of treatment-emergent psychosis. In patients with PD, medication-induced psychosis may occur by itself, or may worsen psychotic symptoms intrinsic to PD. In patients with prominent psychosis but relatively mild motor symptoms, alternative diagnoses (e.g., diffuse Lewy body disease) should be considered before selecting a treatment approach. In patients where the psychosis appears to be related to treatment with dopaminergic agents, the best strategy is to reduce the dose of these medications as much as possible. Where such treatments are not feasible, or for treatment of psychosis due to PD itself, atypical antipsychotics appear to be the most prudent treatment choice.

Depression in PD appears to be related to impairment of noradrenergic and serotonergic function, and may be more common in patients with relatively greater left hemisphere pathology. As such, serotonergically and noradrenergically active antidepressants appear to be reasonable choices for the treatment of depression in PD. By contrast, affective lability appears to be a consequence of alterations in dopamine, serotonin, or both, and tends to respond more fully to agents that increase the activity of either or both of these neurotransmitters. Anxiety in PD also appears to be related to disturbances in serotonin, and seems to be most responsive to treatment with selective serotonin reuptake inhibitors.

Psychological disturbances in PD are common consequences of an illness that produces progressively worsening disability. Although many patients cope with such problems well, both acute and chronic difficulties in coping should not be dismissed as understandable and should prompt referral to a counselor with experience in the psychotherapy of patients with PD.

17

Alcoholism and alcohol-related disorders

Introduction

Alcoholism is a persistent problem in most countries of the world. In the United States, approximately 7–10% of the adult population is estimated to suffer from addiction to ethyl alcohol (Vaillant, 1995), a substance of legal use in several beverage forms. It is a particularly pressing clinical problem in that alcoholics experience a number of physical, neurological, and neuropsychiatric illnesses as a direct result of heavy and uncontrolled drinking over extended periods of time. While conditions relating only to the established and the putative effects of alcohol on the central nervous system are discussed in this chapter, alcoholic persons consistently make up about 14–20% of admissions to private hospitals, about 30–35% of those entering university or municipal teaching hospitals and about 50% of those being treated in the medical, surgical and psychiatric inpatient facilities of the Department of Veterans Affairs health care system (Beresford & Gomberg, 1995). Neuropsychiatric conditions involving ethyl alcohol and its effects are among the most common conditions that most clinicians will see in their practices. Alcoholism itself, like many of the syndromes related to it, is capable of mimicking a great number of other medical and neuropsychiatric conditions and provides perhaps the ultimate example of a clinical entity that requires careful attention to differential diagnosis. For a long time, the criteria used to make this diagnosis were a matter of the individual proclivities of the treating clinician. Since the 1970s, however, the diagnostic criteria for this behavioral illness have received validation sufficient to allow clinicians to diagnose alcohol dependence formally, as will be discussed below. In its many forms and complications, alcoholism remains a clinical challenge as well as an intellectually complex problem for the research efforts of twenty-first century medicine.

Background

Pharmacologically, ethyl alcohol, or ethanol, is a two-carbon molecule capable of passing through the blood–brain barrier because it is soluble both in water and in fat. It has a range of effects on neural structures and systems, some of which will be discussed in this chapter as they pertain to clinical neuropsychiatric problems. The range of effects is so large that ethanol itself was regarded for many years more as a contaminant in biological systems than as an agent with specific actions. Ethanol's principal effect on most neural structures is that of a depressant or sedative agent with a short duration of action; the exact mechanisms for this effect are not well understood. At the molecular level, some effects have been observed that may offer an explanation for this behavioral effect of ethanol. For example, most investigators agree that ethanol acts as an agonist in the neuronal inhibitory system mediated by gamma-aminobutyric acid (GABA) system although fewer might agree on the mechanism involved. Clinically, this view offers the best current explanation as to why agents that facilitate GABA-ergic neurotransmission (e.g., benzodiazepines) effectively manage the ethanol withdrawal syndrome. Ethanol's effects on other neurotransmitter systems, where it characteristically disrupts normal functioning, elude the test of practical usefulness at the present time. Among these are its effects on systems mediated by N-methyl-D-aspartate (NMDA), and on neurotransmitters such as acetylcholine, serotonin, norepinephrine, and dopamine, as discussed below.

As we will see from the discussions of this chapter, the heavy focus of basic research on the neuropharmacology of the drug and its actions has resulted in a view of alcohol dependence as referring principally to the effects of ethanol on the specific mechanisms by which normal neuronal communications are breeched. While this line of thought may ultimately solve the etiological riddle of alcohol dependence, it is important to keep in mind the other actions of ethanol. One of these is its long established ability to disrupt cell membrane coherence in biological systems. While this effect is small and does not apparently alter neuronal transmission – a half degree Fahrenheit of fever provides the same effect with no result on transmission – it may be that this phenomenon's principal pathological role has to do with ethanol's effect on white matter, that is, on the glial cells that facilitate transmission, rather than on the neurons themselves. As will be discussed below, both white matter degeneration (glial) and gray matter loss (neuronal) appear to play separate roles in the clinical presentations of alcohol dependence and its destructive sequelae.

Along this same line of thought, the neuroendocrine effects on the brain consequent upon chronic, heavy ethanol use may also be an area in which subtle actions add up with time (Beresford et al., 1999).

Before going further, it is important to note that some of the material presented herein should be read with some degree of caution, as the history of research in alcoholism records the discovery of many exciting discoveries that as yet have not led to clear answers regarding the etiology or treatment of this perplexing condition. The profound hope for a cure of this devastating condition has driven a desire for a simple etiological answer to a very complex set of questions. The promised answers of ethanol's presumed effects on tetra-hydroxy-isoquinolones (THIQ) as a final or principal path of its addictive actions, and suggestions that the genetics of the dopamine type-2 receptor offer an etiological explanation for alcohol dependence, are only two of the most recent and well known. While these factors may have a role in the susceptibility to developing an addiction to ethanol, current evidence suggests that at best each is only a part of the etiologic puzzle.

While alcohol dependence is largely, if not solely, a human phenomenon, the bulk of our knowledge derives from basic research in animal models. These have, at least for the present, a relatively poor record of overlap with the actual problems of ethanol abuse and dependence found in humans. For example, most of the in vitro and in vivo preparations studied in the recent past have required massive doses of ethanol to achieve a measurable effect, doses well above those capable of being attained by all but the most ethanol tolerant humans, and sometimes beyond even them. Fortunately, newer systems appear to be addressing this problem, promising animal models for alcohol dependence in which the administered doses of ethanol are more comparable to those taken by actively drinking humans (Rodd-Henricks, 2000). Two other examples, the models of genetic sensitivity to ethanol in mice and of response to serotonergic agents that prohibit drinking in rats, have had little crossover with humans, at least to this point.

More recently, some researchers using animal models for various forms of alcohol and drug abuse have espoused a "final common pathway" approach in brain reward systems in order to provide a reductionistic biological system suitable for experiment (Nestler & Aghajanian, 1997). One underlying hope has been to demonstrate that all forms of chemical addiction – irrespective of the type of substance used – may be referable to a common mechanism in reward (or, motivation) circuits in the brain. This model is heuristically useful, but by itself it may be limited in its ability to explain the wide intra- and interindividual variations of effects of potentially addictive substances. At present, knowledge of the neurocircuitry of reward and motivation is very useful for generating new hypotheses; however, it is probably prudent to remain somewhat circumspect regarding the ability of these hypotheses to fully inform clinical observations of alcohol dependent persons. Nonetheless, present knowledge offers a beginning point for considering ethanol toxicity as having observable neuropsychiatric effects and warrants discussion in an effort to increase our understanding of one of the most prevalent addictive disorders affecting millions around the world.

Light to moderate use

In low doses, generally considered as one to two standard drinks (about 0.75 to 1.5 fluid ounces, *c.* 21–42 ml), the principal neurobehavioral effects of ethanol may be regarded as those referable to alterations in function of frontal-subcortical circuits. For example, mild slowing and inefficiency of cognition, emotion, and behavior is a common consequence of mild intoxication. Behavioral disinhibition is perhaps the most obvious consequence of this level of alcohol consumption; one possible explanation for this effect may be that there is a reduction in the ability of the orbitofrontal-subcortical circuitry to effectively restrain limbic mediated drives (those prompting fight, flight, sexual, and appetitive behaviors) when challenged to function despite the presence of alcohol. But ethanol's behavioral effects are probably best thought of as resulting from a broader synergy of several effects. As an example, by placing a major action of alcohol in the several subcircuits involved in motivation (perhaps via its purported ability to increase activity in the ventral-tegmental area-nucleus accumbens pathway; see Chapter 15), low doses of ethanol may initially increase activity in the several frontal-subcortical circuits to which the motivation circuits are related. This may, in part, explain the frequently observed ability of early intoxication to increase in libido, heighten emotionality, and to engage the focus of behavior on emotionally charged objects (or ideas). This latter effect may give the appearance of diminished inhibition, and in a sense this is an accurate description of the mildly intoxicated person's behavior – whether it is truly a consequence of disinhibition or instead an exaggeration of motivation, or both, is debatable. Regardless, the sense of reduced social inhibition lasts in general only briefly and is dose dependent, perhaps with some added input from the centers that mediate psychological expectations of drinking. For some individuals, states of mild intoxication appear to have their greatest effects on behavior, as discussed above, whereas those who are more ethanol sensitive or of relatively older age may also experience motor (reaction time) and cerebellar (coordination) effects.

The occurrence of acute tolerance also warrants comment as a behavioral effect in need of a reasonable mechanistic explanation. Briefly put, acute tolerance refers to the difference between the subjective and behavioral effects of the first dose of ethanol ingested and those that subsequently follow during that same drinking episode. The effect of the first dose is to create the changes described above. This appears to be followed in some way by the various neural systems' responding to a toxic insult such that, when the second dose arrives, the cells and/or circuits involved are better able to meet the physiological challenge. Viewed in its broadest sense, there seem to be an as yet unclear mechanism by which the neurons act to quickly regain and maintain (at least in the context of light to moderate ethanol use) their homeostasis. Alternatively, if mild intoxication involves a destabilization of the glial cell membranes resulting in slowing of the transmission of electrical potentials down the axon, one would have to envision some similarly acute response by the glial cells, again in the service of maintaining normal homeostasis. The extent to which either of these might occur, co-occur, or be joined by some other mechanism remains a mystery. It may be, however, that inquiry in this area can lead to a better means of treating intoxication than those available at present.

Intoxication

As drinking proceeds to the level of legal definitions of drunkenness, generally in the range of 100 mg/dL or greater, cerebral impairment becomes more profound. As studies of professional drivers given increasing doses of ethanol have shown, judgment is affected in a measurable way. So, for example, experienced bus drivers proceeding through an experimental driving course while legally intoxicated demonstrate a willingness to take high-risk chances in driving that they would otherwise not take (Campbell, 1969). This may reflect a heightening of ethanol's effects on the frontal-subcortical circuits noted above, not so much from alteration of impairment of function in any one of them as perhaps from reduced speed and efficiency of communication among them.

It is not that alcohol intoxicated persons can't generate plans of action (dorsolateral circuit) – clearly they can, and sadly do, generate plans such as driving home. It is not that they lack the ability to process socially relevant information (orbitofrontal circuit) – they neither want to be hurt nor to hurt others in an accident. And, its not that they are without emotions (limbic circuits) – they still experience fear, inappropriate euphoria, or both. The problem is not in the absolute cortical functions from which these cognitions, emotions, and behaviors derive. Rather, the problem of defective judgment may likely result from an impaired ability to modulate and integrate all of the relevant and important information in the various frontal-subcortical and limbic-subcortical circuits that is ordinarily needed to develop rational plans. So it is that an intoxicated professional driver understands the task of driving through the experimental course, and is sufficiently motivated to do so, but may suffer an impaired ability to integrate orbitofrontal (not wanting to hurt anyone by risky driving) or the limbic-subcortical information (fear of death or injury) with the idea of guiding the bus through the course. Consequently, it may be that the driver develops and executes a reckless action because he or she is badly deficient in the information needed to plan and execute a sensible action with less risk. Problems of judgment during intoxication may therefore appear more like those that result from disruption of subcortical and white matter functions (speed and efficiency of processing) rather than by impaired cortical functions (i.e., frank loss of cognitive abilities).

At this level too, other effects on cognition become more apparent. One is a mild and reversible impairment of new learning. This suggests involvement of the hippocampal-subcortical-dorsolateral prefrontal network that mediates new learning, although the specific mechanisms by which this network is compromised are not entirely clear. It is conceivable that impairments of new learning arise as a consequence of the neurotoxic effects of alcohol on the structures in this network, alteration of NMDA function involved in long-term potentiation, indirect toxicity via alteration of neuroendocrine functions (and particularly glucocorticoid feedback to the hippocampus), and/or some combination of these and other as yet undetermined mechanisms.

Another commonly noted manifestation is that of impaired cerebellar function. Clinical tests of coordination (e.g., tandem gait, finger-to-nose, assessment for a Romberg sign) are routinely used by police personnel to assess drivers suspected of operating a vehicle while intoxicated, and are thought to indicate impaired cerebellar function. There is some evidence to suggest that among the various cerebellar neurons, Purkinje cells may be particularly sensitive to alcohol, perhaps because they are less able to metabolize ethanol's first metabolite, acetaldehyde (Zimatkin & Deitrich, 1995). Consequently, for these cells a given dose of alcohol exerts a relatively more toxic effect than it does on cells better able to metabolize acetaldehyde.

Looking further down the central nervous system, some persons with levels at or near legal intoxication also notice difficulty in maintaining their wakeful state. This may suggest an effect of alcohol on the ascending activating reticular system, either at the level of the brainstem-diencephalic reticular structures, their white matter projections to the rest of the cerebrum, interference with the receptors for the neurotransmitters projected by this system (e.g., dopamine, norepinephrine, acetylcholine, serotonin) at subcortical and cortical structures, or some combination of these effects.

These phenomena of intoxication caused by light to moderate levels of alcohol use in an otherwise alcohol naïve person, suggests the first principle of alcohol effect or injury to the brain. That is, because of its small molecular size and configuration, ethanol is readily diffused throughout the central nervous system and is therefore capable of injurious effects either through diffuse physiological upset or, as will be seen with chronic heavy drinking, frank structural injury to the brain.

Heavy use

When considering heavy or high doses of ethanol, generally defined as four to five standard drinks (3 to 4.5 fluid ounces, *c*. 85–128 ml, of ethyl alcohol in an hour) or more, sufficient to raise the blood ethanol level above 100 mg/dL, symptoms seen at lower levels of intoxication extend to extreme manifestations in a dose dependent manner. So for example, social disinhibition may rise to extreme behaviors, such as violent, suicidal or self-destructive acts, and may sometimes be confused with behavior seen in other major psychiatric disorders.

High blood ethanol levels may exaggerate impairments in new learning, resulting in transient but dense amnesia, also known as "blackouts." To an observer, the person is awake, attentive and able to converse rationally while in a blackout. However, although arousal and attention remain relatively intact, the person seems unable to encode any of the information to which they attend during the period of the blackout. Consequently, when the ethanol level lowers and the person returns to a non-intoxicated state, they are simply unable to remember any of the behaviors or occurrences during the period of the blackout. Such phenomena account for the stories of persons "waking" in a strange place with no memory of how they arrived there, or being unable to account for their embarrassing behavior at the party of a now former friend.

As intoxication increases, other brain areas suffer the effects of ethanol. Further impairments of cerebellar function may produce gait disturbance, postural instability, and consequently falls. High intoxication levels can lead to impairment of brain stem/ascending reticular activating system functions resulting in loss of consciousness or "passing out," which is often the endpoint of a drinking episode for some alcohol dependence sufferers. Very high levels of acute intoxication presented to an alcohol naïve organism can suppress brain stem activity to the extent that respiratory arrest and death may ensue. An unfortunate example of this is death in an otherwise healthy, alcohol naïve college student who gets into a drinking contest, rapidly imbibing a large amount of spirits or other high alcohol content beverage in a short period of time.

While intoxication and those conditions resulting from it are not clinically negligible, and while knowledge of them is important in the clinical approach to an intoxicated or ethanol poisoned patient, none of the above signs or symptoms are indicative of alcohol dependence or, popularly stated, of alcoholism. Far more subtle and longer lasting neuropsychiatric changes are required before dependence occurs. Current thinking is that neuropsychiatric changes, no matter how poorly understood mechanistically, define the alcohol dependence syndrome and lie at the heart of the clinical term, addiction.

Alcohol dependence

Tolerance

In order to explain alcoholism neuropsychiatrically, one must not only consider brain structure and acute alterations in brain function, but also the natural history or course of alcohol-related brain-behavior relationships. As heavy drinking occurs more frequently, and with greater regularity, chronic tolerance occurs. The brain adjusts to the sedative effects of the ethanol as though the ethanol was no longer perceived as an insult but instead as a necessary part of the homeostatic balance itself. Where, before, the mild behavioral effects, such as social disinhibition, occurred with relatively low doses of ethanol, the ethanol dose necessary to achieve the same effect increases markedly. *Tolerance* is generally regarded as one of the cornerstones for the alcohol dependence diagnosis and may be similar to tachyphylaxis in animal models. Behaviorally, tolerance occasions what may be considered a positive feedback loop: a person who regularly drinks ethanol in order to achieve a specific effect finds that he or she must drink more and more ethanol to achieve the same degree of effect.

Neurophysiological mechanisms to account for tolerance have been difficult to establish fully. They have covered various theories including: (1) adjustment to the neuronal membrane instability ethanol causes; (2) up-regulating pre-synaptic excitatory neurotransmitter release; (3) down-regulating pre-synaptic inhibitory neurotransmitter release; (4) increasing post-synaptic excitatory receptors; (5) inhibiting neurotransmitter re-uptake into pre-synaptic neurons; and (6) increasing pre-synaptic neuronal stores of excitatory transmitters. As mentioned below, evidence for the last of these appears strongest at the time of this writing. Of interest to any neuropsychiatrist, little or no mention of the role of white matter, of glial physiology, appears in most discussions of tolerance.

Withdrawal

As heavy alcohol use extends over time, the central nervous system responds with increasing biological tolerance. When this occurs, present thinking suggests that a new physiological homeostasis has developed, predicated on the presence of alcohol. The ability of the central nervous system to maintain physiological homeostasis in the absence of alcohol therefore appears to be increasingly compromised. As the specific populations of neurons adjust to the alcohol-induced alterations of their activity (see below), they appear to increase their compensatory pharmacodynamic responses to the substance, very likely through several neurochemical mechanisms. As discussed earlier and reiterated below, a very large gap lies between what is known from animal studies of ethanol's effects and the specific clinical manifestations of each. For practical purposes, ethanol's behavioral effect as a short acting central nervous system depressant results in a withdrawal syndrome of central nervous system excitation when it is removed. Most believe that the organism's adaptive mechanisms in creating tolerance persist in the absence of ethanol, but do so in an unbalanced fashion. This results in the classically described alcohol withdrawal syndrome, and may further result in alcohol withdrawal seizures and/or delirium tremens (Table 17.1).

In an alcohol dependent person, approximately 6–12 hours after a rapid drop in the ethanol blood level, autonomic arousal and hyperactivity (tachycardia, tachypnea, fever, hypertension, sweating, tremor, nausea, and vomiting), and anxiety begin to develop. Conceptually, these symptoms are best understood as manifestations of a compromised ability of the central nervous system to maintain physiological inhibition at all levels: cortical; subcortical; and brainstem (including the autonomic system). As withdrawal continues, this ability is further compromised and these symptoms may worsen in scope and intensity. A specific example of this loss of inhibition is the development of marked hyperreflexia and even ankle clonus. In untreated withdrawal, these signs develop over the first 24 to 48 hours after cessation of drinking ethanol, reflect (at least) a substantial loss of upper motor neuron inhibition of lower motor neuron reflexes and (more accurately) central nervous system hyperexcitability more generally, and may herald the incipient occurrence of generalized seizures. To this point in the course of the progression of withdrawal symptoms and in the absence of frank seizures, patients maintain a clear, if not anxious and hyper-aroused, level of consciousness.

If withdrawal is severe, or frequent, or both, the central nervous system may become markedly dysregulated in multiple domains of functioning, resulting in the classic delirium tremens, or shaking delirium. This syndrome is characterized by confusion, delusions, vivid hallucinations, tremor, agitation, sleep-wake cycle disturbance, and increased autonomic activity. All these symptoms are due to the effects of ethanol withdrawal (neurochemical adaptation gone awry) at different levels of the brain. Starting at the level of the brain stem, regulation of autonomic activity may be so impaired as to have been nearly lost – hyper- or hypotension, tachycardia, rapid respiration, altered thermoregulation, and other symptoms may develop and pose serious risks to the patient. Perceptual disturbances (illusions, hallucinations) may develop as a function of autonomous activity of primary sensory cortices (visual, auditory, tactile, gustatory, olfactory), loss of normal sensory gating in the thalamus or hippocampus, or both. The ability to effectively sustain attention to one's surroundings or internal state is compromised, resulting in distractibility and impaired processing of new information. With these functions impaired, higher-level functions (e.g., complex cognition) may be severely compromised, including social judgment, intellectual judgment, reasoning, insight, and problem solving. Perceptual disturbances may then be misinterpreted (resulting in delusions) as the patient's ability to assess the reality of such experiences is impaired. Agitation, including socially inappropriate verbalizations and

Table 17.1. The presentation and course of several problems that commonly occur during alcohol withdrawal

Symptoms	Alcohol withdrawal syndrome (AWS)	Withdrawal seizures	Delirium tremens
Onset	6–12 hours after rapid drop in ethanol blood level	Usually after first 24 hours of AWS	Usually after 72 hours of AWS, up to 10 days, especially if under treated
Prodrome/prognosis	None/past history of severe withdrawal, symptoms despite ethanol in blood, advanced age	Ankle clonus and marked hyperreflexia, past history of withdrawal seizures; head injury	Untreated or under-treated AWS/10–15% death rate when untreated
Symptoms	Anxiety; sweating; tremor; nausea and vomiting	Grand mal, tonic/clonic seizures	Profound delirium (acute confusion); hallucinations: visual, tactile, olfactory, gustatory; extreme increase in vital signs
	Tachycardia (>110); tachypnea; lowgrade fever; hypertension (diastolic >90)		Extreme increase in vital signs
Course	About 7 days	"Seizures come in threes"; rare status	Vital signs return to normal with sufficient medical treatment; cognition may require several weeks
Treatment	CNS sedation	Treat AWS	CNS sedation, usually large doses

Note:
CNS: central nervous system.

aggression, may develop by virtue of impaired neuronal inhibition, responses to hallucinations and delusions, or both.

The seriousness of delirium tremens, which has a death rate of 10–15% without proper treatment, most often results from the profound autonomic dysregulation (resulting in cardiovascular collapse) or secondary complications such as aspiration pneumonia. Treatment consists of providing adequate, usually very large, doses of central nervous system sedative agents, such as benzodiazepines, in order to allow the brain sufficient time to adjust to the normal physiological state to which it must return in the absence of ethanol (discussed in more detail later in this chapter).

Loss of control

When tolerance and withdrawal result in continued heavy drinking, they may eventually result in the person's inability to control alcohol intake. Referred to as the "impaired control" or the "loss of control" phenomenon, the ability to monitor and then to cease drinking once an episode has begun, appears either markedly impaired or lost altogether (Vaillant, 1995). Although a very subtle clinical occurrence, loss of control is a requisite feature of alcohol dependence or, indeed, any other substance addiction. Loss of control is a very complex phenomenon as suggested by its subtle symptomatology, and investigations into its neuropsychiatric substrates have not, thus far, been fully revealing.

Specifically and clinically defined, loss of control refers to an inability to stop drinking once a drinking episode starts. This does not mean that an alcohol dependent person will be unable to refrain from drinking after every taste of alcohol. It does mean that an alcohol dependence sufferer will be unable to limit his or her alcohol intake to a regular and predictable pattern of use for a sustained period of time. Wizened veterans of Alcoholics Anonymous offer neophytes the following test: "Take two drinks, never more than two, never less than two, every day for the next three months. If you can do that, I'll agree that you are not an alcoholic." The loss of control phenomenon makes this an impossible task for most alcohol dependent persons, causing either a relapse of pathological alcohol consumption or prompting the change to complete abstinence from alcohol. Studies of controlled drinking, such as the famous Rand Study of the 1970s (Armor et al., 1978), have demonstrated that the loss of this regulatory ability to control ethanol intake is a permanent loss for the vast majority of those affected by it.

The loss of control phenomenon has lately been given the misnomer of "craving" despite historical use of this term to mean the desires or cues for, or perhaps an obsessive focus on, drinking *between* drinking bouts rather than during episodes. Loss of control and "craving" may be mediated by different neural mechanisms or by the same process; only further research will make this clear. For now, the loss of control phenomenon should be regarded as one of the primary neurobiological processes (if not the fundamental process) that results in ethanol addiction. As such, it represents the primary challenge to understanding the alterations of the central nervous system that result in one of the largest endemic diseases of our time.

Use despite adverse consequences

Tolerance, withdrawal, and the loss of control phenomenon constitute three of the four main groups of symptoms resulting in alcohol dependence. The fourth group results from the effects of the first three – the result of continued, uncontrolled, heavy drinking is generally a social and physical decline. Much of this can be traced to subtle and ongoing impairments in neuropsychiatric functioning, including executive function, social judgment, and motivation. With regard to each, it may be less true that these functions are impaired in the sense of a dementia, but rather that all are recruited in the service of maintaining alcohol-related behaviors to the exclusion of all other social, occupational, and physical concerns.

Neurobiology of alcohol dependence

While ethanol may be usefully regarded as a nervous system contaminant with many effects in many systems, two neurotransmitter systems have received sufficient research attention as to deserve comment. Considering first GABA receptor A (GABA$_A$) system, the regular consumption of large quantities of alcohol has been broadly construed as providing a general sedative effect. However, it is probably worthwhile to consider the type of sedation and its mechanisms further, especially those consistent with the evidence that ethyl alcohol facilitates activity at GABA$_A$ receptors. Given the behavioral effects of larger quantities of alcohol, as well as the role of GABA in the neurocircuitry described in previous chapters (e.g., Complex Cognition, Obsessive–Compulsive Disorder, and Diminished Motivation and Apathy), the impact of heavy ethanol use may be predominantly subcortical, rather than cortical.

Referring to the diagrams that describe the frontal-subcortical circuits and their predominant neurotransmitters in Chapter 4 (see Figure 4.4), GABA pathways (most of which involve GABA$_A$ receptors) are located in predominantly subcortical areas. The effect of significantly augmenting GABA$_A$ receptor activity in these circuits (particularly at the outflow from the basal ganglia to the thalamus) is, in general, one of behavioral inhibition, including a decrease in the speed and efficiency of cognitive processing, but not an absolute loss of cortical cognitive function. This appears consistent with clinical observations that ethanol intoxication by itself does not cause aphasia, agnosia, apraxia, or absolute loss of frontal function, per se. Rather, intoxicated persons become severely slowed in their reaction times and have great difficulty using their cognitive skills effectively. Slowed mental processes of this nature are consistent with GABA effects in the subcortical elements of the frontal-subcortical circuits.

Ethanol also affects the excitatory NMDA/glutamate systems. Chronic ethanol administration results in increased numbers of glutamate receptors in the ventral tegmental area (VTA; see Chapter 15, Diminished motivation and apathy). The effect of this increase appears to be sensitization of the VTA-nucleus accumbens pathway to the presence of glutamate. Although this may not increase the effects of acute administration of alcohol, it may be relevant to the loss of control phenomenon and other addictive behaviors during and after drinking episodes.

Glutamate is a major excitatory neurotransmitter used by the frontal cortices and the thalamus, among other areas. When a drinking person is making use of frontal areas that activate alcohol-related associations, one might posit an increase in the activity of descending glutamatergic afferent connections to the VTA that would subsequently activate the nucleus accumbens, producing two effects. First, there may be an increase in the reinforcement of these associations given their positive effect on this structure, thought to be the "reward" area in the brain. Second, an increase in the motivational state related to pursuit (such as locomotor activity produced by glutamatergic input to the VTA) based on the contents of these associations may occur, resulting in what appears to be a compulsion to find alcohol and drink it, a form of drug seeking behavior. Additionally, the amygdala and the thalamus receive early (essentially pre-conscious) somatic signals that alcohol withdrawal has begun. Receiving such signals, afferents from these areas to the VTA would predictably increase VTA-nucleus accumbens activity, resulting in a similar increase in locomotor/motivation (perhaps manifesting as drug seeking) activity. While these remain only ideas to be studied, such areas of neuropsychiatric inquiry will likely hold useful answers to the puzzles of alcohol addiction and its treatment.

Table 17.2 reviews many of the neuropharmacological actions of ethanol that have been elucidated, largely from the study of rodents and other

Table 17.2. Putative effects of alcohol in the brain at the cellular level and their association with clinical features of alcoholism

Putative site of ethanol action	Clinical manifestation
Increase cell stores of neurotransmitter: a response to ethanol synaptic blocking actions	Possible role in mechanism of chronic tolerance
Enhance neurotransmitter release:	Proposed mechanism of putative "reward" system; possible balance with corticotropin release factor (CRF) and neuropeptide Y (NPY) mediated stress response system
• increases dopamine (DA) release in ventral tegmental area (VTA) and in nucleus accumbens (NAcc), facilitating	
• transmission from VTA to NAcc (Imperato & DiChiara, 1986; Samson et al., 1997; Brodie et al., 1999)	
Synaptic agonism:	
Ligand-gated ion channels (fast transmission)	
• $GABA_A$ receptors (Weiner et al., 1997)	Anticonvulsant properties
• $5HT_3$ receptors (Lovinger & White, 1991; Machu & Harris, 1994; Zhou et al., 1998)	Unknown
• possibly glycine, nicotine receptors (Mihic, 1999)	Unknown
Synaptic Antagonism:	
Ligand-gated ion channels (fast transmission)	
• Glutamate receptors	Unknown
Kainite – ethanol sensitive (Weiner et al., 1999)	
NMDA – ethanol sensitive	
AMPA – ethanol insensitive (Weiner et al., 1999)	
• Alpha-7-nicotine receptor (Aistrup et al., 1999)	Unknown
• ATP (P_2 receptors) (Li et al., 1994)	Unknown
Kinase Activation	
• FYN kinase: enhanced NMDA (Miyakawa et al., 1997)	Unknown
• PKC_{gamma}: antagonize $GABA_A$ (Harris et al., 1995)	
• $PKC_{epsilon}$: enhance $GABA_A$ (Hodge et al., 1999)	
• Protein kinase: enhance $GABA_A$ (Yoshimura & Tabakoff, 1999)	
Corticosteroids: enhance $GABA_A$	Possible hippocampal cell loss: recent memory loss?

Notes:

Abbreviations: DA, dopamine; NE, norepinephrine; 5HT, 5-hydroxytryptamine or serotonin; GABA, gamma-aminobutyric acid; ACh, acetylcholine; NMDA, N-methyl-D-aspartate, kainate, and AMPA, all glutamate receptor subtypes; ATP, adenosine triphosphate; PK, protein kinase. Information courtesy of Thomas Dunwiddie, Ph.D, Professor of Pharmacology, University of Colorado Health Sciences Center, Denver, Colorado.

mammals. Also included in this table is a list of the known clinical manifestations of each neuronal system in humans. The information in Table 17.2 suggests that ethanol acts on a series of neuronal functions directly as well as indirectly. The direct effects include those on all of the primary neuronal functions: (1) neurotransmitter synthesis; (2) neurotransmitter release; (3) post-synaptic excitation; and (4) neurotransmitter re-uptake. At the same time, the right-hand column demonstrates how little is known about the link in humans between ethanol's neural mechanisms of actions and the clinical effects of alcohol. Paraphrasing our University of Colorado colleague, the pharmacologist Professor Thomas Dunwiddie upon whose review Table 17.2 is based (T. Dunwiddie pers. comm.), we have an embarrassment of riches insofar as demonstrating a large number of actions for ethanol in the laboratory. The challenge for the immediate future is to demonstrate which are important in understanding alcohol dependence in humans and which are not.

Alcohol-related illnesses affecting the brain

Illnesses caused, at least in part, by sustained heavy drinking of the sort seen usually, but not exclusively, in the setting of alcohol dependence can be subdivided into two general categories – those occurring because of physiological upset in the central nervous system (CNS) in the absence of structural alteration and those in which structural change appears to be etiologically related to clinical presentation. Of those that will be considered here, delirium tremens and hepatic encephalopathy are generally considered delirious disorders, while Wernicke's encephalopathy, Korsakoff's psychosis, central and extra-pontine myelinolysis, and the controversial alcoholic dementia each appear to involve both functional and structural perturbations of the brain. Underlying these, for the most part, is alcohol dependence itself.

Table 17.3 contrasts the probable CNS structural changes associated with alcohol dependence with those of the other conditions considered in this section. The information contained in this table suggests the possibility that subtle alterations in specific areas of brain tissue may in fact be needed before such profound reactions as delirium tremens can occur or, when present, may limit the resilience of the brain in regaining its normal homeostatic mechanisms, and therefore its functioning, following acute cessation of alcohol consumption. The studies listed suggest that heavy ethanol use, as in alcohol dependence, appears to injure some specific parts of the CNS more than

Table 17.3. Reported structural changes in alcohol dependence and alcohol-related neuropsychiatric conditions

Neuronal or glial loss	Alcohol dependence	Wernicke's encephalopathy/ Korsakoff's psychosis	Delirium tremens	Hepatic encephalopathy	Alcohol dementia	Central/extra-pontine myelinolysis
Frontal/pre-frontal gray matter	All; young age group especially?	Possible	None	none	Loss exceeds age norms	none
Frontal/pre-frontal white matter	Older age group	Possible	None	None	Ventricular/sulcal increase	None
All cortical white matter	All: older age group especially	Possible	None	None	Generalized atrophy	Possible involvement of internal capsule
Subcortical white matter	Older age group	None	None	None	Increased 3rd ventricle	Extending rostrally from pontine lesions
Temporal gray matter	Possible	Possible	None	None	Possible	None
Temporal white matter	Possible and may be related to repeated withdrawal seizure	Possible	None	None	Possible	Possible
Cerebellar/Purkinje cell	Possible; may relate to ALDH isoforms	Midline degeneration	None	None	None	Possible white matter involvement
Diencephalon	None	Midline micro-hemorrhages	None	None	None	Possible white matter involvement
Mammillary bodies	None	Cell loss	None	None	None	None
Pons/brain stem	None	None	None	None	None	Acute central demyelination

others, particularly the elements of the various frontal-subcortical circuits, the cerebellum and the hippocampus.

Since alcohol dependence occurs before each of the other conditions, with the possible exceptions of hepatic encephalopathy or central pontine myelinolysis due to other causes, it is most likely that alcohol dependence sets the stage for the others. For this reason, we review first the evaluation and treatment of alcohol intoxication, withdrawal, and dependence, as the issues considered in these context are requisite elements of the examination and treatment of every patient with any other neuropsychiatric condition due to alcoholism. As in previous chapters, the essential elements of the evaluation include history, physical and neurological examination, mental status examination, laboratory evaluation, and neuropsychological testing. These are discussed more specifically in the context of each of the conditions considered below.

Evaluation and treatment of alcohol dependence

Evaluation of alcohol intoxication

The clinical assessment process may be thought of as a series of steps beginning with acute intoxication and ending in long-term rehabilitation or "recovery." For anyone working with alcohol dependent patients, the most important starting point for any interview is to ask "When was your last drink?" Faced with an intoxicated patient, for example someone brought to an Emergency Room following an automobile accident, the clinician wants to be able to gauge the level of intoxication in a very rough sense in order to sort out symptoms of other acute processes, such as head injury. An awake and alert patient who can describe his or her recent drinking is very helpful, especially when a corroborating third party or family member is present. Breath or blood ethanol determination is also most helpful in this assessment. The presence of stupor or coma, for example, when the blood ethanol level is at 50 mg/dL, or about half the legal intoxication level, suggests that some other pathology is most likely operative. On the other hand, a lucid and conversant patient who says he is starting to feel nervous and whose blood ethanol level is 300 mg/dL, or three times the legal standard,[1] suggests that intoxication occurred at even higher

---

[1] The legal intoxication limit in the United Kingdom, as well as that recently adopted by the federal government of the United States, is 80 mg/dL, while many US states retain the 100 mg/dL standard. For purposes of discussion, we refer to rough approximations in the 80–100 mg/dL range in order to illustrate differences in clinically extreme cases.

levels. This indicates the need for careful attention to withdrawal, which is likely to be severe and will most probably require an aggressive, stepwise detoxification regimen using sedative-hypnotic agents (e.g., benzodiazepines) along with careful monitoring in order to prevent complications such as withdrawal seizures or delirium tremens.

The critical guideline in assessment is to recall that tolerance to ethanol varies widely from one individual to another. One cannot place one's faith in a single parameter such as the blood ethanol level. The history and a physical examination must be done to chart the course of symptoms and their present state. Ethanol intoxication will commonly reveal a disturbed mental state including poor attention, affective lability, and slurred speech. Classic signs of cognitive impairment may also be present such as slowed executive functions, impaired memory, and a relative lack of social propriety. A sizeable number of intoxicated patients may appear to be depressed after having taken a large amount of this central nervous system depressant. Some may describe thoughts or plans of suicide while others may articulate or act out violence towards others.

The neurological examination is likely to bring out other symptoms of acute intoxication, as described in an earlier chapter. These may include cognitive impairment, cerebellar dysfunction (nystagmus, incoordination, ataxia), dysarthria, and an altered (usually diminished) level of arousal. Unless other pathological processes are at work or the patient begins to actively withdraw from alcohol, such symptoms should disappear when the ethanol clears the system. When mental status abnormalities or neurological symptoms persist beyond the period of intoxication, the clinician must advance to the next step in evaluation, and begin to assess the patient for additional alcohol-related (e.g., Wernicke's encephalopathy) or other comorbid (e.g., subdural hematoma) neuropsychiatric conditions.

Treatment of alcohol intoxication

Treatment of alcohol intoxication observes two principles: maintaining physical and medical safety and allowing the body to metabolize ethanol and its first metabolite acetaldehyde, both of which have intoxicating properties. Most intoxicated patients respond to the sedation by "sleeping it off" in a safe place, monitored by family or friends or in the care of public authorities. Those who articulate injurious behavior or who act violently should be monitored carefully and, if necessary, restrained using standard nursing procedures until the violent behavior and/or the period of intoxication has passed. At this point, safety must be continuously re-assessed and appropriate plans made to ensure the health of the patient.

Assuring medical safety at present means delivering supportive care in such a way as to ensure the patient's well being. The standard practice of injecting an intravenous (IV) bolus of glucose into a stuporous and presumably intoxicated patient in the emergency room in order to rule out diabetic hypoglycemia is first preceded by an intramuscular (IM) injection of 10–100 mg of thiamine in order to prevent neuronal damage. Many advocate giving replacement doses of magnesium in order to support neuronal functioning and add water for general hydration. The result of this combined approach in some locales is the "yellow bag" IV solution containing water, thiamine, glucose, and magnesium. In any case, alcoholic patients seen emergently deserve a single IM injection of thiamine to assure access to the vitamin parenterally – gastric erosion and poor absorption of thiamine is a common occurrence in this patient group. Finally, as is noted below, special care must be taken with respect to assessing electrolytes — most notably serum sodium levels — and liver function tests.

At present there is no agent that directly blocks the intoxicant properties of ethanol. In fact, it is not entirely clear as to which of ethanol's myriad effects on the various phases of neuronal system functioning are responsible for what we know phenomenologically as intoxication. Most likely, research will identify a series of effects relating to specific clinical manifestations of multiple systems and various synergies between them. At present, therefore, in the most severe cases where intoxication has resulted in compromise of brainstem function leading to respiratory or cardiovascular collapse, standard treatments are ventilation and the supportive medical procedures mentioned above. In theory, ethanol's actions to facilitate activity at $GABA_A$ receptors should be reversed by administration of a $GABA_A$ receptor antagonist such as flumazenil. To our awareness, one placebo-controlled study of flumazenil use in severe ethanol intoxication suggests that some effect is possible although at doses higher than those needed to reverse benzodiazepine coma (L'heureux & Askenasi, 1991). This agent has not reached common use as an anti-intoxicant, however, possibly because robust GABA antagonism may facilitate the development of seizures. Specific agents for treating intoxication and its effects deserve further investigation.

Evaluation of alcohol withdrawal

As illustrated in Table 17.1, ethanol withdrawal may proceed in relatively discrete stages, each potentially more catastrophic than the last. From time to time new or unusual approaches for each stage of withdrawal are suggested, as for example the more or less recent controversies over whether a "non-medical detox" – waiting out withdrawal without use of sedative agents – can be done safely, or whether withdrawal seizures can be obviated by treating the withdrawal syndrome itself aggressively. The general principle in assessing and treating the alcohol withdrawal syndrome and its complications is to conserve life and limb. For example, those health care systems wishing to employ sedatives to treat withdrawal symptoms only when specific symptoms present are best served by careful surveillance of their patients and rapid transfer of these patients to a medical facility when prodromal withdrawal symptoms first manifest. For this practice to be safe and effective, rather labor intensive monitoring is required to avoid the development of potentially devastating consequences of seizures or delirium tremens and only after such problems develop does one then try to suppress, or just catch up, with the withdrawal process. Similarly, while academic debates concerning withdrawal seizures (i.e., whether withdrawal seizures are self-limiting or are in some way independent of withdrawal) may result in interesting experimental hypotheses for the study of best clinical practices, conservation of health in everyday practice dictates that the alcohol withdrawal syndrome (AWS) should be treated aggressively in the interest of most markedly reducing the risk of seizures.

Evaluation of alcohol withdrawal attends to the symptoms and signs listed in Table 17.1 and discussed above. These fall in two principal areas: subjective report of symptoms and clinical (physical and mental status signs) an increasingly hyperexcitable CNS. As with tolerance, individual variations in the alcohol withdrawal syndrome are wide and not every patient will have every symptom, or sometimes even a majority of them. Increasing anxiety, rising and/or fluctuating vital signs, and prominent signs of reduced upper motor neuron inhibition are each indicators of alcohol withdrawal syndrome and may be used independently as target symptoms when using sedative-hypnotic medications. These latter signs, typically reflected by hyperreflexia and ankle clonus, and muscle fasciculations may be regarded as serious warning signs of an incipient seizure. A previous history of withdrawal seizures or delirium tremens, or the development of symptoms and signs of alcohol withdrawal while ethanol is still in the blood stream also predict a severe course of acute ethanol withdrawal. The effect of advanced age on alcohol withdrawal is somewhat more subtle: two studies done to date have both noted that the AWS seems to be more easily controlled medically but that it lasts longer than in young persons (Beresford & Gomberg, 1995). All of these factors require investigation in each patient.

Treatment of alcohol withdrawal

At present, treatment of alcohol withdrawal includes use of sufficient amounts of a CNS depressant or sedative-hypnotic agent (typically benzodiazepines, although anticonvulsants are sometimes also used as adjuncts) to eliminate the symptoms and signs of withdrawal. When used, gradual reductions of the daily dose of these agents follow effective amelioration of the target symptoms of withdrawal. With such treatment, particularly when agents with relatively long half-lives (e.g., chlordiazepoxide) may be used safely, the treatment of alcohol withdrawal will generally be complete in about seven to ten days. As the extent of tolerance varies widely, the severity of AWS can vary as widely if not more so. Therefore, proper treatment of alcohol withdrawal necessitates titration of the chosen medication with respect to the disappearance of the target symptoms, not simply instituting a standing dose of medication and expecting it to be effective. Alcohol withdrawal is a dynamic process with its own momentum and that momentum can increase if CNS hyperexcitability proceeds unchecked. Aggressive treatment at the beginning from the onset of alcohol withdrawal is necessary if untoward sequelae, such as medical crisis or death from partially treated delirium tremens, are to be avoided.

At the same time, the goal of treatment is relief of symptoms and signs, not stupor or coma. The patient should be comfortable with vital signs in the normal range and no clonus or hyperreflexia; he or she should not be made to be unarousable and consequently even more vulnerable to aspiration pneumonia.

Among the several agents that may be usefully employed in the treatment of alcohol withdrawal, benzodiazepines are most commonly used and are widely available. A few of these agents and their most commonly used dose ranges for the treatment of alcohol withdrawal are listed in the Table 17.4. Titration, however, is still the key to treatment. We have seen some patients who required as much as 700 mg of chlordiazepoxide in the first day to ameliorate the symptoms and signs of alcohol withdrawal without inducing either loss of

Table 17.4. Agents used to treat alcohol withdrawal syndrome (mg ranges of maximum daily dose)

Drug	Day 1	Day 2	Day 3	Day 4	Day 5	Day 6–10
Chlordiazepoxide	300–400	200	100	As needed	Off	Off
Diazepam	80	60	40	20	Off	Off
Lorazepam	8–10	4–6	3–4	2–3	1–2	1

consciousness or even somnolence. In general, the long acting agents are preferable except when hepatic failure is present. In that instance, an agent such as lorazepam, which requires only glucuronide conjugation (sometimes referred to as "serum metabolism") and excretion, should be used. A short to intermediate acting agent such as this, however, necessitates more frequent doses, closer monitoring, and longer use over the seven-day course since the body does not store it.

As a final note, some advocate giving anti-adrenergic agents (e.g., beta-blockers or alpha$_2$-agonists) to relieve tremor and other symptoms of alcohol withdrawal. While this may reduce the peripheral manifestations of autonomic hyperactivity, it does very little to reduce the generalized CNS hyperexcitability that sometimes leads to seizures and that may induce a propensity to more severe and easily developed future episodes of withdrawal. It is with this consideration in mind that we suggest that anti-adrenergic agents generally be considered adjuncts, not definitive agents of choice, in the treatment of alcohol withdrawal.

Evaluation of alcohol dependence

When an individual reaches the point of deciding against further alcohol use, and manages to maintain an alcohol-free life for a period of several months, subtle forms of healing in the CNS begin to appear. After chronically drinking what may be considered a corrosive substance to the CNS, the brain appears to be capable of returning to pre-morbid levels of functioning if structural damage involving cell death (neurons, glia, or both) has not occurred. This period of healing is sometimes referred to as extended withdrawal. In fact, it appears to be a more active process and it may involve re-establishing the circuits of the brain that are required to reclaim relatively fuller function.

Longitudinal outcome studies have shown, however, that the ability to return to a controlled style of alcohol use does not appear to be one of them (Armor et al., 1978; Vaillant, 1995) – once loss of control occurs, it appears to effect, in most persons, a permanent change that maintains this behavior. How this is mediated in the brain is not yet fully understood.

The first step in the evaluation is to assess the patient for problems in the domains noted earlier: tolerance, withdrawal, loss of control, and use despite adverse consequences (medical, psychological, social/legal). In the process of taking the history leading to diagnosis, the clinician defines several items of some prognostic value including an assessment of the patient's social stability and resources and several factors that assess personal resources. These include the patient's ability to structure his time without involving drinking as an activity, the existence of a knowledgeable personal relationship with another human who accepts the patient but rejects his or her drinking, the sources of hope and improved self-esteem in the patient's life, and lastly, any untoward consequence that follows immediately on resuming drinking (Vaillant, 1995). Vaillant observed that patients who could effect two or more of these latter four factors were likely to maintain extended abstinence; those with one or none were much less likely to be successful in this regard.

Once it is clear that the patient's condition merits a diagnosis of alcohol dependence, one must then evaluate the patient's readiness to receive this diagnosis. The extent of the patient's ambivalence in accepting the diagnosis can generally be assessed by his or her response to a non-judgmental delivery of the diagnosis as a medical opinion. For patient's whose ambivalence prevents acceptance of the diagnosis and its treatment implications (i.e., abstinence from alcohol) there is at present very little evidence to suggest that forced treatment produces changes in alcohol use that last beyond the period of mandated treatment. At present, our ability to treat patients successfully requires the full cooperation and collaboration of the patient and hinges on his or her willingness to continue with treatment even in the face of continued ambivalence or distress.

Treatment of alcohol dependence

A review of the many treatment approaches to alcohol dependence is well beyond the scope of this chapter. However, a few brief comments may set the stage for readers interested in pursuing this topic in more detail. Behavioral treatments for alcohol dependence, at present, revolve around assisting our patients to martial their internal and external resources in the interests of abstinence, ideally, and continued health. Patients are encouraged to change alcohol-related behaviors, including breaking contact with associates that encourage their drinking, giving up past-times in which alcohol plays a major role, not visiting places in which they customarily drink, giving up other motivationally charged objects with which they associate drinking, and so on. They must be encouraged to develop new routines or associations (substitutes) to fill the gap in their life created by the absence of alcohol; for many, Alcoholics Anonymous will serve them in this fashion. Although there is no universal agreement about the usefulness of twelve-step programs (e.g., Alcoholics Anonymous) among patients or physicians, these programs can be very helpful to patients willing to engage in their strictly proscribed methods. Their families and friends must be recruited into the treatment plan, providing support and encouragement for behaviors and routines that promote abstinence from alcohol, setting firm limits (sometimes ultimatums) on any relapse in drinking, and uncompromisingly providing consequences for any deviation from the treatment plan. While this topic is broad and could serve as the subject for another book, the works of Vaillant and others offer clinically useful guides to this area of treatment (Vaillant, 1995).

At the time of writing, only two medicinal agents exist for the treatment of alcohol dependence: disulfiram and naltrexone. Disulfiram, a beta-hydroxylase inhibitor, probably has little direct effect on the neuropsychiatric systems that subsume chemical addiction, although this possibility has not been ruled out. Its primary use is as an aversive agent – if ethanol is ingested by a person with a therapeutic blood level of disulfiram, a very unpleasant reaction characterized by profound nausea, vomiting, hypotension, palpitations and headache ensues. Patients are warned of these effects before beginning it and must agree to take it voluntarily or at the insistence of a court. For many, the potential biological effects of disulfiram are complemented by its additional (if not actually primary) role as a reminder not to drink. As a sole ingredient in alcohol dependence recovery in voluntary patients, its usefulness appears limited to only a few months.

Naltrexone, an opiate receptor antagonist, is hypothesized to reduce the reinforcing properties of alcohol by limiting the effects of alcohol on endogenous opiate systems (possibly via the opiate/dopamine interactions in the neurocircuitry subserving motivation) that may mediate alcohol's "reward" properties. As with treatment using disulfiram, published studies suggest that treatment with naltrexone in the absence of a focused program of alcoholism recovery has limited usefulness against relapsing into alcohol dependence.

With such a therapeutic program in place, however, naltrexone exerts a demonstrable effect in lessening the severity of ethanol-use relapses, especially within the first three months of treatment, the duration of most of the published clinical trials (Litten & Allen, 1998). This may be the best empirical explanation for why agents such as disulfiram or naltrexone alone are capable of only short-term improvement in alcohol dependence – long-term recovery must work in a much larger context, one in which recovery is measured in decades rather than weeks or months.

At the time of this writing, other medications for alcohol dependence treatment are being actively investigated. It is hoped that increasing knowledge of the neurobiology of alcohol dependence will ultimately yield more consistently effective short- and long-term treatments for this very destructive disorder.

Evaluation and treatment of Wernicke's encephalopathy and Korsakoff's psychosis

Wernicke's encephalopathy and Korsakoff's psychosis refer to the seminal descriptions of neurological and mental impairment related to alcohol first articulated by Wernicke (Wernicke's encephalopathy) and Korsakoff (Korsakoff's psychosis) at the end of the nineteenth century. The original symptom complex of Wernicke's encephalopathy included a generalized confusional state, ophthalmoplegia, nystagmus and ataxia of variable presentation and inconsistent resolution. In some cases, patients fail to recover memory, almost to the exclusion of clear deficits in other areas, and may develop a state of profound and irreversible memory impairment for new information and, to some degree, previously acquired information, as well as momentary or fantastic confabulation. This latter syndrome is sometimes described by its older (and somewhat misleading) eponym, Korsakoff's psychosis, but is most accurately described as the alcohol amnestic syndrome.

Etiologically related both to ethanol use and thiamine deficiency, the development of these conditions has been dramatically reduced in most industrialized countries by both primary prevention (e.g., thiamine supplementation in food products) and secondary prevention (e.g., adequate education of emergency medical personnel) measures. Wernicke's encephalopathy now most commonly presents with confusion and cerebellar signs such as lateral nystagmus and ataxic gait; ophthalmoplegia, although sometimes seen in severely affected patients, is much less common in modern clinical practice. Similarly, the alcohol amnestic syndrome most commonly presents as impairment of new learning; dense retrograde amnesia and fantastic confabulation are now relatively uncommon features of this condition as is the originally described state of global confusion.

Table 17.5 lists the classically described triad of eye, cerebellar, and cerebral signs seen in Wernicke's encephalopathy. The neuropathological studies of Victor et al. (1971) relate these signs to neuron and myelin destruction in the floor and walls of the third ventricle extending to the upper part of the pons, most frequently including the locus coeruleus, the central gray area of the midbrain and the sixth cranial nerve nuclei. Similarly, they observed neuron and myelin loss in most areas of the cerebellum and especially in the vermis and the flocculi. Purkinje cells in the affected areas appeared particularly vulnerable to injury. The overall damage to the cerebellum led to the conclusion that the disease process interrupts both afferent and efferent signals to the cerebellum resulting in ataxia and other signs of cerebellar dysfunction.

The neuropathological associations with the short-term memory deficit of alcohol amnestic syndrome, however, are less clear. The authors identified neuronal and glial injury in the neocortical areas in about half of their cases and hippocampal damage in about one-third of the cases. Most striking was that there was wasting of the medial areas of the mammillary bodies in all of their cases. This led to the conclusion that severe injury to this region between the hippocampus and the hypothalamus might account for the memory impairment. A more recent study (Shear et al., 1996) using magnetic resonance imaging (MRI) volumetric measurement and memory testing in affected patients has not confirmed this association, prompting reconsideration of this matter. As Table 17.5 illustrates, other investigators have also observed brain changes consistent with neuronal death relating to the combination of alcohol use and thiamine deficiency in many areas of the brain, including prefrontal cortex, hippocampus, subcortical structures, and even the corpus callosum. Which of these observed findings is or is not principally due to the Wernicke–Korsakoff neuropathological process continues to be a source of scholarly debate in the research literature (see under Alcohol dementia, below).

Evaluation of Wernicke's encephalopathy

The evaluation for Wernicke's encephalopathy follows from the description of the problem above. In most cases, the history should support the presence of alcohol dependence and poor nutrition, and in ideal cases information establishing a recent ingestion of glucose in the setting of probable thiamine deficiency may be elicited. Physical and neurological examinations should demonstrate a lack of signs and symptoms of full-blown acute alcohol withdrawal, although a minority (15%) of patients will demonstrate mild symptoms of alcohol withdrawal (Adams et al., 1997a). In most patients, confusion (inattention, impaired memory and orientation, impaired executive functions, apathy), cerebellar dysfunction (most prominently gait disturbance), and ocular abnormalities (bilateral lateral gaze nystagmus, accommodative impairment, or bilateral lateral rectus palsy) are the predominant features of this condition. As noted earlier, however, the type and severity of these symptoms shows significant inter-individual variation. Although patients may be somnolent, they are usually easily aroused and at least briefly engaged in the examination. With rapid treatment (parenteral thiamine and adequate nutrition) the confusion generally clears to a remarkable degree; without treatment, the patient's condition progresses from confusion and drowsiness to coma and eventually to death (usually in one to two weeks). Although a very small group of patients initially present with only memory deficits, this mode of presentation is unusual and may simply represent a group that has survived the initial Wernicke's encephalopathy prior to being brought to medical attention and has since progressed to the alcohol amnestic syndrome.

Evaluation of the alcohol amnestic syndrome (Korsakoff's psychosis)

By definition, this disorder involves a relatively isolated impairment of memory with relative preservation of other cognitive functions. Therefore, evaluating the patient for alcohol amnestic syndrome requires that: alcohol withdrawal delirium be ruled out; the patient is no longer in the midst of Wernicke's encephalopathy; no additional severe cognitive impairments are present and suggesting another neuropsychiatric disorder (e.g., traumatic brain injury, subdural hematoma, stroke, alcohol dementia); and the patient appears to have reached a level of recovery in which memory impairment is the dominant (if sometimes only) clinical feature.

In addition to the evaluations noted above, then, the focus of the examination for alcohol amnestic syndrome is a thorough and rigorous mental status examination. While anterograde memory (new learning) is markedly impaired among patients with this condition, retrograde memory (that for previously acquired information) may also be severely impaired. Although patients will typically have more severe loss of anterograde memory than of retrograde

Table 17.5. Symptoms and signs of five alcohol-related neuropsychiatric conditions

Symptoms and signs	Wernicke's encephalopathy/ Korsakoff's psychosis	Delirium tremens	Hepatic encephalopathy	Alcohol dementia	Central/extra-pontine myelinolysis
Acute confusion	++	++++	++++ (late stage)	±	+++
Residual cognitive impairment	++	±	None	++++	±
Impaired registration	++	+++	++	++	0
Impaired working (short-term) memory	+++	+++	+++	+	±
Non-auditory (visual) hallucinations	0	++++	±	0	±
Auditory hallucinations	0	±	0	±fixed	0
Ophthalmoplegia	++++	++	++	0	0
Ataxia/cerebellar dysfunction	++++	++	++	±	+
Motor weakness	0	0	+(wasting)	0	++++
Autonomic hyperactivity	0	++++	0	0	0
Increased liver indices	0	0	++++	0	0
Structural lesions on MRI	±mammillary degeneration	0	"atrophy"	"atrophy"	Demyelination in pons extending to subcortical structures+++

Notes:

Symbols indicate the relative strength of the neuropathological findings in these conditions: 0, not seen; ±, variably seen; + to +++, seen, with the latter symbol suggesting nearly pathognomonic findings.

MRI, magnetic resonance imaging.

memory (a pattern sometimes referred to as that of Ribot's law), Adams et al. (1997a) note that these patients do commonly have marked impairments for all such information. As the patient recovers from the initial onset of the disorder, some improvement in retrograde memory may occur, but the extent of this recovery is highly variable.

Patients with alcohol amnestic syndrome are also commonly observed to confabulate answers to questions. This process probably does *not* represent a volitional attempt to fill in the gaps created by their memory impairment. Instead, confabulation probably represents difficulty fully retrieving the information needed to answer the question and/or juxtaposing related associations in such a fashion that novel and factually untrue (or at least incomplete) responses are generated. Though fantastic and grandiose confabulations are sometimes seen, momentary confabulations (those that seem to represent partially correct responses) are more common.

With regard to the remainder of the mental status examination, level of arousal and attention should be normal, as should language. Praxis and recognition should be normal. Complex cognitive functions, particularly social appropriateness and motivation, should be relatively spared. Executive functions that are dependent on memory (including conceptual set shifting and complex organizational tasks) may be impaired. Patients with prominent cognitive impairments in areas of cognition that extend beyond memory and its executive function correlates may merit the diagnosis of alcohol dementia in the view of many practitioners, as discussed below.

Treatment of Wernicke's encephalopathy and the alcohol amnestic syndrome

Generally stated, treatment requires thiamine, restoration of adequate nutrition (including B vitamins), and abstinence from ethanol. In the presence of the acute Wernicke's encephalopathy seen for the first time in a medical setting, parenteral thiamine is the first, best step in definitive therapy. An intramuscular injection of 100 mg will suffice in most cases. Excess vitamin will be metabolized or excreted and, as with all vitamins, thiamine and B complex vitamins must be replaced daily with oral doses, unless there is evidence of severe gastric malabsorption (in which case intramuscular or intravenous replacement may be required). When the condition is still at an early stage and reversal is possible, eye signs generally respond first with resolution of the ophthalmoplegia or nystagmus within the first day. Remaining cerebellar signs follow and should clear within several days to a week. The confusional state or the more common recent memory deficit may take longer to return to normal. Resumption of drinking and thiamine depletion may each worsen pathological progression. Most agree that three to six months of good nutrition and no alcohol are required for maximum benefit.

In their follow-up series of patients treated in this way, Victor et al. (1971) observed that about 25% of their patients improved markedly, 50% improved somewhat, and the remaining 25% suffered symptoms that were neither better nor worse after treatment. Their experience has proved the norm for the most part and probably reflects the fact that the extent of neuronal death is the underlying critical factor limiting improvement. Of particular note is the observation that Wernicke–Korsakoff patients did not worsen unless ethanol and thiamine depletion returned. In the great majority of cases the conditions do not appear to follow the pattern of inevitable decline seen in other forms of dementia.

Evaluation and treatment of delirium tremens

While delirium tremens (DTs) was discussed in some detail earlier in this chapter (in the context of its potential progression in the course of withdrawal from sustained, heavy use of ethanol), we wish to highlight it here because of its clinical dangerousness and its relation to the other forms of severe CNS dysfunction. DTs still occurs frequently, even in settings where those suffering from active alcohol dependence are receiving treatment. This includes most general, public, and teaching hospitals. The best estimate of frequency comes from a cooperative study in the Department of Veterans Affairs system (Kaim & Klett, 1972) that reported a 5% prevalence of DTs; this is a high frequency in any case, but especially so when estimates suggest that the active drinking rate among inpatients in that system is about 25%. Left untreated, or only partially treated, DTs carries a mortality rate of 10–15%, with deaths due to uncontrolled hyperactivity of the central and autonomic nervous systems resulting in death from any of several causes, including hypertension, stroke, cardiac arrhythmia, cardiac ischemia, electrolyte imbalance and hyperpyrexia, to name a few. Viewed as a hyperactive, hypermetabolic state, DTs has the potential to exacerbate most forms of underlying systemic illness hastening death or severe morbidity from these other causes.

Viewed as a complication of alcohol dependence, DTs almost never occurs early in the progression of alcohol dependence and, to the best of our knowledge, never without the forewarning of the AWS. Among patients who eventually develop DTs, the prodromal withdrawal syndrome is generally not subtle and can include most of the symptoms and signs listed in Table 17.1. Some suggest that the AWS results in a "kindling" process, analogous to that sometimes discussed with respect to seizure and/or bipolar disorders, in which the occurrence of withdrawal symptoms facilitates the further occurrence of such symptoms, leading to a worsening of the syndrome with successive episodes. Whether this is the case is difficult to say since, theoretically at least, the great majority of actively drinking alcoholic persons suffer at least some, albeit subtle, withdrawal symptoms nearly every day and only a relative minority progress to severe symptoms. A kindling process may be applicable to the DTs since the occurrence of one episode appears to be the best predictor of subsequent episodes. There may also, however, be underlying structural or other alcohol-induced alterations in the CNS that assist this process.

DTs may occur any time from the third to about the tenth day following the rapid drop in ethanol blood level, which is usually coincident with cessation of alcohol consumption. This time course accounts for the not uncommon call to the neuropsychiatrist from the surgical floor on the second postoperative day to assist with a patient whose last drink was the day before his operation. The patient, whose alcoholism history was either hidden or ignored, now appears confused, hallucinating, and with rising vital signs. Later onset, such as that around one week to 10 days, may occur as a consequence of the withdrawal progression or, more commonly in clinical settings, represents a breakthrough of symptoms when partial treatment of alcohol withdrawal proves insufficient to avert the development of DTs. As noted above, the process itself is regarded as a pathophysiological upset, to an extreme degree, of neuronal functioning. It is generally not regarded as evidence of structural injury to the CNS of the sort that can be visualized on MRI, although forms of structural injury from other causes may be apparent. As a result, the goal of the clinician is for the complete reversal of the symptoms and signs of DTs through proper evaluation and treatment.

Evaluation of delirium tremens

The DTs are rightfully considered a medical emergency and may also constitute a psychiatric emergency from the point of view of the safety of everyone involved, as when a confused patient becomes agitated and combative. In a clinical setting, the first step in the evaluation therefore is to ensure the safety of patient and caregivers by assessing the level of agitation and employing measures to ensure safety (e.g., in some cases, physical restraints) in a manner outlined in standard nursing procedures present in most facilities. When DTs develop outside a hospital setting, emergency personnel should be enlisted to promptly transport the affected patient to an acute care medical facility. As a general rule, if the etiology of the presenting delirium is at all unclear, sedative agents should not be immediately administered, as they may obscure the evaluation of patients for other causes of acute confusion (e.g., traumatic brain injury, subdural hematoma) in which assessment level of consciousness is needed to determine the severity and course of the condition.

With safety assured, clinical assessment can focus on the clinical history and on the presenting symptoms: confusion, agitation, tremor, hallucinations, and unstable vital signs. In most cases, the history obtained directly from the patient may not be entirely reliable, and other information should be sought from a third party who knows the patient or from medical records of prior encounters. When possible, the clinician should establish the course of events, the prior history of withdrawal or other ethanol related events, and the presence or absence of other diseases or conditions. The last element of the history includes, in particular, asking about recent trauma (and especially head trauma); comorbid disorders of the brain, psychiatric conditions; intercurrent abuse of or dependence on other substances; and a history of medical conditions, especially common conditions that might result in delirium, such as endocrine, metabolic, and infectious diseases. These areas represent the primary differential causes of acute confusion with hallucinations and abnormal vital signs (see Chapter 12, Delirium). Questions about prior withdrawal should include past contact for withdrawal treatment, the occurrence of seizures and prior episodes of DTs. If available, a description of the course of the last may be especially helpful in predicting the course of the present episode.

Finally, as in the withdrawal syndrome itself, it is important to attempt to determine the time of the last heavy and sustained alcohol use and the onset of symptoms. For example, if the patient had been drinking heavily until the day before, DTs fades in the differential in favor of toxic, metabolic, infectious, or traumatic etiologies for the delirium. Also, later onset of symptoms appears to suggest a longer course of disability and treatment.

The mental status examination usually first reveals a profound attention deficit in which the patient cannot focus on the interview or can do so for only brief periods. Affect is often labile and speech may be incoherent. Simple orientation questions may lead to inconsistent or nonsensical answers – most patients can state their name correctly but not the place or the date, and may mistake their present surroundings for others (mistaking the unfamiliar hospital setting for one more familiar, such as home, work, or a hotel). Immediate recall and short-term memory are usually very difficult to test, owing to lack of sustained attention. This is particularly true of the complex cognitive functions, as they are heavily dependent on intact functioning of more basic cognitive functions (e.g., attention).

Hallucinations are a prominent part of the syndrome and often occupy the remnants of attention that the patient can assemble. They occur predominantly in the visual domain, although tactile, auditory, gustatory, and olfactory hallucinations may sometimes also occur. In general, DTs result in visual (snakes, elephants, gnomes), or tactile (bugs crawling on the skin) perceptual abnormalities. Patients suffering hallucinations whose cognition is, for the most part, intact are possibly suffering from a major psychosis, such as bipolar or schizophrenic disorder, from a medical condition (e.g., hyperthyroidism, corticosteroids), or a toxic state from a non-ethanol source such as hallucinogens. The presence of auditory hallucinations suggests the same differential. This should not be confused with what some have called "alcoholic hallucinosis" that generally refers to more or less permanent auditory hallucinations that occur in a non-delirious state. These hallucinations tend to take the form of self-deprecating or threatening voices (Benson & Gorman, 1996). At present, these hallucinations are believed to result from apparently permanent neural damage due to the effects of sustained, heavy drinking, to repeated withdrawal, or to some combination of these and perhaps one or more other conditions, such as head trauma or drug use.

The physical examination begins with the assessment of vital signs, which may reveal extreme fluctuations of heart rate, respiratory rate, blood pressure, temperature, or some combination of these. Such abnormalities, along with the mental confusion, tremor, and hyperreflexia, serve as the target symptoms for treatment. They are also critical in sorting the differential diagnosis as for example when the blood pressure is high but the pulse is low, suggesting increasing intracranial pressure from head trauma or other cause, or in the opposite case when pulse is high and blood pressure is low, suggesting bleeding and shock. Similarly, fever in the absence of hypertension (or in the presence of hypotension) might indicate an infectious process (or sepsis) and therefore a search for its location and cause.

The neurological examination should include a careful screening for other causes of delirium, as in funduscopic examination for evidence of increased intracranial pressure, lateralizing signs on the elemental examination, and then also the above noted signs consistent with DTs (e.g., tremor, hyperreflexia including ankle clonus). More specific tests of sensation and cerebellar functions are difficult to assess reliably in acute DTs since these require the patient's conscious cooperation. The tremor is typically present both at rest and on volitional movement. Hyperreflexia and ankle clonus, often extreme in both cases, is commonly viewed as the consequence of reduced upper motor neuron inhibition attendant to this form of delirium.

Laboratory assessment should include standard hematological and biochemical parameters with special attention to liver function tests, electrolytes, and altered white blood cell counts that might suggest acute infectious conditions or immunological compromise predisposing to delirium by other acute infectious causes (e.g., acquired immunodeficiency syndrome). As discussed in the next section, elevated liver enzymes may suggest the use of non-hepatically metabolized sedatives during treatment of acute alcohol withdrawal; abnormal serum chemistries may suggest the need for rehydration, and careful correction of disturbances (e.g., hyponatremia, which requires a relatively slower correction to avoid central pontine demyelination). Neuroimaging should be strongly considered, as many patients may not be able to reliably offer a history of head trauma, and the sequelae of such injuries (e.g., traumatic hematomas) may be fatal or severely debilitating if not detected early. Electroencephalography (EEG) may be useful to distinguish this form of delirium from others in some cases, particularly when the classic delirium tremens EEG findings of fast low-voltage activity are present.

Treatment of delirium tremens

Prior to thoughts on treatment, it is useful to recall that the DTs can be avoided in the great majority of cases by proper treatment of the AWS, especially in those with a prior history of DTs, withdrawal seizures or just severe withdrawal symptoms. An ounce of prevention in this area is worth several pounds of cure.

The two general aims of treatment are quieting the CNS and supporting the function of the other systems of the body. Treatment for the first is, in principle, the same as that of the less severe alcohol withdrawal syndrome – give sufficient CNS sedative to reverse the agitation and confusion and to lower the vital signs to normal levels. Most medical texts suggest the use of medium to long acting benzodiazepine agents in an aggressive treatment approach beginning when the diagnosis is first made. Some suggest giving intravenous lorazepam in intermittent intravenous boluses or in a continuous intravenous drip with increasing doses until the vital signs have returned to normal levels. Others accomplish the same effect with oral doses of agents such as chlordiazepoxide, diazepam or other long-acting agents. There are limits to both approaches.

While intermittent intravenous administration of lorazepam may relieve the vital signs more quickly, because of its short to medium length of action (half-life of about 8–10 hours) its effects will wear off quickly; attention must therefore be constant with respect to the frequency and amount given and its clinical effects. In general, intermittent administration of ultra-short acting agents, such as midazolam, should probably be avoided because their very short duration of action risks leaving the DTs uncovered between administrations. Both issues may be mitigated to a large degree by continuous intravenous administration; however, this approach risks oversedating patients with excessive doses of these medications.

By contrast, use of the longer acting orally administered agents will result in a more gradual withdrawal process once a sufficient dose level for control of the agitation and vital signs has been achieved in the first 8–12 hours. Titration at the beginning requires careful attention since these agents require about one to two hours after each dose to achieve a clinically useful effect. An initial oral dose followed by re-evaluation and dosage adjustment every two hours is usually needed. However, many patients with delirium tremens may have comorbid gastritis and/or bleeding, both of which may interfere with the absorption of these agents following oral administration.

In either case, whether using short- or long-acting intravenous or orally administered, under-treatment must be avoided. This requires careful attention to the total dose needed within the first 8–12 hours to control the symptoms, followed by stepwise dose reduction as the symptoms wane. Some use the presence of clearing sensorium or of somnolence as an indication to reduce the dose from that needed acutely. When dose reduction begins, a relapse of confusion or subjective complaint of tremulousness, or an increase in vital signs, indicates returning to a higher dose and reducing more gradually.

With regard to specific patient groups, in general, elderly persons will require lower acute sedative doses than younger people but will need longer to recover in the tapering phase, thereby requiring a higher total dose of the sedative agent. The traditional dictum with regard to doses for elderly persons, "start low and go slow," applies here in part. Lower starting doses are advisable but aggressive treatment in the acute phase is no less warranted. Patients with concurrent liver failure should probably be treated with "serum metabolized" agents (e.g., lorazepam); since these agents are primarily metabolized by glucuronidation and sulfonidation, they are typically better tolerated by patients with impaired liver function than are agents that require more complex metabolism. Elderly patients or those with gastric erosion should not be given oral chlorazepate since absorption will possibly be impaired. Similarly, use of intramuscular long acting benzodiazepines usually results in poor or erratic absorption and should be avoided.

With respect to the use of other agents affecting the CNS during treatment of DTs, very low doses of antipsychotic agents, such as 1 to 2 mg of haloperidol or 0.25 mg of risperidone, may reduce perceptual disturbances such as hallucinations and illusions. There is some, albeit relatively low, risk of lowering seizure threshold with these agents; however, this risk must be weighed against the benefit of reduced psychosis and agitation gained by their use. Patients with a history of prior seizures from any cause should be treated with the benzodiazepines exclusively, if possible. Some have recently suggested anticonvulsants, such as valproic acid, as useful primary or adjunctive agents but this has yet to be demonstrated as superior to the anxiolytic sedatives.

Last, supportive care for DTs should involve admission to an intensive care unit during the acute phase of the syndrome. Support entails proper nutrition and hydration, including thiamine, magnesium, electrolytes, and glucose as noted above. Nursing care may be necessary for a period longer than that required for treatment of the acute delirium, as full cognitive recovery, and therefore a safe return to independent functioning, may often be delayed beyond the period of the acute delirium. This is especially true in older patients or in those who have suffered previous episodes.

Evaluation and treatment of hepatic encephalopathy

As illustrated in Table 17.5, this condition refers to an acute loss of complex and some basic cognitive abilities in the presence of elevated tests of liver function. Since about 15% of alcohol dependent persons suffer liver failure during the course of this condition, hepatic encephalopathy is often a consequence of alcoholism, although an indirect one. Recent investigation (Schomerus & Hamster, 1998) suggests that the delirious process of hepatic encephalopathy is independent of other ethanol CNS effects, a suggestion that counters some of the current clinical wisdom. Similarly, a long held belief was that the pathophysiological mechanism of hepatic encephalopathy was disruption of neural transmission by high levels of circulating ammonia due to impaired protein metabolism in the liver. While this factor may play a significant role in the genesis of the encephalopathy, the actual mechanism or mechanisms remains less definitively understood. Controlled studies of reversal of some severe forms of hepatic encephalopathy, including deep coma, by the $GABA_A$ antagonist, flumazenil, suggest possible GABA involvement in this form of delirium (Gyr et al. 1996).

Evaluation of hepatic encephalopathy

As with any acute confusional state, the assessment of hepatic encephalopathy requires the careful attention to history, physical and neurological examinations, and mental status examination as described in Chapter 12 (and therefore not repeated here). By definition, laboratory tests of hepatic function, particularly the bilirubin and the transaminases, are the principal chemical indicators of the extent and type of hepatic failure. The bilirubin correlates roughly with mental status change only at very high levels, however, and the transaminases may be raised one hundred fold with little concomitant change in mental status, as seen in combined ethanol and acetaminophen overdose cases. It is best, therefore, to recognize the presence of liver failure but to focus on changes in the mental state when attempting to diagnose hepatic encephalopathy. Further, the term itself carries different meanings for different people. To the gastroenterologist, it may mean a state of confusion just short of stupor and coma. To the neuropsychiatrist, however, it means a demonstrable loss of cognitive function such as may be seen in any delirium.

In mild to moderate cases, mental status examination often reflects difficulty with concentration and complex attention, affective lability, difficulty with short-term memory, calculations, and other aspects of complex cognition such as abstraction, problem solving, judgment, and insight. As in most deliria, not every patient will have problems in all of these cognitive functions. Note too that in the setting of alcohol dependence, problems in these areas may be easily mistaken for intoxication, depression, or Wernicke's encephalopathy. With the exception of an immediate breath or blood ethanol determination and a screen for addictive substances in those with substance dependence histories, these diagnostic considerations should be suspended until the underlying exacerbation of the liver disease can be reversed and the patient evaluated a second time. As liver failure progresses or as hyperammonemia rises to perilous levels, the moderate changes in mental state may worsen to outright confusion and disorientation and may progress to stupor and to coma.

The neurological examination generally reveals non-lateralizing changes consistent with delirium, including findings such as tremor, hyperreflexia and occasionally ankle clonus, nystagmus, and primitive reflexes. In more severe cases, fasciculations (sometimes most obvious in the tongue although also present elsewhere) and asterixis ("liver flap") may also be observed.

Noting the possible exception of an alcoholic person with hepatic encephalopathy who has had a liver transplant, most patients with hepatic encephalopathy do not require neuroimaging unless the clinician suspects some other injurious process such as stroke or head trauma. In some cases, EEG may be useful – hepatic encephalopathy is associated with a characteristic (although not pathognomonic) finding, triphasic waves (also referred to as blunt spike and wave, pseudoparoxysmal spike and wave). While this EEG pattern is most commonly seen among patients with impending or frank hepatic coma, and may also be seen among patients with other encephalopathies, when present in a patient with a severe delirium due to hepatic failure it may help support this diagnosis.

Treatment of hepatic encephalopathy

Treatment of the underlying hepatic crisis will reverse hepatic encephalopathy in all but the last stages of liver failure. Commonly, a low protein (low nitrogen) diet and the prescription of lactulose will control the ammonia levels and allow the encephalopathy to clear. As in other examples of alcohol-related illnesses, abstinence allowing for the healing and subsequent obviation of alcoholic hepatitis will result in extended good hepatic and thereby cognitive function. One series documents such improvements as continuing for as long as 18 months (Lucey et al., 1992).

When these measures prove insufficient, the clinician may try a very low dose of a neuroleptic as in other delirious states, with the prior cautions regarding alteration of seizure threshold also occurring in this situation. At this point, use of other psychoactive medicines should be avoided, especially benzodiazepines, since they may exacerbate or mask symptoms of the delirium. If needed in extreme cases, as for example when a patient's wishes with respect to heroic medical care must be assessed, flumazenil, mentioned above, may be tried. Systematic trials (Gyr et al. 1996; Barbaro et al., 1998a,b) suggest that flumazenil may transiently reverse hepatic encephalopathy to some degree in about 20% of severely ill patients. Since it appears that the dose needed for reversal varies from patient to patient and because the seizure risk is high in alcoholic patients, a very low starting dose is suggested. Depending on the effect, the dose may thereafter be increased. Flumazenil's half-life is short, about one hour for most people, and in the event of overdose of this agent its effects can be inhibited competitively by agents that facilitate action at $GABA_A$ receptors (e.g., benzodiazepines, such as midazolam or lorazepam).

Evaluation and treatment of alcohol dementia

Clinicians who diagnose and treat the damage to the CNS resulting from alcohol dependence have long had the uneasy sense that there was more to chronic ethanol-induced brain injury than that attributable entirely to Wernicke's encephalopathy or Korsakoff's psychosis. Cutting (1979, 1982), Lishman et al. (1987), Lishman (1990), and others suggested that there might be room to consider direct ethanol injury to the brain, that is, an alcohol dementia. The principal reason for this came from the observation that some alcohol dependent individuals experience marked cognitive impairment in multiple domains of function, not just memory. At the same time, they and others noted that persons so affected generally do not experience a progressive cognitive decline, such as that observed in patients with Alzheimer's disease. Instead, some of these patients demonstrate a static or even slowly improving dementia following cessation of alcohol consumption and after acute withdrawal is over.

Computed tomographic (CT) scan studies in the 1970s and 1980s revealed apparent support for the notion of alcohol dementia by revealing atrophic changes (sulcal widening and ventricular enlargement) in the brains of alcohol dependent patients. These findings were hailed as indications of an underlying dementing process caused by alcohol, at least until subsequent studies noted that the atrophic changes mostly reversed themselves after three to six months of abstinence and that the apparent atrophy was not associated with concomitant loss of intellectual functioning on neuropsychological testing. Since that time, controversy regarding the legitimacy of the concept and diagnosis of alcohol dementia has persisted, with some authors suggesting that Wernicke–Korsakoff pathophysiological processes entirely account for any overt "dementia" due to alcohol and others asserting that ethanol itself produces sufficient neural or glial injury so as to produce an alcohol dementia. Some have sought to solve the puzzle by proposing specific criteria for alcohol dementia involving course, concurrent peripheral neuropathy, and other such clinical observations (Smith & Atkinson 1995; Oslin et al., 1998). These, however, do not address what amounts to a fundamental problem of the neuropathology that distinguishes between Wernicke's encephalopathy, Korsakoff's syndrome, and direct ethanol-induced brain injury.

Nonetheless, inquiry has proceeded with the advent of new techniques, such as MRI volumetric analysis, neuronal counting and others. Table 17.6 lists the studies done in the past 10 years that address the pathology of alcohol dementia with an eye to structural changes in the brains of alcohol dependent persons. First, it will be noted that changes appear to occur both to neuronal populations (gray matter) and to glial cells (white matter). Second, these investigations appear to support the notion of regional vulnerability to alcohol-related injury, particularly the frontal cortex, subcortical white matter, thalamus, hypothalamus and probably hippocampus. While these observations do not solve the controversy, they suggest that damage may be more widespread than that reported for Wernicke's encephalopathy and also that investigations should consider damage both to neurons and to glial cells as having a role in the process. At the same time, those few recent studies in which neuropsychological testing and brain structure investigations appear to converge suggest that there may indeed be correlations between specific neuropathological changes and specific brain functions. The most convincing of these at present is the relationship of prefrontal gray and white changes and the impairment of executive functions.

Evaluation of alcohol dementia

Practically speaking, we are a long way from advancing beyond the original diagnostic conceptualization of alcohol dementia. In general, patients will demonstrate cognitive impairments that extend beyond those of alcohol amnestic syndrome, meaning that if memory impairment is present it is not present as the dominant or only feature. Many of these patients demonstrate problems with executive function, reduced speed and efficiency of processing, and may resemble patients with white matter/subcortical dementias from other causes (e.g., multiple sclerosis). However, since there is, as of yet, no universal agreement on the existence of alcohol dementia there are of course no clearly accepted definitions of the disorder itself. Further research is needed to clarify both whether there is an alcohol dementia and, if so, how best to characterize it clinically.

Therefore, alcohol dementia is, at this time, a diagnosis of exclusion. The differential includes that discussed in Chapter 13 and is extensive. Special attention should be given to the exclusion of the alcohol-related illnesses mentioned in this section, with the addition of Marchiafava–Bignami disease. In this condition the corpus callosum degenerates, largely through injury to the glia and to the interhemispheric axons, resulting in a partial disconnection between the two cerebral hemispheres. While some argue that it is, and others that it is not, another example of the neuropathology related to Wernicke's encephalopathy, its clinical presentation is very subtle and nearly always occurs in the presence of other injuries to the brain such as those listed in Table 17.6. The result is that callosal degeneration generally presents as part of a larger picture of cognitive impairment rather than as a specific group of obvious clinical symptoms unique to it.

Physical examination, unfortunately, is no more specific for this entity except insofar as to rule out the other ethanol related conditions and sequelae mentioned in this chapter. While some believe that the classically described peripheral loss of sensation due to alcoholism (alcohol neuropathy) is part of the degenerative process and should be counted as part of the alcohol dementia syndrome, the association between cognitive and sensory loss requires further investigation before both can be claimed as resulting from direct ethanol neurotoxicity.

Treatment of alcohol dementia

In the absence of more specific diagnostic criteria, it is difficult to describe specific treatment. As discussed in Chapter 13, some patients may receive a maximum use benefit from agents that boost one or another of the intact neural systems. Some with behavioral disturbances attendant to their dementia, particularly agitation precipitated by delusions or hallucination or that is otherwise very severe, may be helped by dopamine blocking agents, either in the form of the typical antipsychotics or some of the atypical antipsychotics (e.g., risperidone). Others may be helped by cholinesterase inhibitors recently available in this country for use in other forms of dementia, although there is no literature to support this treatment at the time of this writing. Still others, as discussed in the section on central pontine myelinolysis, may potentially be

Table 17.6. Recent studies of alcohol-induced brain injury

Study	"Alcoholic" N	Control N	Method	Gray matter loss	White matter loss
Jernigan et al., 1991	28	36, matched	MRI	Cortical Subcortical	Diencephalon Caudate Dorsolateral frontal and parietal cortex Mesial temporal lobe
Hansen et al., 1991	5 dogs		Neuropath	Temporal cortex	Temporal and frontal cortex
Mutzell, 1991 (subgroup of heavy drinking plus "hepatotoxic" drug use)		195, non-alcoholics	CT	Cortical	Cortical and subcortical
Mutzell, 1992	211	Above	CT	Cortical	Cortical and subcortical
Mann et al., 1992	14 females 51 males		CT		
Ronty et al., 1997 (brain trauma subjects)	15	41	CT		CSF volume increase
Jensen & Pakkenberg, 1993	11	11, matched	Neuropath: Neuron counts	No difference	Subcortex
Pfefferbaum et al., 1993	28 males	85 males			Ventricular and sulcal volume > age expectation
Di Sclafani et al., 1995	14 elderly males resident	11, matched	MRI	No difference	No difference
Sullivan et al., 1995	47	72	MRI	Temporal cortex	Subcortex
Emsley et al., 1996	19 Korsakoff 17 non-amnesic	23	MRI	Subcortex	Subcortex

Study	Sample		Method	Region	Findings
Sullivan et al., 1996	11 w/seizures	35 seizure free			Temporal and frontal-parietal cortex; Frontal-parietal cortex only
Kril et al., 1997	14 • 4 W–K syndrome • 4 Wernicke's alone • 6 non W–K		Neuropath: neuron counts	Superior frontal	Frontal • cortex, subcortex, medial temporal • same as above
Sullivan et al., 1998	62	71, schizophrenia 73, non-alcoholics	MRI	Cortex	Alcoholics only
Pfefferbaum et al., 1998	16: 5 year follow-up	28	MRI	Anterior superior temporal	
Dao-Castellana et al., 1998	17		FDG-PET	(cortical hypometabolism)	
Oishi et al., 1999	15 non-Marchiafava Bignami	15 matched	MRI Xenon-CT	(decreased flow: cerebral cortex, thalamus, putamen)	Callosal wasting
Baker et al., 1999	?? thiamine deficient		Neuropath	Purkinje cell loss	vermis

Notes:

W–K syndrome, Wernicke–Korsakoff syndrome; MRI, magnetic resonance imaging; CT, computed tomography; FDG-PET, flurodeoxyglucose-positron emission tomography helped by stimulants, or perhaps by antidepressant agents. At present, there is very little clinical research to enlighten this subject.

At the same time, supportive treatment, especially abstinence from alcohol and adequate nutrition, is critical to reducing the likelihood of continued deterioration and/or facilitating improvement. Effecting abstinence from alcohol in persons with alcohol dementia is often a greater challenge than that faced by most non-impaired alcohol dependent people. Standard behavioral treatment of alcohol dependence requires the ability to learn and develop new, more adaptive, coping strategies that reduce the likelihood of relapsing alcohol dependence. These abilities may be compromised by alcohol dementia, and may thereby reduce the likelihood of achieving abstinence from alcohol in these patients. Additional environmental structure, such as long-term residence in a nursing home or domicillary, where behavior can be monitored may be needed to afford the sort of stability that facilitates recovery. Disulfiram may be useful in such patients as well, so long as there is sufficient cognition as to allow for a clear understanding of the consequences of drinking while on that medication. To our knowledge, naltrexone has not been tried in this patient group although it may potentially be of use.

Evaluation and treatment of central pontine myelinolysis

If Wernicke's encephalopathy and Korsakoff's psychosis reflect a process of neuronal death, and alcohol dementia suggests both neuronal (gray matter) and glial (white matter) degeneration, central pontine myelinolysis (CPM) appears to be predominantly, if not purely, a white matter disease. This relatively infrequent condition was so named because of the apparent lysis of the myelin sheaths insulating the nerve fibers of the central pons. CPM is most likely the result of large, rapid shifts in serum osmolality, as seen in rapid correction of hyponatremia, hyperglycemia, or as may be attendant to otherwise occult electrolyte disturbances in chronic alcoholism. The myelinolysis may extend rostrally to include basal ganglia structures, especially the caudate, putamen, thalamus and medical temporal structures. Lesions in these areas may disrupt the function of frontal-subcortical circuits, including the dorsolateral prefrontal, lateral orbitofrontal, and anterior cingulate circuits. The result may be a clinical picture that looks very much like a dementing process involving the frontal lobes, with slowing and inefficiency of cognition, impaired social propriety, and markedly decreased motivation and energy.

As Table 17.5 suggests, the evaluation seeks to differentiate CPM from the other conditions listed as frequent in alcohol dependent patients. While confusion and cerebellar incoordination are common to other ethanol-related syndromes, motor weakness and hyponatremia, with or without a recent or immediate history of rapid correction, are generally not. These two findings, when present in the group of symptoms, indicate the necessity of neuroimaging to assess for CPM, with MRI being the preferred modality (over CT imaging) given its sensitivity to white matter pathology and superior ability to image the brainstem.

Treatment for this condition at present requires slow correction of the hyponatremia, good nutrition and the lack of ethanol, in the hope of myelin healing or regeneration. The few reports of follow-up MRI studies suggest that the white matter lesions are very slow to return to a normal state, if in fact they ever do so. However, the persistence of white matter lesions does not necessarily entail unchanging and persistent neurological and neuropsychiatric impairments. In areas of demyelination, assuming relative sparing of axons themselves, sodium channel upregulation may occur along the axon between the previous locations of the nodes of Ranvier; this upregulation permits more effective propagation of action potentials along the now unmyelinated axon, and may be the basis by which functional recovery occurs, when it does.

At present there is no known treatment for the myelinolysis itself. We recently reported a case, however, in which we successfully treated the acute neuropsychiatric manifestations caused by extrapontine myelinolysis (caudate and putamen, in this case) using low-dose methylphenidate (Bridgeford et al. 2000, in press). Use of this stimulant markedly improved impairments of executive functioning, social propriety, and motivation. This experience suggests that the neuropsychiatric sequelae of extrapontine myelinolysis may be more amenable to treatment than has been previously suggested. Whether such treatment might extend to other white matter illnesses related to ethanol use remains to be investigated.

Summary

Alcohol dependence remains a multi-faceted clinical challenge for all health care disciplines and especially for the neuropsychiatrist. Viewed most broadly, the following guidelines offer the best hope for those suffering from alcoholism and its effects. Alcohol dependence, itself a series of neuropsychiatric phenomena, can be reliably diagnosed and successfully treated. Current evidence suggests that many of the central nervous system changes caused by alcohol dependence itself are at least partly reversible with abstinence from ethanol. Acute events, such as the forms of ethanol withdrawal, can be treated successfully if medical treatment is aggressive and well-informed. Structural changes in the brain that can be attributed to chronic degenerative processes, such as Wernicke's encephalopathy and alcohol dementia, can either be improved with good nutrition and abstinence from ethanol or limited in their deterioration by the same means. Careful neuropsychiatric evaluation is necessary when cognitive loss is present in any form to guide the development and consideration of the extensive differential diagnosis and to assist the development of a working diagnosis and treatment plan.

18

Traumatic brain injury

Introduction

The term brain injury is applied to a variety of clinical problems in the scientific literature. Some authors include all head injury, including facial, cranial, and brain injuries, in their definitions. Since it is possible to have a head injury without having a brain injury, and *vice versa*, such groupings make interpretation of this literature quite challenging. Others, while limiting discussion to brain injury only, include such diverse etiologies as stroke, tumor, toxic/metabolic disturbance, infection, and mechanical disruption, again leading to some difficulty in learning the pathophysiology and neuropsychiatry of *traumatic* brain injury alone. For the purposes of this chapter, our discussion of brain injury will be focused on closed (non-penetrating) traumatic (mechanical) brain injury only. Our reasons for so doing will become clearer in the next section, but it is sufficient for now to assert that closed traumatic brain injury (TBI) is the most common form of this problem, and also to suggest that the pathophysiology and neuropsychiatric sequelae of closed mechanical brain injury are different from those of not only stroke, tumor, or infection, but also those due to open brain injuries.

TBI is a common problem in the United States. A conservative estimate of brain injury (mechanical type) occurrence rate is 200 per 100 000 persons per year. This translates into approximately 500 000 individuals suffering a new TBI per year in the United States. Estimating the actual frequency and severity distribution of TBI is complicated by the fact that many patients (particularly those with mild TBI) do not present to hospital emergency services and therefore may not be included in TBI surveillance studies upon which most such estimates are based. Fife (1987) reviewed data from the National Health Interview Survey for 1985–87 and concluded that only 16% of persons injured present to a hospital for evaluation; in other words, five out of six persons with a TBI (most of whom are mildly injured) are not included in estimates of the incidence of TBI. From a practical standpoint, clinicians therefore should not take an immediately skeptical view of the veracity of an individual patient's report of a significant TBI based only on his or her failure to be evaluated in emergency room or hospital setting at the time of injury.

These issues aside, the best estimates of the distribution of TBI by severity suggest that mild TBI occurs most frequently (80%), and that moderate injuries (10–13%) and severe injuries (7–10%) are less common. The method used to determine this distribution of TBI severity is most often derived from studies using the Glasgow Coma Scale (GCS; Teasdale & Jennett, 1974), although other useful methods are available and widely used to assess TBI severity (see under Evaluation later in this chapter). Of those injured, 3–8 per 100 admitted to a hospital as a result of TBI will die, and approximately 85 000 individuals will develop persistent neurological deficits and functional disability as a result of their injuries (Kraus & Sorenson, 1994). The likelihood of developing some degree of persistent neurological disability following both moderate and severe TBI is quite high (approximately 66% and 100%, respectively). How often persons with mild TBI develop persistent impairments is less clear, although estimates suggest a range of 10–20%, depending on how mild TBI is defined (see under Evaluation).

The most common causes of TBI are falls, motor vehicle accidents, assaults, and recreation/sports-related injuries. The epidemiological data suggest that TBI is bimodally distributed according to age, with the highest occurrence of TBI in the late teens and early twenties and a second period of high frequency after age 65. Risk factors for TBI include male gender (ratio of 2–3:1), alcohol use (involved in about 50% of all TBI), and lower socioeconomic status.

TBI accounts for only about 1% of deaths in the United States per year, but results in significant morbidity and cost. Morbidity associated with TBI may include the development of delirium, dementia, postconcussive syndrome, personality changes, and aggressive-, mood-, anxiety-, and psychotic disorders. Seizure disorders are also a significant and not an infrequent sequelae of TBI. Averaged for all levels of severity and outcome, the lifetime cost of morbidity associated with TBI is approximately $85 000 per person (1985 estimate). Extrapolated to account for cost of acute and chronic care, and also other direct and indirect costs, 1992 estimates of the economic burden of TBI suggest a total cost of nearly 49 billion dollars, with approximately 65% of the total cost accrued by those who survive such injuries.

Table 18.1. The major mechanisms by which mechanical trauma produces brain injury

| Primary injury mechanisms | | Secondary injury mechanisms | |
Biomechanical	Cytotoxic	Intracranial complications	Systemic
Crush (compression)	Cytoskeletal injury	Traumatic hematomas	Hypoxia/hypercapnia
Direct impact (contusion)	Axonal swelling	Cerebral edema	Anemia
Acceleration/deceleration	Disturbance of cell metabolism	Hydrocephalus	Electrolyte disturbance
Translation, rotational, and angular acceleration	Ca^{2+} and Mg^{2+} dysregulation	Increased intracranial pressure	Infection
Micro-explosive injury (cavitation)	Free radical release		
Diffuse axonal injury	Neurotransmitter excitotoxicity		

Pathophysiology

While mechanical brain injury occurs in the context of either open (penetrating the cranium and dura) or closed (non-penetrating) injuries, these two injury types tend to differ in their effects on brain tissue. In general, open injuries tend to produce more focal and discrete damage, whereas closed injuries tend to be more diffuse (i.e., often there is no clear single focus of injury) as a function of the biophysics involved. As suggested in the preceding section, the pathophysiology and subsequent consequences of these two injury types are therefore predictably different. Since closed injuries are more common, the pathophysiology presented here will focus on the biophysics relevant to closed TBI.

The pathophysiology of TBI may be divided into two components: primary (cerebral biomechanical and cytotoxic) effects and secondary (systemic) complications due to metabolic perturbations (Table 18.1). The primary effects of TBI include biomechanical injury resulting from crushing or acceleration/deceleration forces and cytotoxic damage that immediately follows biomechanical disruption. These primary biomechanical effects impart their effect on the brain instantaneously (or nearly so) at the time of injury. Although the neuropathological consequences of these injuries may be limited by some primary prevention measures (e.g., helmets, automobile air bags, seat belts, etc.), at present there are no effective therapies to reverse the effects of such injuries once they occur. There are some promising avenues of intervention for some of the cytotoxic consequences of and systemic conditions complicating TBI, but at present available interventions are somewhat crude in their mechanisms (e.g., regulation of cerebral P_{CO_2} and cerebral perfusion pressure, volume resuscitation with hypertonic saline, control of infection, etc.).

As research improves our understanding of the pathophysiology of TBI, the strategies for limiting the severity and permanence of the neurological damage imparted by TBI are likely to be more effective. However, since not all people follow these primary prevention strategies consistently, and because many patients may not receive effective and expeditious treatment of their injuries, it is very likely that some patients will continue to develop persistent and disabling neuropsychiatric problems following TBI. Therefore, we will consider these components of injury in some detail to provide a framework for understanding how such injuries affect the brain and how they may contribute to the development of the neuropsychiatric sequelae of TBI.

Biomechanical injury

Goldsmith (1966) suggested that biomechanical injury to the brain may be divided into three types: (1) static or quasi-static force loading (e.g., crush injury); (2) impact of the skull with another object (and consequently of the brain with the skull) at an appreciable velocity; and (3) sudden (impulsive) movement of the head independent of an impact (e.g., whiplash). The first of these injury types is somewhat uncommon (e.g., the head being pressed or squeezed in such a way that both the skull and then brain are compressed and subsequently injured) and will not be considered in detail here. The second and third types of injury are much more common, and involve the application of contact and inertial forces to the head and brain.

Contact forces are those causing one object to physically strike another and inertial forces are those resulting from sudden acceleration or deceleration. The principal inertial forces are translation and rotation. Translational force occurs when the force vector passes in a straight line through the center of mass of the brain. Rotational force occurs due to application of force to the brain outside its center of gravity, resulting in rotation of the brain around its center of mass. Simply as a function of the mechanics of most injuries, translational force rarely occurs without some degree of rotation, and *vice versa*. For pure translational force to occur, the brain would need to move in a perfectly straight line as a consequence of an ideally placed force applied through its center of mass – this is not a typical or realistic situation, as most injury forces are applied at least somewhat off-center (coronally, sagittally, or axially) and thereby establish some rotational force. Therefore, in most injuries both translational and rotational forces are applied, and together they create potentially damaging levels of angular acceleration (discussed below).

To understand the effects of these forces on the brain, it is important to note the tolerance of brain tissue to certain types of movement. In general, the brain tolerates compressive strain reasonably well, owing to its high content of virtually incompressible fluids. Tensile strain (created by stretching tissue) is less well tolerated and shearing strain (created when one tissue slides against another) is tolerated more poorly still.

When the skull is moved or stopped abruptly, movement of the brain lags behind due to that fact that it is substantially more elastic than the skull. This delayed movement has several consequences. First, movement of the brain continues in a straight line until it impacts the inner surface of the skull, possibly resulting in contusion if the velocity of this impact surpasses the ability of the tissue to withstand the compressive strain produced. Additionally, as this movement occurs the elastic brain tissue stretches, and damage may ensue if the tensile strain exceeds the brain's tolerances. Further, as the brain moves along the skull, and as different brain regions move at different rates with respect to one another (due to differences in gray–white elasticity) shearing strain develops and produces additional injury. All of this occurs following a single sudden movement of the brain within the skull, whether from direct impact to the skull or sudden acceleration/deceleration.

Given the elastic nature of the brain, after it impacts the skull on one side it may rebound to some degree and move in the opposite direction until it impacts the skull on the opposite side. These impacts are repeated through several oscillations, putting the cortex at risk for multiple contusional injuries, particularly to areas in which bony ridges, protuberances, or fossae place limits on full movement of a particular brain region (e.g., basal and polar temporal and frontal regions). In the simplest sense, this is one basis for the classic coup (injury at the site of impact) and contre coup (injury opposite the site of impact) pattern seen with more severe TBI.

Although many clinicians, TBI patients, and laypersons focus on the point and force of contact when discussing TBI, both issues are less relevant to the pathophysiology of TBI than inertial forces, and particularly angular acceleration. The relatively greater importance of angular acceleration is a consequence of the brain's relatively poor tolerance of tensile or shearing strains, and relatively greater tolerance for compression. As noted earlier, when a combination of translational and rotational forces is applied to the head, angular acceleration develops. As the center of angulation becomes closer to the center of mass of the brain, an increasing proportion of the angular acceleration is contributed to by rotation. Rotation is particularly damaging to brain tissue because it creates tensile and shearing strains both at the surface of and deep within the brain. These strains injure areas where there is limited structural (i.e., bony or meningeal) support and where free rotation is limited, such as the pial vessels and bridging veins, gray–white junctions of the cortex and subcortical structures, hypothalamus, fornices, corpus callosum, and midbrain (e.g., ascending reticular activating system). High velocity angular acceleration of short duration appears more easily to injure superficial structures (such as blood vessels) while longer durations of angular acceleration appear to have a greater effect on deeper structures.

Diffuse axonal injury is a principal and serious consequence of long duration with intertial forces producing tensile and shearing strains, and may produce significant morbidity via disruption of the connections between lower brain structures and their higher, modulating cortical counterparts. For example, when such strains injure connections between the ascending reticular activating system and the rest of the brain, frank loss of consciousness (LOC) may result. When the brain is subjected to more limited but still significant strains, structural or functional disruption of the connections between brainstem, diencephalic, subcortical, and cortical areas may occur and produce alteration of consciousness, post-traumatic amnesia, or confusion (i.e., causes the injured person to become "dazed and confused").

Another contributor to both diffuse axonal injury is micro-explosive, or cavitation, injury. The occurrence of cavitation injury in closed TBI is probably the pathophysiological event that most clearly distinguishes it from open TBI. Cavitation injury occurs as a function of the shifts in pressure and volume occurring within the closed intracranial cavity at the time of impact or acceleration/deceleration. In a closed system, the ideal gas law (an expanded statement of Boyle's law) applies. Recall that the ideal gas law states that $PV = \eta RT$, where P = pressure, V = volume, η = moles of material, R = the gas constant, and T = temperature. When brain tissue moves within the closed intracranial space following impact or acceleration/deceleration, a pressure gradient develops along

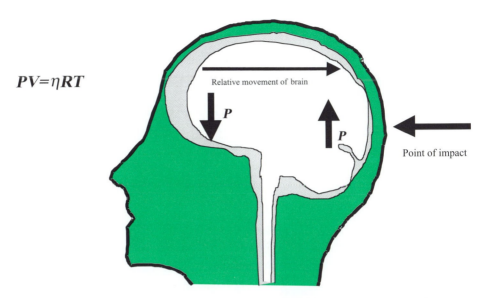

$$PV = \eta RT$$

Relative movement of brain

P

P

Point of impact

Figure 18.1 A simplified application of the ideal gas law (an expanded version of Boyle's law) to understanding microexplosive injury in closed traumatic brain injury. As the impact moves the skull, movement of the more elastic brain tissue lags behind, increasing pressure near the point of impact (coup) and decreasing pressure in the area opposite the point of impact (contre coup). *P*, pressure; *V*, volume; η, moles of material; *R*, gas constant, *T*, temperature.

the line of movement such that pressures are relatively positive at the point of compressive strain (coup) and relatively negative at the opposite side of the brain (contre coup) (Figure 18.1). Recall that there is an extremely thin extracellular fluid layer between neurons and along the axons. When this thin fluid layer is subject to a sudden decrease in pressure at the contre coup site, it undergoes a transient aqueous-to-gaseous shift ("micro-explosion") (Figure 18.2). Since the gas both accommodates the reduced pressure and also fills the relatively reduced volume at the contre coup site, the pressure dynamics within the intracranial space remain balanced according to the ideal gas law. Because gas occupies more space than fluid, the structure of the tissue in which the gas "cavitations" occur is disrupted. Such pressure gradients also affect microvasculature, injuring capillary endothelium and resulting in small, focal hemorrhages. Only when the intracranial space remains closed do the consequences of this phenomenon obtain robustly. Therefore, the occurrence of such microexplosive injury and the occurrence of diffuse axonal injury in excess of focal

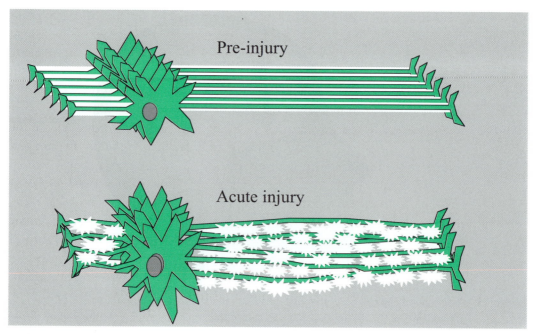

Figure 18.2 An illustration of micro-explosive, or cavitation, injury. The white spaces between the axonal and dendritic projections in the pre-injury diagram represent extracellular fluid layers in the contre coup tissue. In the acute injury state, a sudden drop in pressure causes the extracellular fluid to transiently shift to gaseous state, thereby distorting the anatomy of the axons and dendrites. This is believed to be one of several major mechanisms producing diffuse axonal injury.

cortical injury both distinguish the pathophysiology of closed TBI from its open counterpart.

Cytotoxic injury

Cytotoxic factors also contribute to TBI. Cytotoxic agents are both released and formed at the time of impact, initiating a cascade of metabolic events that furthers neuronal injury. As described in the preceding section and illustrated in Figures 18.1 and 18.2, biomechanical forces alter the neuronal architecture, thereby disrupting cellular function. Where the biomechanical forces distort the axonal cytoskeleton, they impair transport of materials from the neuronal soma to the terminus of the axon. The distortion of the axonal cytoskeleton may be understood as forming a "dam" within the axon, resulting in axonal swelling proximal to the dam. This swelling distorts the axon, and may result in lysis of the axon at the point of cytoskeletal injury. Disruption of the axonal membrane not only releases the content of the axon into the surrounding tissue, but more generally perturbs the function of the entire cell, resulting in collapse of the neuronal soma and Wallerian degeneration of axon towards the neuronal soma, and in some cases leads to death of the neuron.

Such disturbances in neuronal structure and metabolism dysregulate the influx and egress of calcium and magnesium, facilitating the production and release of neurotoxic free radicals as well as the release of neurotoxic neurotransmitters and excitatory amino acids. Loss of ion control across the plasma membrane results in degradation of ion gradients, cellular energy failure, and necrosis. For example, increases in intracellular calcium (flooding in from the more calcium-rich extracellular compartment) cause activation of lipases/proteases and development of free radicals (destroying the cell), and production of arachidonic acid. Arachidonic acid is converted to prostaglandins and leukotrienes, which subsequently cause a decrease in blood flow. This leads to ischemia, more membrane disruption, and continued injury. Similarly, intracellular magnesium levels drop with membrane disruption, affecting ATPase, cofactor synthesis, and mitochondrial respiration.

Release of neurotransmitters also sets this destructive cascade in motion. For example, disruption of the blood–brain barrier during TBI permits influx of peripheral acetylcholine into the central nervous system (CNS). Increase in acetylcholine results in behavioral suppression (decreased level of consciousness) mediated by an inhibitory acetylcholine system in the rostral pons, and changes in the permeability of cell membranes throughout the CNS result in worsened ion homeostasis. Other neurotransmitters also play a role in the development of neuronal injury, but the mechanisms are not as well known. When excitatory amino acids (e.g., glutamate, aspartate, kainic acid, NMDA, and homocysteic acid) and neurotransmitters (e.g., acetylcholine) are released outside the controlled confines of synapses of the cells in which they are usually contained, they act as endogenous cytotoxins and, in combination with free radicals, produce additional injury to surrounding neurons thereby perpetuating this cycle of increasing injury.

Intracranial complications

The secondary effects of TBI are global intracranial processes that develop as consequences of both biomechanical and cytotoxic injury. Such secondary processes include traumatic hematomas, cerebral edema, hydrocephalus, and increased intracranial pressure, and are most often associated with relatively severe injuries. However, in some individuals (particularly the elderly) these problems may develop even with apparently mild mechanisms of injury. Recall that high velocity angular acceleration of short duration, as occurs in a fall, appears more easily to injure superficial structures such as pial vessels and bridging veins, increasing the risk of traumatic hematomas, particularly among elderly patients in whom these tissues may be more fragile at baseline. At present, these secondary complications are relatively more amenable to therapeutic intervention than are the biomechanical or cytotoxic mechanisms of injury, and limiting their severity may lessen the likelihood of neurological and neuropsychiatric sequelae.

Traumatic hematomas

Traumatic hematomas result from lacerations of the cerebral vasculature caused by either bony injury or tensile and shear strain, and may manifest as epidural, subdural, or intracerebral lesions. All of these lesions are potentially life-threatening. Importantly, the risk of developing traumatic hematomas is not limited to the time of acute injury, but persists for several days after the initial insult: vessels previously tamponaded by edema and vasospasm may deteriorate, and blood flow through injured vessels may increase as cerebral edema decreases, both of which pose risks for the formation of new hematomas despite apparent progress towards recovery.

Epidural hematomas form in the space between the dura and the skull, and about 90% are associated with skull fractures. Typically, rupture of the middle meningeal artery or bleeding from epidural veins or sinuses lacerated by the adjacent skull fracture results in bleeding into the epidural space. Although these hematomas may be fatal if not treated expeditiously, chronic neurological and neuropsychiatric sequelae are unlikely if there is no underlying cortical contusion and if they are evacuated promptly. Subdural hematomas most often result from laceration of cortical ("bridging") vessels over the lateral convexities of the brain, which then bleed into the subdural space.

Generally, subdural hematomas form as a consequence of high magnitude acceleration forces, and as such they are frequently associated with injury to the underlying brain tissue (including diffuse axonal injury). Therefore, they tend to be associated with more long-term morbidity than epidural hematomas. This is especially true when intervention requires not only evacuation of the hematoma, but also resection of necrotic underlying brain tissue. Intracerebral hematomas result from rupture of blood vessels within the brain substance, and are most often the result of depressed skull fractures, missile wounds, or deep shearing injuries. They tend to develop at the border zone between regions supplied by the anterior and middle cerebral arteries and are associated with significant neurological and neuropsychiatric impairment.

Cerebral edema

Cerebral edema is best thought of as an increase in total brain water following injury, and may have vasogenic and/or cytotoxic etiologies. The principal danger posed by acute cerebral edema is increased intracranial pressure, cerebral herniation, and death. Vasogenic edema results from traumatic disruption of the blood–brain barrier, permitting movement of water into the extravascular space. Hyperventilation lowers P_{CO_2}, leading to vasoconstriction, reduction of blood flow, and may help attenuate the extent of vasogenic edema. Achieving a balance between appropriate vasoconstriction and that capable of producing further injury is paramount, and is probably best accomplished by maintaining P_{CO_2} at approximately 35 mm Hg (Kelly, 1999). Intravenous hypertonic saline during fluid resuscitation and bolus infusions of hyperosmolar agents (mannitol) may be used to absorb extravascular fluid into the vascular space and reduce acute cerebral edema. Prolonged use of hyperosmolar agents may complicate the patient's condition, however, as they can filter into the extravascular space, leading to increased edema, increased intracerebral edema, and further deterioration. Cytotoxic edema develops when cell damage leads to diffusion of water from the intracellular to the extracellular space. At present, there is no effective method by which to arrest the formation of cytotoxic edema.

Hydrocephalus

Acute hydrocephalus develops when outflow of cerebrospinal fluid from the ventricular system is obstructed, either as a consequence of mechanical blockage of the ventricular system or blockage of absorption at the arachnoid villi by blood or other foreign substances. Acute hydrocephalus poses a serious risk of herniation and death. Chronic hydrocephalus is associated with dementia, which may be at least partially reversible if intervention occurs early and before permanent parenchymal damage.

Increased intracerebral pressure (ICP)

Increased ICP is often the end product of many of the above processes. It occurs when the increased pressure exceeds the autoregulatory capacity of the CNS. Ordinarily, the CNS is capable of regulating pressure within the system both as a whole (Cushing response) and also between compartments. When these autoregulatory mechanisms fail, pressure increases exponentially. The most damaging result of increased ICP is herniation, including subfalcine (cingulate), transtentorial, and tonsillar types.

Subfalcine (cingulate) herniation refers to lateral translation of a lobe or hemisphere below the falx cerebri. This type of herniation is generally well tolerated, though if severe anterior cerebral artery compression occurs, subsequent ischemia of the mesial frontal areas (anterior cingulate region) may produce devastating neuropsychiatric consequences (see Chapter 15). Transtentorial (uncal) herniation refers to caudal displacement of the basal portions of the temporal or frontal lobes (and in the worst cases the midbrain) through the tentorium. This results in brainstem distortion, vascular occlusion, and decerebrate rigidity. Tonsillar herniation refers to caudal displacement of the medulla and cerebral tonsils through the foramen magnum. This displacement is most problematic, as it compresses the brainstem against the occipital bone, which disrupts the function of the vagal motor nuclei, causing loss of the vasomotor and respiratory control centers and death.

Systemic complications

Systemic complications include hypoxemia, hypotension, hypercapnia, anemia, hypernatremia, hypoglycemia, and infection, all of which may develop as a function of the above described mechanisms of injury, as consequences of trauma to other parts of the body, or iatrogenically. These complications are more often associated with relatively severe brain injuries, and are likely to have the greatest effect on regions of the brain with relatively high metabolic requirements (thereby fostering the development of post-traumatic deliria in the acute injury setting). Prolonged systemic complications may severely compromise the function of these sensitive areas, thereby contributing to the profound chronic problems with arousal, attention, memory, and other cognitive, emotional, and behavioral abilities seen in the most severely injured patients.

Neuropsychiatric sequelae of TBI

Traumatic brain injury may produce a variety of neuropsychiatric problems, including impaired cognition, depression, mania, affective lability, irritability, anxiety, psychosis, and the postconcussional syndrome. These problems develop frequently, and produce significant morbidity among TBI survivors. The literature addressing the etiology of these problems is a contentious one, particularly as regards the neuropsychiatric sequelae of mild TBI. Some authors posit strong, predictable, neurobiological relationships between TBI and neuropsychiatric problems, while others seem to suggest that much of the neuropsychiatric morbidity associated with TBI (and particularly mild TBI) is largely the result of pre-morbid psychiatric problems, maladjustment to injury, or compensation seeking and frank malingering. It does appear that pre-TBI psychiatric disorders may be exacerbated by such injuries, and that TBI may impose some limitation on treatment response in a previously treatment-responsive patient. Whether one regards the development of neuropsychiatric problems following TBI as resulting from neurobiological changes, emotional and psychological reactions, or a complex interaction of these factors, it is clear that such problems do develop, interfere with recovery and rehabilitation, and require treatment.

Despite the common occurrence of these symptoms following TBI, there are relatively few rigorous studies that provide clear guidance regarding appropriate management. Complicating matters, many of the symptoms with which patients present, and which clinicians often use to make psychiatric diagnoses, may be primarily related to brain injury rather than comorbid psychiatric disturbance (e.g., fatigue, sleep disturbance, weight change, diminished libido, etc.). The symptomatic overlap between the somatic effects of TBI and those attributable to neuropsychiatric pathology confounds diagnosis and substantially increases the complexity of evaluation and treatment.

Given that the neuropsychiatric sequelae of TBI are neither singular in type nor uniform in presentation or response to treatment, evaluating and treating so affected patients is challenging. The evaluation and treatment of impaired cognition, depression, mania, anxiety, aggression, and psychosis due to TBI are often discussed separately, an approach derived from the psychiatric literature in which ostensibly distinct clinical phenotypes warrant independent consideration. However, TBI patients often develop symptoms and syndromes that cross conventional diagnostic boundaries (e.g., comorbid anxiety, depressed mood, and aggression), making it difficult to translate a diagnosis-specific treatment approach into clinical practice with many TBI survivors. Additionally, many of the treatment strategies, pharmacological or otherwise, used in the treatment of neuropsychiatric problems after TBI are not diagnosis-specific – a single agent may be usefully employed to treat several problems.

Given these considerations, in this section we offer a brief description of currently recognized secondary psychiatric syndromes due to TBI, and then describe the evaluation and treatment of these problems in a symptom-targeted, rather than diagnosis-targeted, fashion. Although we will not reiterate this point in each section, it should again be noted that primary psychiatric disorders may not only be exacerbated by a TBI, but also may substantially complicate the evaluation and management of post-TBI neuropsychiatric disorders.

Delirium

Delirium directly due to TBI is a syndrome of transient and reversible disturbance of consciousness, change in cognition, and/or alteration of perception that has onset at the time of injury. The term delirium is rarely used in the TBI literature; instead, terms such as states of impaired consciousness, posttraumatic amnesia, altered consciousness, and acute confusional state are more often used. Unfortunately, many of these terms are, at best, poorly defined, making interpretation and application of the literature difficult. Of these terms, posttraumatic amnesia seems most like delirium, with both containing the essential feature of a period of clouded consciousness in the immediate post-TBI period that precedes the attainment of full orientation, continuous awareness, and ongoing memory in persons recovering from head injuries. However, delirium really refers to a problem that extends well beyond impaired new learning (see Chapter 12), involving also alterations in the level of consciousness, attention, other aspects of cognition (language, praxis, gnosis, executive function, motivation, and comportment), perceptual disturbances (illusions and hallucinations), emotion (especially affective lability), and behavior. With this in mind, posttraumatic amnesia may be identified as one feature among the many symptoms of delirium due to TBI.

The exact mechanisms by which posttraumatic delirium is produced are not completely understood, as is true for any delirium. The pathophysiology of TBI reviewed in the preceding sections does suggest a number of likely contributors, most of which are most easily understood in the context of relatively severe TBI. First, injuries in which there is high magnitude and sustained angular acceleration induce significant tensile and shearing strains that damage both superficial and deep cerebral structures, and/or induce cellular dysfunction that perturbs the normal activity of neurons and neuronal networks. These factors alone can produce diffuse axonal injury of sufficient severity to disrupt the ability of lower (brainstem) centers to provide adequate activating tone to diencephalic, subcortical, and cortical structures, the consequence of which is reduced arousal and globally impaired cerebral functioning, or even coma. When viewed on a continuum of severity, lesser degrees of injury may be understood as producing lesser degrees of dysfunction more consistent with a delirium. At a point closer to the normal end of this continuum, one might see the sort of posttraumatic amnesia associated with mild TBI, in which other cognitive impairments (such as various impairments in complex cognition) are mild if present at all. The secondary cerebral and systemic complications of TBI (cerebral edema, increased ICP, dysregulation of cerebral blood flow, hypoxia, etc.) may also compromise cerebral function as suggested earlier, thereby contributing to (or causing) posttraumatic delirium. These factors are probably more relevant to deliria following severe TBI than to those associated with lesser degrees of injury.

Severe TBI may produce delirium that persists for weeks to months. Lesions in the brainstem (as suggested above) are especially associated with protracted symptoms, as are basal ganglia and basal forebrain lesions. Additionally, left (dominant) hemispheric lesions have been associated with longer duration of delirium than right hemispheric lesions.

The treatment of delirium due to TBI is essentially the same as for delirium from any other cause – work-up and treat the underlying cause(s) to the greatest extent possible, and institute supportive pharmacological and environmental strategies to treat the neuropsychiatric symptoms (see Chapter 12). Although longer duration of coma (particularly that greater than two weeks) roughly correlates with poorer outcome, the relationship between duration of delirium due to TBI and functional outcome is not entirely clear. In general, if the duration of delirium (or PTA) is relatively short, a more favorable outcome is likely. However, if the duration of coma, delirium, or PTA is protracted, and if there are significant comorbid medical and psychosocial problems during either the acute or post-acute injury periods, recovery may be markedly slowed and/or incomplete.

Dementia

As with all other dementias (see Chapter 13), dementia due to TBI is a syndrome of acquired and persistent impairment in multiple areas of cognitive function, without disturbance of consciousness, due to the direct physiological effects of TBI that produces significant impairments in functioning. Distinguishing dementia from delirium due to TBI is a particularly difficult task, as the usual caveats about attention being relatively normal in dementia may not apply particularly well to this population – given the potentially permanent injury to lower (brainstem and diencephalic) areas caused by TBI, relatively permanent alterations of arousal and attention may be part of the clinical presentation of these patients. Since large scale permanent injuries to deep cerebral structures are more strongly associated with severe TBI, the dilemma between diagnosing a chronic confusional state (delirium) and severe dementia due to TBI is not one that will often be faced by the neuropsychiatric clinician in an outpatient office, and may be to some degree moot in any case. However, the principal remains the same with less severely injured patients, and clinicians should not be surprised by the presence of some degree of attentional difficulties, slowness of thought, and even mild hypoarousal in addition to impairments of memory, executive functioning, emotion, personality, and behavior among patients with dementia due to TBI.

Dementia due to TBI is truly a mixed dementia, both within and between patients, and the types and severities of the various cognitive impairments associated with this condition vary according to the sites and severities of injury in a given patient. Although it is tempting to regard mild TBI as producing a clinical picture most like white matter dementia, recent studies (Thatcher et al., 1997, 1998a, 1998b) suggest that even in mild TBI diffuse injury to both gray and white matter contributes to symptom formation and electrophysiological abnormalities. This having been said, the preceding section on pathophysiology suggests that some relatively specific structural and neurochemical disturbances are predictable sequelae of TBI. Among the various possible sites of cortical injury, the frontal lobes (particularly all prefrontal cortices and the frontal poles), the anterior and medial temporal cortices, and the white matter underlying and connecting these areas to subcortical and other cortical association areas are particularly vulnerable to injury. This vulnerability is a consequence of their proximity to underlying bony protuberances or ridges and the constraints on free translation and rotation these bony structures place on these areas (Figure 18.3).

Additionally, neurochemical disturbances may develop both as a result of the apparent lower tolerance for TBI of some systems (e.g., acetylcholine, glutamate) and the involvement of other systems in the areas most commonly suffering structural compromise due to TBI (e.g., mesocortical and mesolimbic dopamine, norepinephrine, and serotonin projections). Consequently, functions referable to these areas are predictably impaired, including executive function, motivation, social behavior, emotional regulation, personality, speed and efficiency of information filtering and processing, sustained and complex attention, and memory (typically, retrieval is more impaired than encoding).

Similar impairments may follow milder injuries, and may be of sufficient functional import to warrant a dementia diagnosis. These cases are often perplexing for clinicians, patients, families, and the medicolegal system, as some find it more difficult to accept the veracity of deficits apparent on the clinical interview and evaluation without overt evidence of lesions on neuroimaging studies or gross electrophysiological abnormalities. The discrepancy between symptoms and imaging or electrophysiology is more likely a function of the relative insensitivity of most current neuroimaging and electrophysiological studies to the diffuse and relatively subtle sequelae of mild TBI than an accurate reflection of a lack of injury in these persons. As the tools for evaluating these patients become increasingly sophisticated and available (e.g., PET, SPECT, MRS, QEEG), it is likely that our ability to corroborate subjective symptoms and neuropsychological impairments with the sort of "objective" evidence in which many patients and insurers are often exclusively interested will improve greatly. In the meantime, and as noted in Chapter 9 and our other discussions of neuropsychological testing, a pattern of deficits consistently supporting dysfunction referable to the areas predictably injured by TBI despite good effort by the patient can provide sufficient objective evidence of dysfunction due to TBI both to substantiate the patient's complaints and to design appropriate treatments.

The evaluation and treatment of dementia due to TBI is similar to that suggested for dementias of other etiologies – determination of etiology, environmental manipulation, medications, and social/medicolegal interventions (see Chapter 12). Dementia following TBI may be a result of other injury-related complications, including hydrocephalus, chronic subdural hematomas, posttraumatic endocrine disturbances (e.g., hypothyroidism), or the pseudodementias of depression or anxiety. As a result, patients with dementia following TBI require careful evaluation and treatment for these and other potentially reversible etiologies of cognitive impairment, and in all cases these patients should undergo neuroimaging, preferably using MRI.

The prognosis of dementia due to TBI depends on its etiology and on the time elapsed since injury. Many patients with cognitive impairment following

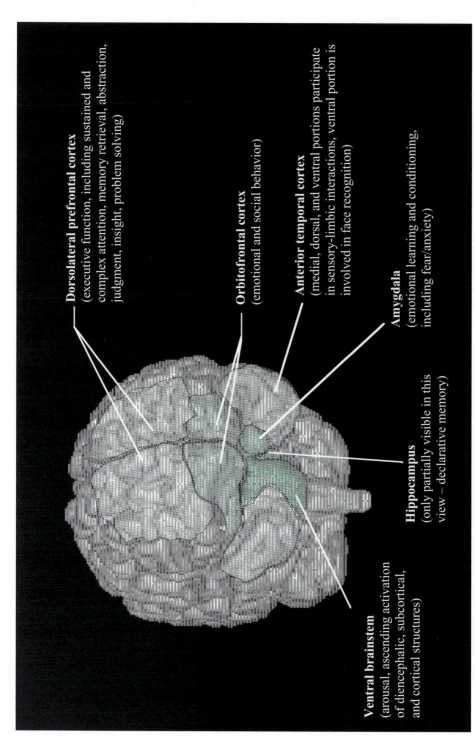

Dorsolateral prefrontal cortex
(executive function, including sustained and complex attention, memory retrieval, abstraction, judgment, insight, problem solving)

Orbitofrontal cortex
(emotional and social behavior)

Anterior temporal cortex
(medial, dorsal, and ventral portions participate in sensory-limbic interactions, ventral portion is involved in face recognition)

Amygdala
(emotional learning and conditioning, including fear/anxiety)

Hippocampus
(only partially visible in this view – declarative memory)

Ventral brainstem
(arousal, ascending activation of diencephalic, subcortical, and cortical structures)

Figure 18.3 Anterior view of the brain highlighting the cortical areas that are particularly vulnerable to traumatic brain injury. These areas are particularly vulnerable as a result of their proximity to underlying bony structures that excessively limit their movement and/or abrade the cortical surfaces during traumatic brain injury. When injured, functional impairments may result in dementia.

TBI will improve substantially during the first year following injury, including not only those with mild TBI but also some with moderate and more severe injuries. However, the extent of spontaneous recovery of cognitive function among patients with significant structural damage is often disappointingly incomplete. Guided by neuropsychological testing, identifying remaining areas of cognitive strength may facilitate functional improvement through the use of compensatory strategies.

Although patients are often concerned about prematurely developing Alzheimer's disease as a result of their TBI, the relationship between these two disorders is still incompletely understood. It does appear that patients with a genetic vulnerability to Alzheimer's disease (those with one or more copies of the apolipoprotein E-ε4 allele) may be more likely to develop this disorder at an earlier age following a TBI than similarly vulnerable patients who do not experience a TBI (Mayeux et al., 1993, 1995; Nicoll et al., 1995; Friedman et al., 1999). It does not appear that TBI is an independent risk factor for developing Alzheimer's disease specifically (Mayeux et al., 1993; Mehta et al., 1999), although certainly there is an incontrovertible risk of developing a dementia due to TBI alone. The strength of these relationships between TBI, Alzheimer's disease, and the genetic vulnerability (or possibly protection in the case of apolipoprotein E-ε2 allele) requires further investigation.

Mood Disorders

Mood disorders are often significant problems for patients after TBI. Depression occurs in as many as 60% of patients post-injury (Busch & Alpern, 1998). Dysthymia is also common among these patients, with a prevalence of at least 10% during the first year post-injury. These disorders may be transient problems lasting only weeks following TBI, but on average most of these patients develop depression of several months duration (on average, about four months, lasting up to 12 months in some patients; Robinson & Jorge, 1994). The timing of major depression following TBI does not, unfortunately, reliably indicate the strength of the relationship between the injury itself and the development of a depressive disorder. Although many patients develop depression immediately following TBI, a cohort of patients may develop delayed-onset depressions that are not clearly phenomenologically or biologically different from those with early-onset depression. Regardless of the timing of onset, the DSM-IV (American Psychiatric Association, 1994) criteria for these disorders, which rely on both subjective symptoms and objectively observable changes in mood and behavior, appear adequate to identify these disorders in TBI patients.

Studies have not thus far consistently supported the hypothesis that patients developing depression after TBI have significantly higher rates of pre-injury depression, although there is certainly some suggestive evidence that this may be the case. It is true, however, that pre-existing depressive disorders may be more severe or difficult-to-treat by TBI. While the nature of the relationship between prior psychiatric disorder and post-TBI mood disorders requires further study, at present it seems fair to say that pre-existing psychiatric disorders, poor social adjustment, and social dissatisfaction pre-injury pose an increased risk of developing depression following TBI.

Robinson & Jorge (1994) suggest that the pathophysiology of depression due to TBI may be understood as an effect of the dynamic neurotransmitter and neurohormonal changes produced by TBI, and their suggestion is consistent with our discussion of the neurobiology of emotion in Chapter 5. The presence of left anterior (dorsolateral prefrontal and basal ganglia) lesions correlates most strongly with major depression. Interestingly, this association appears to be more robust for transient depressions (<3 months) that develop during the post-acute period following TBI than for more longstanding depressions. One possible explanation for this finding is that acute disruption of ascending noradrenergic or serotonergic projections to these areas caused by diffuse axonal injury may recover to some degree and/or there may be upregulation of receptors for these neurotransmitters during the first few months following the injury. The mechanisms by which prolonged or delayed-onset depressions develop following TBI are less clear, but are likely to involve a more complex interaction between neurobiological and psychosocial factors.

Mania has been reported following TBI, and may occur in as many as 10% of TBI patients. As with depression, the DSM-IV criteria appear adequate for making this diagnosis. The rate at which these patients develop a true bipolar course, as opposed to developing only a secondary manic syndrome, has not been extensively studied and the true frequencies of bipolar illness in these patients are not known. Mania due to TBI does not appear to be associated with severity of injury, the degree of physical or cognitive impairment, personal or family history of psychiatric disorder (including bipolar disorder), the availability of social support, or the level of social functioning. However, there is an association between the development of epilepsy (partial complex seizures) and the development of secondary manic syndromes following TBI.

As suggested by the review of the neurobiology of emotion presented in

Chapter 5, patients with mania due to TBI have a significant frequency of lesions involving the temporal basopolar or orbitofrontal cortices, particularly in the right hemisphere. Robinson & Jorge (1994) suggest that functional changes in reticulolimbic or limbic-cortical aminergic inhibitory systems, and/or the aberrant regeneration pathways during recovery from TBI, may play a role in the genesis of secondary manic syndromes due to TBI.

Definitive treatment studies of depression and mania due to TBI are lacking, but case reports and case series suggest that the treatment of these problems is, in general, largely the same as that offered to patients with phenomenologically similar primary psychiatric disorders. There are, of course, a few caveats regarding the selection of treatment that warrant consideration that are discussed in more detail in the next section of this chapter.

Anxiety disorders

Anxiety symptoms and syndromes may develop following TBI, and represent significant problems for the patient, family, and caregiver in both acute and chronic stages of recovery. Epstein & Ursano (1994) reviewed the literature from 1942 to 1990 and concluded that significant anxiety develops in nearly 30% of TBI patients during the first five years (and generally during the first six months) following injury. Anxiety may first manifest as an acute stress disorder, and if not adequately addressed it may further develop into full post-traumatic stress disorder. Specific anxiety disorders, including phobic disorders, panic disorder, generalized anxiety disorder, and even obsessive–compulsive disorder (OCD), may also result from TBI. Anxiety may also present as a diffuse and non-specific symptom, and is often a feature of the post-concussive syndrome.

The etiology of anxiety following TBI is complex and may result from neurobiological factors, psychosocial factors, or some combination of both. Based on our discussion of emotion in Chapter 5, we would predict that anxiety should develop more often as a result of injury to the right frontal lobe than from injury to the left frontal lobe. This prediction is based on the relative hemispheric asymmetry of emotion, with the left-side mediating emotional "activation" (either euphoria, mirth, or non-specific excitement as in anxiety) and the right-side mediating "inhibition" (as in depression). Consistent with this view, Grafman et al. (1986, 1996) report that right frontal injuries are more likely to produce "edginess" in the acute post-injury period that later develops into anxiety. The occurrence of OCD is similarly interesting in light of our previous presentation of this problem, since right orbitofrontal cortex and caudate nucleus dysfunction are implicated in the pathogenesis of both primary and secondary (including post-TBI) OCD. The development of OCD following injury to right frontal-subcortical circuitry also supports the suggestion that the right hemisphere may play an important role in the regulation and inhibition (stopping) of thoughts and behaviors initiated and maintained by the left frontal-subcortical circuits.

The treatment of anxiety due to TBI should combine both psychotherapeutic, behavioral, and psychopharmacological strategies, though the balance of these approaches will inevitably vary depending on the specific type of anxiety the patient suffers. When medications are used, particular care must be taken to avoid using agents that predictably worsen cognitive and memory problems or that may precipitate paradoxical agitation (e.g., benzodiazepines). For example, buspirone and propranolol may be preferable in such patients, as both tend to produce relatively fewer additional cognitive side effects than more traditional anxiolytics such as the benzodiazepines. For additional information on pharmacological strategies, see under Treatment in this chapter.

Psychotic disorders

Psychosis due to TBI is a relatively uncommon problem, although the relatively scant literature regarding this problem makes any assertions regarding the true frequency of this problem impossible at this point in time. Davison & Bagley (1969) estimated the 10–20 year incidence of psychosis following brain injury as at least two to three times higher than that of the general population, with the observed rates in the literature up to the time of their review ranging from 0.07–9.8%. Achte et al. (1991) found an even higher rate (750 out of 3000, or 25%) of paranoid disorders following moderate to severe TBI.

Phenomenological descriptions of TBI and psychosis are meager and discrepant. Complicating the interpretation of these reports is variability in the patient populations (civilian or military, adult or child) and injury type (severe or minor, open or closed, blunt or penetrating). Additional difficulty interpreting such reports stems from the failure of authors to use specific diagnostic criteria in their descriptions, variable methods of evaluating cases (chart review, patient interview, or family interview), and questionable reliability of the evaluator (psychiatrist or non-psychiatrist). Lack of consistent definitions of psychosis, particularly as regards symptom type, frequency, and severity, substantially limits our ability to meaningfully integrate the contents of these reports and make inferences about their implications.

Pathophysiological explanations of TBI and psychosis are similarly scarce. A multifactorial pathophysiology is often suggested, including direct trauma and tissue damage, interaction with effects of previous brain insults (substance abuse, perinatal damage, epilepsy and other brain disease), genetic predisposition, co-morbid physical impairments, and environmental factors. Clinicopathological correlates such as electroencephalography (EEG) and computed tomography findings are described in some reports, which suggest that these patients may be more likely to demonstrate bilateral pathology than the more left-sided pathology often associated with schizophrenia. However, left temporal lobe abnormalities on magnetic resonance imaging evaluation of two patients with schizophrenia-like psychoses associated with cerebral trauma have been reported (Buckely et al., 1993). Although the pathophysiological relationship between TBI and psychosis is uncertain, it has been our experience that delusions and hallucinations are more often associated with severe TBI than with milder TBI, that these problems are not simply the result of delirium or post-traumatic epilepsy, and that they are often extremely difficult to treat effectively.

Treatment guidelines for TBI and psychosis are also uncertain, although the usual approach is to treat the psychosis with antipsychotic medications. In general, atypical antipsychotics are preferable as they are less likely to interfere with cognition and motor function, and are less likely to produce tardive dyskinesia. Common clinical experience suggests these patients do not respond as robustly to standard treatments of psychosis as do patients with schizophrenia. Based on anecdotal reports of benefit, neuroleptics, anticonvulsants, clonazepam, lithium, and beta-adrenergic antagonists are all potentially useful, but there have been no properly controlled double-blind trials to assess therapeutic efficacy of antipsychotic medication for psychosis due to TBI.

Aggression

Irritability and aggression are relatively common sequelae of TBI, and present significant problems and even danger to TBI survivors, their families, and their caregivers. Up to 96% of patients with TBI exhibit agitated behavior during the acute injury period, although overt aggression often resolves within the first two weeks post-injury. However, many patients will experience persistent irritability and episodic dyscontrol for many years (if not indefinitely) following

TBI. In the DSM-IV, irritability and aggression due to TBI are categorized under Personality Change due to TBI, aggressive type. Silver & Yudofsky (1994a) strongly disagree with this categorization, as aggression and other neuropsychiatric problems following TBI are far more specific than the term "personality change" suggests, and instead advocate application of a diagnostic label specific to the clinical problem, namely aggression. This distinction is more than a semantic issue. Recognition of this problem as a specific disorder promotes increased accuracy of evaluation, diagnosis, and treatment, and avoids the unfortunate countertransferences that are often generated when a "personality disorder" diagnosis is inappropriately applied or misunderstood by other careproviders.

The neurobiological bases of post-TBI aggression follow logically from the information presented in Chapters 4 and 5. Hypothalamic injury may result in dysregulation of "fight or flight" reactions mediated through neuroendocrine and autonomic responses. Specifically, lesions to the ventromedial hypothalamus produce nondirected rage with stereotypic behavior (scratching and biting). The hypothalamus is vulnerable to injury via diffuse axonal injury due to its extensive connections to the rest of the limbic system. Within the limbic system (and especially the medial temporal lobe), damage to the amygdaloid complex may result in activation (subictal seizures or hyperexcitability) of the amygdala which may result in rage reactions to otherwise emotionally trivial stimuli. Similarly, damage to the orbitofrontal cortex (which receives and modulates much of the limbic input to the frontal lobes) may result in disinhibition of emotional and motor responses that manifest as assaultiveness. Using our metaphor of the orbitofrontal lobes as the "limbic police," injury to this area results in dysfunction of the police forces and may permit the development of "limbic anarchy" where impulses are unrestrained and a lack of concern for the rights of others may develop. Such aggression and assaultiveness following TBI are sometimes referred to as "acquired sociopathy," and this label is consistent with the present method of understanding the implications of orbitofrontal injury.

Multiple neurotransmitter systems are involved in aggression. As discussed in Chapter 5, serotonin, norepinephrine, dopamine, acetylcholine, and GABA systems are felt to have prominent roles in influencing aggressive behavior. Serotonin, which has been associated with violence in other contexts, may be reduced following TBI, although data are as yet not conclusive. Similarly, excess dopamine may facilitate aggression and excessive norepinephrine can increase anxiety and agitation, but there is little reason to suspect that TBI results in clinically significant and prolonged elevation of these neurotransmitters per se. Instead, TBI-related reductions of acetylcholine and GABA (gamma-aminobutyric acid) may limit the ability of remaining frontal-subcortical circuits to regulate the action of dopamine and norepinephrine on limbic and paralimbic targets effectively. It is very likely that there is no single neurobiology of aggression due to TBI, as aggression may be a final clinical consequence of many forms of prefrontal, limbic, and paralimbic dysfunction.

The multiplicity of pharmacological treatments for aggression due to TBI is consistent with this view of the relevant neurochemistry. The strategies available seek to reduce aggression via augmentation of existing and beneficial neurotransmitter systems or blockade of systems implicated in the production of aggression, and often combination strategies are required. These treatments are described in the following section of this chapter. Behavioral treatments and psychoeducation of the patient and family are also important components of the comprehensive treatment of aggression.

Personality changes

Personality changes are one of the most significant problems faced by individuals with TBI and their families. These changes may range from subtle shifts in self-concept and interpersonal style to dramatic and clinically problematic alterations in the TBI survivors' sense of self, comportment, and behavior. Frequently described personality changes include those seen in "frontal lobe syndromes," especially impulsivity, lack of sense of self, lack of empathy, and inability to self-monitor. Though dramatic "reversals" of premorbid personality may occur (for example, a previously extroverted individual suffers dense bilateral injury to the dorsolateral prefrontal and anterior cingulate cortices, rendering him profoundly apathetic), more modest changes or even amplification of pre-injury traits are by far more common.

As stated in Chapter 6, personality is the enduring pattern of thinking about, feeling about, and relating to oneself and one's environment. From this vantage point, all of the preceding neuropsychiatric sequelae of TBI can be understood as altering personality. Hence, the combination of neurobiological, psychological, and social changes that are produced by TBI may cause either transient or permanent alterations in personality, and consequently some patients will be diagnosed with either "personality change" or Axis II personality disorders. Such diagnoses are, however, rarely helpful to the patient, and among caregivers such labels often produce unnecessary confusion, stigmatization, and resistance to participating in the care of these patients. With this in mind, we agree with the perspective offered by Silver & Yudofsky (1994a) described above, that specific problems in cognition, mood, and behavior should not be subsumed under the unnecessarily broad category of personality change in lieu of a more meaningful and specific description of the patient's problems. Although recognizing the effect of TBI on personality may be useful in the psychotherapy of a TBI survivor and in academic endeavors like this text, clinical care should focus on specific problems (e.g., dementia, depression, aggression, etc.) rather than global issues like personality.

Localization of personality to any single brain region is an impossible endeavor, as personality by definition involves functions (e.g., cognition, emotion, and behavior) that are predicated on the activities of multiple selective distributed networks (see Chapter 6). Nonetheless, it is clear that changes in frontal and temporal lobes function and the effects of diffuse axonal injuries strongly contribute to the personality changes that typically accompany TBI. In severe injuries, alterations in dorsolateral prefrontal and anterior cingulate circuits may result in overt losses of intellectual capacity and drive. However, milder injuries may also affect the function of these areas, resulting in an experience of intellectual "dullness" or "fuzzy thinking," and a sense of diminished mental or social interest and energy. Orbitofrontal circuit injuries can, as discussed in the preceding section on aggression, result in irritability, irascibility, and affective lability. Damasio (1994) has also suggested that such injuries may profoundly affect social behavior, resulting in inappropriateness, childishness, and a lack of an ability to appropriately integrate the contextual relevance of thought, emotion, and behavior. Medial temporal injury, particularly to the amygdala, may also affect emotional responding and emotional learning, resulting in placidity or an apparent absence of the ability to appreciate the emotional relevance of internal or external stimuli (e.g., the Kluver–Bucy syndrome). Independent of significant cortical contusion, diffuse axonal injury may "unplug" neural networks from one another, resulting in functional impairment of specific selective distributed networks and their interactions with one another. All such changes result in alterations in the TBI survivor's thoughts, feelings, and reactions to self and the environment, or personality.

There are no specific pharmacotherapies for personality alterations due to TBI. However, pharmacological or behavioral treatments of specific problems (e.g., apathy, impaired cognition, etc.) caused by TBI may secondarily effect beneficial personality changes. Less overt problems may require attention also – many TBI survivors will describe distress over the change in their personality, particularly their sense of self. Psychotherapy is entirely appropriate for these patients, and may greatly facilitate their adjustment to disability (or other problems) resulting from their injury. Psychotherapy should also place emphasis on education, cognitive rehabilitation, and involvement of the patient's family/supports in the process of coming to terms with illness.

Postconcussive syndrome

Postconcussive syndrome (PCS) is a contentious and much debated diagnosis, but does require at least some comment in this context. PCS refers to a group of symptoms that follow TBI, which are most often organized into three categories: cognitive (decreased memory, attention, and concentration); somatic complaints (headache, fatigue, insomnia, dizziness, tinnitus, sensitivity to noise or light); and affective complaints (depression, irritability, and anxiety). Although this group of symptoms may follow TBI of any severity, they are most often discussed in the context of mild brain injury (GCS = 13–15). In the immediate post-injury period, 80–100% of patients will describe one or more of these symptoms. Most studies suggest that a significant number of patients will be symptom-free at one month, and the majority (approximating 90%) will be symptom-free at 12 months. A small number (conservatively estimated at 10%) will remain persistently symptomatic with PCS, resulting in long-term disability.

There has been wide debate about the role of disability compensation and litigation in the development of the postconcussive syndrome. However, the studies suggesting a positive correlation between the development of symptoms and litigation are fraught with methodological difficulties, including sampling bias (medicolegal referrals) and imprecise inclusion criteria (poorly defined postconcussive syndrome). At present, it is clear that some individuals with this syndrome exist, and that for these individuals PCS becomes a chronic problem independent of medicolegal concerns.

The pathophysiology of PCS is not well understood, although diffuse axonal injury is often suggested as the prime contributor to this problem. As mentioned earlier, more recent studies of these patients suggest that both gray and white matter alterations are present in persistently symptomatic mild TBI survivors (Thatcher et al., 1997, 1998a,b), and electrophysiological abnormalities in these patients are unlikely to be accounted for by white matter injury alone (Thatcher et al., 1989, 1991, 1999; Arciniegas et al., 1999, 2000a). Given the neuroimaging and electrophysiological evidence, and the multiple and distributed neuroanatomic underpinnings of the various symptoms of PCS, the most likely neurobiological explanations for this condition are those that conceptualize this problem as the consequence of diffusely distributed injuries that subtly impair the speed and efficiency of neural processing. Other factors, such as primary or secondary neuropsychiatric problems (e.g., depression, anxiety, affective lability), physical or neurological impairments, psychosocial, and medicolegal issues, may also contribute to the presentation in some cases.

Treatment of postconcussive syndrome is largely empiric, as therapeutic efficacy studies are lacking at present. In general, a symptom-targeted approach is warranted, and often times it is therefore quite complicated. Where present, identifiable problems such as depression, anxiety, irritability, and impaired cognition should be treated before ascribing such problems to PCS and making any predictions about the likelihood of their becoming long-term problems. Psychoeducation regarding the pathophysiology, typical sequelae, time course, and potential recovery/persistent deficits should be given to the patient and family, validating the patient's complaints without fostering persistent illness behavior.

Evaluation and treatment of the neuropsychiatric sequelae of TBI

Recognition of these secondary neuropsychiatric syndromes and their differences in presentation and treatment response from both each other and also primary psychiatric syndromes can guide appropriate management and care of these patients. The evaluation and treatment of patients with TBI requires a multidisciplinary approach that includes neuropsychiatrists, neuropsychologists, neurologists, physiatrists, speech, occupational, and physical therapists, neuro-ophthalmologists or neuro-optometrists, counselors, peers, and family. For the purposes of this text we will narrow our focus to the elements of the evaluation most relevant to neuropsychiatrists and offer suggestions for treatment of the neuropsychiatric sequelae of TBI reviewed in the preceding section. More comprehensive descriptions of the evaluation and treatment are offered elsewhere; for additional information, readers are referred to several excellent textbooks in this area, including Silver et al. (1994), Rizzo & Tranel, (1996), and Marion (1999).

Evaluation: initial TBI severity

In some circumstances, neuropsychiatrists are involved in the evaluation and treatment of patients with TBI in the acute injury setting. More commonly, neuropsychiatrists become involved in the care of the patients during the post-acute or late period following TBI. The neuropsychiatrist may sometimes be the first clinician to identify a TBI of clinical significance, particularly in the patient presenting with a neuropsychiatric problem that is either atypical in character or in treatment response in a patient with a history of a remote "mild" TBI. Regardless of the timing of neuropsychiatric involvement, a basic understanding of the methods of determining initial TBI severity and TBI outcome is needed to facilitate interpretation of the clinical history, to evaluate the likelihood of a relationship between a reported head or brain injury and neuropsychiatric problems, and to communicate effectively with the patient's careproviders.

Before ascribing the neuropsychiatric problems experienced by a patient to the effects of TBI, establishing that a physiologically significant injury occurred is paramount. In patients with severe injuries, the injury history will often be fairly obvious and well documented. However, patients with "mild" injuries may not have a documented injury at all, and the neuropsychiatrist may therefore be faced with the challenge of retrospectively determining the initial TBI severity without the benefit of either documentation of the injury itself or even reliable collateral sources of information (e.g., witnesses to the injury or its immediate neuropsychiatric effects). Consequently, a familiarity with the methods by which one may validly interpret the history as supportive of the occurrence of a physiologically significant TBI is essential.

The most commonly used method of determining initial TBI severity in the acute injury period is the GCS (Teasdale & Jennett, 1974). The GCS assesses neurological functioning along three dimensions: motor response, eye opening, and verbal response. Each dimension is assigned a score (minimum = 1, maximum = 4–6 depending on the category) based on the spontaneity and appropriateness of responses and/or activity in that category, offering total score range of 3–15 points. Injury severity is categorized by this scale as mild (GCS = 13–15), moderate (GCS = 9–12), or severe (GCS = 3–8).

While the GCS is a useful descriptor of injury severity, many patients are not assessed according to these criteria by virtue of either failing to present to an emergency room at the time of injury (as is true for many, if not most, mild TBI patients) or failure of emergency medical personnel to assess the patient using this method (also more commonly true for "mildly" injured patients). Additionally, the ability of the GCS to fairly represent the patient's injury severity depends on the timing of the assessment: if the patient is assessed at the scene of the accident (within minutes) the score will relatively accurately reflect the severity of the injury. The GCS continues to be particularly useful for assessing more severe injuries even if the assessment is delayed, as these patients typically continue to demonstrate significant deficits in motor response, eye opening, and verbal response. However, patients with mild or moderate injuries may often recover to a score of 15 before they are evaluated and assigned a GCS score, which may lead subsequent providers (and insurers) to misunderstand a physiologically and functionally significant injury as a trivial and inconsequential one.

Fortunately, several alternative methods of assessing TBI severity are available and widely used to classify injury severity, including several based on the duration of post-traumatic amnesia (PTA). PTA is best defined as the period of dense impairment of new learning (anterograde amnesia) surrounding the acute injury (Russell & Smith, 1961). Although patients may superficially appear "normal" following mild TBI, their attention and encoding of the events they are experiencing may be impaired, resulting in permanently impaired recall of those peri-injury events. During the period of PTA, these patients may also be confused, irritable or affectively labile, demonstrate impaired judgment and insight, and insist that they are "fine" and able to be released from the hospital. The phenomenon is similar to an alcoholic blackout, in that both represent a physiologically significant insult to the brain transiently disrupting the ability to encode new information but does not eliminate completely one's ability to interact with the environment. Both are suggestive of deliria, though neither is commonly described as such. Importantly, this phenomenon is not assessed by the GCS, and a person can score a 15 on this scale while still densely amnestic.

The duration of PTA varies to some degree with the severity of initial injury (it is typically longer with more severe TBI) and the impairment in new learning becomes less dense as the patient recovers. Patients will often describe an absolute loss of memory for a period of time immediately surrounding the injury (brief retrograde and anterograde amnesia), followed by islands of partial and disconnected memories for events occurring as their attention and new learning begin to normalize. Towards the end of the period of PTA, patients report increasingly detailed and connected memories such that they become able to recall *subsequent* events, but not the initial injury, in reasonable (if still incomplete) detail. The severity of and recovery from PTA can be assessed in an ongoing fashion during the acute and post-acute injury period with validated and reliable instruments such as the Galveston Orientation and Amnesia Test (GOAT; Levin et al., 1979).

The GOAT assesses remote and recent memory on a 100-point scale, including personal remote memory (name, place of birth, place of residence), memory of the injury, and orientation (e.g., time and place). Recognizing that recovery of memory is gradual, patients who score less than 65 points are classified as in the period of PTA, those scoring 65–75 points are borderline amnestic, and those scoring greater than 75 points are considered to be through the period of PTA. Importantly, 75 points is not normal, it is simply "normal enough" to establish a reasonably (if still only partially) coherent set of new memories. The GOAT is easily administered, and is more likely to be sensitive to the relevant impairments experienced by patients with mild and moderate injuries than is the GCS.

As with the GCS, determining the initial TBI severity using the GOAT relies upon its application by emergency and medical personnel at the time of injury. While hospitals and emergency services particularly interested in TBI assiduously assess PTA in this fashion, many others do not. Further, since many "mildly" injured patients may not present for evaluation during their period of PTA, this information is not consistently available to help clinicians determine initial injury severity at a later date. Consequently, clinicians may be required to retrospectively estimate the severity of TBI.

Several methods of retrospectively determining TBI severity are available. Retrospectively determining the duration of post-traumatic amnesia is very difficult, as many patients cannot offer an accurate account of the duration of PTA simply as a result of being amnestic for the event. One may be able to estimate duration of absolute PTA based on the time between the last event remembered before the injury and the first memory recalled after the injury. As with the GOAT, it is important to then assess the duration of time before the patient can recall *subsequent* events in reasonable (although not necessarily complete) detail. Using this method, initial TBI severity may be operationally defined as mild (15 minutes to 1 hour PTA), moderate (1–24 hour PTA), or severe (>24 hours PTA). For example, if the unwitnessed injury (e.g., a motor vehicle vs. tree accident) took place in the morning and at a location 30 minutes away from the nearest emergency service, the patient's first memory is of being in the computed tomography (CT) scanner of a hospital 45 minutes away from the scene of the accident, and the patient has no continuous memory of events until being at home later that evening, one might reasonably infer a PTA of mild-moderate severity. In this method, determining whether or not a loss of consciousness (LOC) occurred is both unnecessary and logically impossible – an amnestic patient cannot accurately report on a LOC that occurred while he or she was amnestic.

More formal methods of retrospectively determining the significance of a "mild" TBI are also available, though no uniformly accepted criteria has emerged. The American Congress of Rehabilitation Medicine (1993) suggests that a mild TBI may be defined by the occurrence of one (or more) of the following events: (1) any LOC; (2) any PTA; (3) any alteration of consciousness produced by the event ("dazed and confused"); or (4) focal neurological deficits of any duration. If any of these occurs, a "mild" TBI may be diagnosed. If the LOC is longer than 30 minutes, the GCS after 20 minutes is less than 13, or the PTA is greater than 24 hours then a moderate–severe injury may be diagnosed. While useful, these criteria may have the unintended consequence of classifying patients with acute stress reactions ("dazed and confused") as having a mild TBI where no physiologically significant brain injury has occurred.

Ruff & Jurica (1999) recently proposed a refinement of these criteria that classifies mild TBI into three categories based on LOC, PTA, and neurological symptoms. In their proposal, they suggest mild TBI be classified as Type I if there is a period of altered or lost consciousness of brief (<5 minutes) duration, PTA of 1–60 seconds, or any neurological deficits; Type II if there is a definite LOC of less than 5 minutes, PTA of 1 minute to 12 hours, or any neurological deficit; and Type III if there is a LOC of 5–30 minutes, PTA > 12 hours, or any neurological deficit. These authors suggest that these criteria may usefully establish a minimum criteria for determining that a physiologically significant brain injury has occurred. Unfortunately, they do not clarify the sorts of neurological events that are classified as deficits (e.g., do they include dizziness, headache, incoordination, and tinnitus, or is the intended referent hemiparesis, aphasia, or some other more severe problem?). As such, these criteria should be regarded as useful but entirely preliminary.

The DSM-IV offers research criteria for the Postconcussional Disorder, and suggests that the occurrence of a significant cerebral concussion may be inferred when there is a LOC, a period of PTA, or the development of post-traumatic seizures. Some authors have misinterpreted both the examples cited in the research criteria (LOC > 5 minutes, PTA > 12 hours) and the criteria themselves as strict diagnostic criteria for mild TBI, where their intent is instead the proposal of a set of criteria for a common consequence of TBI, namely postconcussional disorder. Although it is certainly reasonable to diagnose a mild (or even more severe) TBI when these criteria are fulfilled, they are indeed far too conservative to merit routine clinical application. Hence, these criteria should not be used in clinical settings at this time.

Evaluation: TBI outcome severity

While determining the initial TBI is necessary to decide whether or not a physiologically significant injury occurred, the clinical and functional outcomes from any such injury are ultimately the issues that prompt patients and their families to seek neuropsychiatric evaluation and treatment. As with initial TBI severity, there are several methods of formally grading outcome with which one should be familiar, if for no other reason than they are necessary for communicating with other care providers, insurers, and attorneys.

The Glasgow Outcome Scale GOS (Jennett & Bond, 1975) is the simplest and most frequently used assessment of TBI outcome. The GOS ranks outcome on a scale of 1 to 5 (1 = death, 2 = persistent vegetative state, 3 = severe disability, 4 = moderate disability, 5 = good recovery), and is a generally accepted measure of global outcome in this field. The principal problems with this scale are its relatively ambiguous definitions for moderate and good recovery, and a relatively low ceiling to pass before meeting the definition of "good" outcome – although able to perform basic activities of daily living, live independently, make independent use of transportation services, and communicate effectively with others, these "good" outcome patients may have significant neuropsychological and neuropsychiatric problems.

The Rancho Los Amigos Scale (RLAS) (Hagen et al., 1972) provides a more detailed method of determining outcome severity. The RLAS ranks outcome on a scale of 1 to 8 (1 = coma, 8 = purposeful, appropriate, but still symptomatic), and the highest outcome category characterizes the moderately to mildly impaired TBI patient more accurately than the GOS. However, while neuropsychiatric (cognitive, emotional, and social) impairments are mentioned as potential problems, their effect on functioning is not well defined. In other words, most of the mild–moderately impaired TBI patients seen in neuropsychiatric practice will all fit the definition of level 8 outcome on the RLAS, and treatment interventions that result in improvement will not be reflected on this scale. For this reason, we suggest that the assessment of TBI outcome use both the RLAS and also the Global Assessment of Functioning

Scale (GAF) (American Psychiatric Association, 1994) to both define TBI outcome severity and also to assess functioning on a familiar scale that will be more sensitive to neuropsychiatric changes and benefits derived from treatment.

While familiarity with and use of initial severity and outcome grading methods is needed, it is important to note that the relationship between initial TBI severity and outcome is not straightforward. Prolonged coma, extended (i.e., greater than two weeks) PTA, hemorrhage, skull fracture, older age, and significant comorbid injuries predict relatively poorer outcome, but remarkable recoveries may occur regardless of these factors. By contrast, surprisingly severe symptoms and disability that appear to be out of proportion to the degree of initial injury but are not adequately accounted for by superimposed psychological, social, or economic/medicolegal factors. Additionally, two relatively well-matched individuals may have remarkably different outcomes from similarly severe mechanisms of injury, suggesting that there may be other, as yet poorly understood, vulnerability factors (e.g., apolipoprotein E genotype, or other genetic vulnerability factors) that contribute to TBI outcome. With this in mind, we feel that it is important to give patients the benefit of the doubt with respect to their report of a relationship between an apparent head or brain injury and the development of neuropsychiatric problems. Even in cases where symptoms are best attributed to "psychological overlay" or "emotional factors," or even malingering, the problems with which these patients present merit careful evaluation and will frequently require treatment even if they are not direct neurobiological consequences of TBI.

Evaluation: a suggested approach

Establishing the diagnosis follows from a thorough assessment of the patient, guided by an integration of clinical findings and their implications for the differential diagnosis. When the history and clinical evidence support the diagnosis of TBI, and additional neuropsychiatric problems are present, an evaluation should be undertaken.

If the clinical history does not support the occurrence of a physiologically significant TBI, clinical attention should be directed towards the differential diagnosis of the specific neuropsychiatric problem with which the patient is presenting (e.g., depression, mania, anxiety, dementia, etc.), and an assessment of the patient's reason for focusing on the "injury" as an etiology for his or her current problems should be pursued. Clinicians should be careful about balancing an objective scientific approach to diagnosis with a consideration of the meaning and defensive purpose that is attached to the "injury" by such patients. Abruptly confronting some patients with a "lack of credible evidence" to support a TBI diagnosis has the potential to worsen those patients whose belief in the TBI explanation of their problems serves an important psychological (defensive) function. It is prudent to explore the patient's ability to entertain other possible explanations for their problems and their coping skills more broadly as part of the evaluation, to begin to reinforce other coping skills or interpretations gently, and to avoid abruptly stripping them of this temporarily necessary (albeit maladaptive) defense.

At a minimum, the neuropsychiatric evaluation of a patient with a TBI should include these elements.

(1) *History*, patient report should be combined with witness reports and records (where available) documenting the injury history (GCS, GOAT, etc.). In the absence of additional information, a retrospective assessment of injury history should be obtained using one of the methods described above. The temporal relationship between the injury and onset of neuropsychiatric symptoms is particularly important – a close correspondence between injury and acute onset of cognitive symptoms (at least) is expected. In cases where patients experienced significant physical symptoms as a result of their injury (e.g., headache, pain, etc.), or where medications (e.g., narcotics, benzodiazepines, or other commonly prescribed medicines) obscure the experience of cognitive impairment, patients may not become aware of cognitive problems until they attempt to resume their usual daily activities (e.g., work, activities of daily living, etc.). When symptoms occur, a static or slowly improving set of cognitive, emotional, and behavioral problems is expected. The development of increasing or progressive impairments is not typical and should prompt consideration of another cause of neuropsychiatric impairment.

A history of predisposing factors, including in particular pre-morbid psychiatric conditions, social or occupational dysfunction, and neurological problems, should be obtained. The role of the injury in exacerbating or altering the course of such problems should be determined. Any evidence suggesting co-morbid medical conditions requires particular attention, especially if it includes cardiovascular disease, hypertension, diabetes, inflammatory diseases, or other illness that may directly or indirectly further compromise brain function.

The severity of outcome needs to be established using the methods described above. If significant neuropsychiatric problems are present, assessment of type and severity should be undertaken using standardized scales such as the GAF, the Neuropsychiatric Inventory (Cummings et al., 1994), the Neurobehavioral Rating Scale (Levin et al., 1987), the Overt Aggression Scale (Brooke et al., 1992), and the like. These scales usefully quantify current problems and may be used to carefully assess response to treatment.

(2) *Physical and neurological examinations,* careful physical and elemental neurological examinations are important for determining the presence of physical disabilities that require ongoing or additional attention (e.g., cervical or lumbar pain, vestibular or visual problems, gait disturbance, incoordination, etc.). Even in the absence of such findings, the presence of abnormal primitive reflexes or other neurological "soft signs" (e.g., motor function, motor symmetry, laterality, sensory function, spatial orientation, and language) may provide evidence of impaired brain function. Standardized assessments of "soft" or subtle signs are available for use in this portion of the assessment (Denckla, 1985).

(3) *Mental status examination,* a thorough examination, including both general and cognitive portions (see Chapter 9), is essential. On the general mental status examination, assessment of emotion, including anxiety and irritability, should be a priority and the suspicion for emotional dysregulation (either depression or affective dysregulation) should be high.

With regard to cognition, screening tests such as the mini-mental status examination (MMSE) are notoriously insensitive to the cognitive impairments associated with TBI. Therefore, a normal MMSE should not be regarded as evidence of a lack of cognitive impairment – a more detailed assessment of attention, memory, and executive function should be performed. Tasks of complex attention (Trail Making Test A and B), word list generation, alternating sequences, visual constructional tasks, and memory tasks focused on the manner, quality, and speed of information retrieval are particularly useful in the examination of these patients. However, when consistent and significant impairments on the MMSE are demonstrated they should be regarded as quite concerning, particularly given the relative insensitivity of this test in this population.

(4) *Laboratory examination,* patients with moderate or severe TBI often undergo neuroimaging studies during the acute and post-acute period

following injury, and these films should be reviewed (where available). As suggested in the chapters on neuroimaging and dementia, we suggest that every patient with significant cognitive impairments should undergo a structural neuroimaging study (preferably using MRI) at least once during their evaluation. The rationale for this suggestion is not simply academic curiosity. If significant cerebral contusions or diffuse white matter injury are demonstrated on such studies, one may more assuredly consider the injury to be relatively severe even where the mechanism of injury might not have predicted such severity. Additionally, such findings should prompt additional caution regarding the use of and potential adverse effects of many medications, and may be used to set realistic goals for maximal improvement in the late period following injury. Conversely, a truly normal scan may be used to realistically encourage patients to continue pursuing efforts towards greater recovery and to reassure patients that such is possible.

As many patients with mild TBI will not be studied during the acute injury period, the evaluation in the late period following injury may be the first opportunity to perform such studies. Careful interpretation of the results of this imaging is appropriate, as many will be read as "normal" even when subtle but clinically relevant abnormalities are present. Clinicians are encouraged to review scans themselves and with the neuroradiologists, as this is the best way to ensure that formal interpretations are informed by the relevant clinical correlations. As suggested previously, more detailed methods of analysis using gray–white matter threshold intensity determination or volumetric analysis may reveal abnormalities not readily apparent on standard clinical interpretation. Functional studies such as PET (positive emission tomography) or SPECT (single photon emission computed tomography) may also be useful, although their application to TBI diagnosis is not well established. Use of such studies is, at present, only appropriately performed and interpreted in centers that have expertise in both the technology and its application to this population.

The issue of whether quantitative electroencephalography (QEEG) should be performed is a contentious one. Advocates of this technology suggest that it may reveal patterns of abnormal physiology that are both sensitive and specific to TBI, including mild TBI. At present, this tool is largely regarded as one for research purposes, but it may clarify the diagnosis when there is question about the veracity of the TBI history.

Finally, reversible causes of neuropsychiatric problems should be performed as in any other evaluation, including studies for reversible dementias and medical causes of depression (TSH, B12, folate, RPR, ESR, HIV, etc.).

(5) *Neuropsychological evaluation*, this is particularly useful when additional information on the pattern and the extent of cognitive impairments is needed to clarify the diagnosis and guide treatment planning. A neuropsychological assessment directed at specific aspects of cognition and psychological functioning may help refine the differential diagnosis (e.g., more clearly distinguishing between subcortical and cortical patterns, or assess the potential contribution of depression or anxiety to clinically observed deficits and functional impairments). Further, the results of testing help identify areas of relative strength that can be supported when developing a treatment plan for both patient and family (e.g., medication regimens, compensatory behavioral strategies).

Treatment

Treating the neuropsychiatric sequelae of TBI is a challenging task, and usually requires a multimodal approach. A detailed discussion of all aspects of treatment is well beyond the scope of this book, but a few general principles are important to keep in mind. To reiterate a point made earlier in this chapter, whether one regards the development of neuropsychiatric problems following TBI as a consequence of injury-related neurobiological disturbances, emotional and psychological reactions to trauma and physical injury, or as the product of a complex set of many such factors, it is clear that post-TBI neuropsychiatric problems do develop, interfere with recovery and rehabilitation, and require treatment.

Despite the high frequency of neuropsychiatric problems following TBI, there is a relative paucity of TBI-specific treatment studies available to guide treatment selection. Consequently, the vast majority of currently available treatments for the neuropsychiatric sequelae of TBI are based on those used to treat phenotypically similar psychiatric disorders. In general, such treatments are helpful to TBI survivors, although certain categories of medication appear to be less well suited to TBI patients due to their side-effect profiles (see below).

Also, as stated previously it is generally true that the neuropsychiatric sequelae of TBI are neither singular in type nor uniform in presentation or response to treatment – TBI survivors often develop symptoms and syndromes that cross conventional diagnostic boundaries (e.g., comorbid anxiety, depressed mood, aggression, and cognitive impairment). As a result, translating diagnosis-specific treatment approaches into clinical practice with many TBI survivors is a challenging (if not unrealistic) task. Many of the treatment strategies, pharmacological or otherwise, used to treat neuropsychiatric problems after TBI are not diagnosis-specific – a single agent may be usefully employed to treat several problems (see Table 18.2). Therefore, we will depart from the usual method of discussing treatment with respect to a specific diagnostic category (e.g., depression, mania, anxiety, aggression, psychosis, and so on), and instead briefly present treatment options by modality and the problems for which they may be most useful.

Psychotherapy

Psychotherapy (e.g., supportive, individual, cognitive–behavioral, group, and family) is an important component of treating any neuropsychiatric problem following TBI. As stated previously, the tasks in psychotherapy include adjustment to neuropsychiatric, neurological, and physical disability by both the patient and the family, re-establishing a cohesive sense of self, and also addressing additional psychological, social, and medicolegal issues that commonly occur after TBI. In general, these issues are best addressed by a clinician familiar with not only TBI, but also with the complex psychosocial issues (including medicolegal problems) specific to TBI. Of the many references available, we recommend *Psychotherapy of the Brain-Injured Patient: Reclaiming the Shattered Self* (Miller, 1993) as a guide to the theory and practice of psychotherapy for these patients.

Second, patients and families should be encouraged to become involved with local TBI support groups. Local and statewide Brain Injury Association chapters exist in most areas of the United States, and offer peer-level psychological support and advocacy for patients and families. Many such local associations also have knowledge of TBI professionals in their area, and may be able to facilitate connecting TBI survivors and their families to the professional and community resources they need. Additionally, many local associations can assist patients and families in navigating what are often times confusing systems of service provision that may otherwise present barriers to accessing the care that they need. Several local associations also sponsor peer- and self-advocacy programs designed to foster the brain-injured individual's return to independent living and continued self-advocacy to the greatest extent possible given his or her post-injury capabilities.

Neuropsychological and cognitive remediation therapies

The importance of neuropsychological evaluation and treatment for cognitively and behaviorally impaired brain-injured patients cannot be overstated – it is an essential element of treatment. The fundamental principle of most current neuropsychological and cognitive remediation treatments is to facilitate the recovery of cognitive and behavioral functions to the greatest extent possible via the development of compensatory strategies that make use of the individual's cognitive and behavioral strengths. In essence, the person learns to use their strengths to compensate for his or her deficits. For example, patients with working memory and memory retrieval deficits but good language skills are frequently taught to develop note-taking skills, to use "reminder alarms" on their watches, and to use dictaphone or digital recorders to compensate for their memory impairments. Many patients jokingly refer to their notebooks, daytimers, and other such devices as "peripheral brains," but nonetheless find these strategies extremely useful.

In general, these therapies should be practical, problem-focused, relatively short-term in duration, and realistic in light of the patient's deficits. While task-specific therapies are needed early in treatment, incorporating skills that permit compensatory strategies to be applied to more general situations is a necessary component of treatment. Such therapies should be performed by a neuropsychologist (and/or associated staff) experienced in the treatment of TBI patients. In many cases, counselors, occupational, physical, and speech therapists must be called upon to serve as psychotherapists as part of their interaction with these patients. The importance of incorporating the basic principles of psychotherapy (re-establishing a sense of self, sense of competence, and adjusting to disability) during rehabilitation is paramount – these sessions are often intensely anxiety provoking as a result of the direct confrontation of disability that they entail. Since many of these therapists will have the highest frequency and duration of contact with the patient, they are often in the best position to perform some aspects of psychotherapy and should be supported in performing this role.

Additionally, these treatments are most effective when they are explicitly tied to real-life situations and challenges, and when the family and other caregivers, friends, employers, and so on are able to be engaged in the development and reinforcement of such compensatory strategies. Additionally, good functional recovery is also contingent upon the development of compensatory skills in family members and significant others – when the TBI patient encounters a situation that thwarts their compensatory skills, others in the patient's life should become able to respond appropriately to the emotional or behavioral problems that such failures frequently precipitate. To that end, some rehabilitation centers and services also provide in-home evaluations, which are critical to designing compensatory strategies that are a good fit with the patient's home environment.

Medications

When medications are prescribed, cautious dosing (start-low and go-slow) and empiric trials with continuous reassessment of symptoms using standardized scales and monitoring for drug–drug interactions are essential. As a general rule, medications with significant antidopaminergic and anticholinergic properties should be assiduously avoided, and benzodiazepines should be used sparingly, if at all. Although TBI patients may be particularly susceptible to adverse effects of psychopharmacological medications (e.g., seizures with tricyclic agents, impaired cognition with carbamazepine, psychosis with L-dopa/carbidopa, etc.), at times dosages similar to those used to treat idiopathic psychiatric illness may be required and well-tolerated. Again, the method of dose titration should be very gradual, both to avoid untoward and intolerable side effects and also because many patients become wary of medication interventions after negative experiences. When a single medication does not provide adequate relief of symptoms or cannot be tolerated at therapeutic doses, an alternative strategy is to augment the effect of one medication using a second low-dose agent with a different mechanism of action.

With regard to medication therapies for the neuropsychiatric sequelae of TBI described in this chapter, disappointingly few randomized, double-blind, placebo-controlled studies are available to guide treatment selection. One of us recently published an evidence-based review of psychopharmacology in TBI, which interested readers may find useful for selecting treatments (Arciniegas et al., 2000b). As a means of quickly summarizing this review, Table 18.2 presents a set of recommendations for treatment of the neuropsychiatric sequelae of TBI based on the published literature, and Table 18.3 outlines the typical dose ranges and schedules of these medications when used to treat the neuropsychiatric sequelae of TBI.

Table 18.2. Medications that may be used in the treatment of neuropsychiatric problems following traumatic brain injury (TBI). This list includes only those medications for which there are reports in the TBI literature

	Depression	Affective lability and/or irritability	Mania	Psychosis	Agitation or aggression	Anxiety	Apathy	Cognition	Risk of adverse events
Nortriptyline	++	+	−					−	+
Desipramine	++	+	−					−	+
Amitriptyline	+		−		+++			− −	+++
Protriptyline	+	+	−				++	−	+
Fluoxetine	+++	+++	−		++				++
Sertraline	+++	+++	−		++				+
Paroxetine	++	+++	−		++				+
Lithium	+	+	+		++			−	+++
Carbamazepine		+	++		+++			−	++
Valproate		++	+++		+++				+
Benzodiazepines						+		− −	+++
Buspirone	+	++			+	+			+
Typical Antipsychotics				++	+		−	−	+++
Atypical Antipsychotics				+++	+		−	−	+
Methylphenidate	++	++			++		++	++	+++
Dextroamphetamine	++						++	++	+
Amantadine	+	++			++		+	+	
Bromocriptine			−	−			++	+	+
L-dopa/carbidopa			−	−			+	+	+
Beta-blockers	−				+++		−	−	−
Donepezil							−	+	+

Notes:

(+), potential benefit; (−), potential adverse effect. (Adapted from Arciniegas et al., 2000b.)

Table 18.3. Medications and their dose ranges and typical dosing schedules commonly used in the treatment of the neuropsychiatric sequelae of traumatic brain injury

Medication	Adult Dose Range (mg/day)	Typical Dosing Schedule
Nortriptyline	25–150	Qhs
Desipramine	25–300	Qhs
Amitriptyline	25–150	Qhs
Protriptyline	15–60	QAM
Fluoxetine	10–40	Q AM or Qhs depending on medication-related activation or sedation
Sertraline	25–200	Q AM or Qhs depending on medication-related activation or sedation
Paroxetine	5–50	Q AM or Qhs depending on medication-related activation or sedation
Lithium	150–1500	QD to TID
Carbamazepine	200–1000	QD to TID
Valproate	125–1500	QD to TID
Buspirone	15–90	TID to QID
Haloperidol	0.5–5	QD
Risperidone	0.5–4	QD
Olanzapine	2.5–10	QD
Methylphenidate	5–60	BID to TID
Dextroamphetamine	5–60	BID to TID
Amantadine	50–400	QD to BID
Bromocriptine	2.5–20	TID
L-dopa/carbidopa	10/100–25/250	BID to QID
Propranolol	80–400	BID to QID
Donepezil	5–10	QD

Notes:

QAM, every morning; QD, each day; Qhs, at bedtime; BID, twice daily; TID, three times daily; QID, four times daily.

Summary

Traumatic brain injury is a common problem and one capable of producing a host of neuropsychiatric problems. Closed mechanical TBI is most conducive to diffuse cerebral injury via the combination of pathophysiological process created by primary biomechanical and cytotoxic processes and secondary complications of brain and multisystem trauma. Determining the significance of any given injury to the brain is a challenging task, particularly in mildly injured persons who do not come to medical attention in the acute injury period. In all cases, the occurrence of a definable loss of consciousness, period of post-traumatic amnesia, alteration in consciousness, or focal neurological deficit caused by the injury should suffice as minimum criteria establishing a physiologically significant insult to the brain. Further assessments of the injury should seek to determine the extent of such problems, their duration, and course towards recovery. Assessment of outcome from TBI should be based on a comprehensive view of cognitive, emotional, behavioral, physical, and functional recovery.

The neuropsychiatric sequelae of TBI include delirium (usually limited to the acute post-injury period), dementia, mood-, psychotic-, anxiety-, and aggressive disorders, and postconcussional syndrome, among many others. The relationship between TBI and neuropsychiatric problems is complex. First, pre-TBI psychiatric disorders may be exacerbated by such injuries and may be risk factors for the development of post-injury neuropsychiatric problems and functional impairment. Second, TBI itself may produce neuropsychiatric problems as a direct consequence of injury to the brain. Third, depression, anxiety, pain, fatigue, sleep disturbance, seizures, and other post-TBI problems may result in functional impairment that subsequently adds to these problems and begins a vicious cycle of increasing neuropsychiatric symptoms and functional disability. Finally, medicolegal issues and stresses may add to the list of problems faced by TBI survivors, and further complicate their post-TBI conditions.

In general, evaluation and treatment of neuropsychiatric sequelae following TBI should seek to assiduously define the problems, attempt to ascertain the nature of their relationship to the injury, and finally seek to effect functional recovery regardless of the nature of the problem. A multidisciplinary approach is suggested, and should include a combination of psychotherapy and education, symptom-target psychopharmacological interventions, compensatory strategy building, and other rehabilitative treatments.

Bibliography

Aarsland, D., Larsen, J. P., Lim, N. G., et al. (1999). Olanzapine for psychosis in patients with Parkinson's disease with and without dementia. *Journal of Neuropsychiatry and Clinical Neurosciences,* 11, 392–4.

Achte, K., Jarho, L., Kyykka, T. & Vesterinen, E. (1991). Paranoid disorders following war brain damage. Preliminary report. *Psychopathology,* 24, 309–15.

Adams, R. D., Victor, M. & Ropper, A. H. (1997a). Dementia and the amnestic (Korsakoff) syndrome. In *Principles of Neurology,* 6th edn, ed. R. D. Adams, M. Victor & A. H. Ropper, pp. 417–34. New York: McGraw-Hill Company, Inc.

Adams, R. D., Victor, M. & Ropper, A. H. (1997b). *Principles of Neurology,* 6th edn. New York: McGraw-Hill.

Aistrup, G. L., Marszalec, W. & Narahashi, T. (1999). Ethanol modulation of nicotinic acetylcholine receptor currents in cultured cortical neurons. *Molecular Pharmacology,* 55, 39–49.

Akkerman, K., Carr, V. & Lewin, T. (1992). Changes in ego defenses with recovery from depression. *Journal of Nervous and Mental Disease,* 180, 634–8.

Akkerman, K., Lewin, T. J. & Carr, V. J. (1999). Long-term changes in defense style among patients recovering from major depression. *Journal of Nervous and Mental Disease,* 187, 80–7.

Albucher, R. C., Abelson, J. L. & Nesse, R. M. (1998). Defense mechanism changes in successfully treated patients with obsessive–compulsive disorder. *American Journal of Psychiatry,* 155, 558–9.

Alexi, T. & Azmitia, E. C. (1991). Ethanol stimulates [^{3}H]5-HT high-affinity uptake by rat forebrain synaptosomes: role of 5-HT receptors and voltage channel blockers. *Brain Research,* 544, 243–7.

American Academy of Neurology (1989). Assessment: EEG brain mapping. *Neurology,* 13, 1100–1.

American Congress of Rehabilitation Medicine (1993). Definition of mild traumatic brain injury. *Journal of Head Trauma Rehabilitiation,* 8, 86–7.

American Electroencephlographic Society (1987). Statement on clinical use of quantitative EEG. *Journal of Clinical Neurophysiology,* 4, 75.

American Psychiatric Association (1994). *Diagnostic and Statistical Manual of Mental Disorders,* 4th edn. Washington, DC: American Psychiatric Association.

American Psychiatric Association (1997). Practice guideline for the treatment of patients with Alzheimer's disease and other dementias of late life. *American Journal of Psychiatry,* 154, S1–S39

American Psychiatric Association Task Force on Quantitative EEG Techniques (1991). Quantitative electroencephalography: a report on the present state of computerized EEG techniques. *American Journal of Psychiatry*, **148**, 961–4.

Andersen, G., Vestergaard, K. & Riis, J. O. (1993). Citalopram for post-stroke pathological crying. *Lancet*, **342**, 837–9.

Andersen, G., Ingeman-Nielsen, M., Vestergaard, K., et al. (1994). Pathoanatomic correlation between poststroke pathological crying and damage to brain areas involved in serotonergic neurotransmission. *Stroke*, **25**, 1050–2.

Andersen, G. (1995). Treatment of uncontrolled crying after stroke. *Drugs and Aging*, **6**, 105–11.

Andersson, S., Krogstad, J. M. & Finset, A. (1999). Apathy and depressed mood in acquired brain damage: relationship to lesion localization and psychophysiological reactivity. *Psychological Medicine*, **29**, 447–56.

Andrews, G., Tennant, C., Hewson, D. M. & Vaillant, G. E. (1978). Life event stress, social support, coping style, and risk of psychological impairment. *Journal of Nervous and Mental Disease*, **166**, 307–16.

Ankarcrona, M., Dypbukt, J. M., Orrenius, S., et al. (1996). Calcineurin and mitochondrial function in glutamate-induced neuronal cell death. *FEBS Letters*, **394**, 321–4.

Arciniegas, D., Adler, L., Topkoff, J., et al. (1999). Attention and memory dysfunction after traumatic brain injury: cholinergic mechanisms, sensory gating, and a hypothesis for further investigation. *Brain Injury*, **13**, 1–13.

Arciniegas, D., Olincy, A., Topkoff, J., et al. (2000a). Impaired auditory gating and P50 nonsuppression following traumatic brain injury. *Journal of Neuropsychiatry and Clinical Neurosciences*, **12**, 77–85.

Arciniegas, D. B., Topkoff, J. & Silver, J. M. (2000b). Neuropsychiatric aspects of traumatic brain injury. *Current Treatment Options in Neurology*, **2**, 167–86.

Armor, D. J., Polich, J. M. & Stanbul, H. B. (1978). *Alcohol and Treatment*. New York: Wiley.

Audesirk, G., Cabell, L. & Kern, M. (1997). Modulation of neurite branching by protein phosphorylation in cultured rat hippocampal neurons. *Developmental Brain Research*, **102**, 247–60.

Auzou, P., Ozsancak, C., Hannequin, D., et al. (1996). Clozapine for the treatment of psychosis in Parkinson's disease: a review. *Acta Neurologica Scandinavica*, **94**, 329–36.

Baker, K. G., Harding, A. J., Halliday, G. M., et al. (1999). Neuronal loss in function zones of the cerebellum of chronic alcoholics with and without Wernicke's encephalopathy. *Neuroscience*, **91**, 429–38.

Barbaro, G., Di Lorenzo, G., Soldini, M., et al. (1998a). Flumazenil for hepatic encephalopathy grade III and IVa in patients with cirrhosis: an Italian multicentre double-blind, placebo-controlled crossover study. *Hepatology*, **28**, 374–8.

Barbaro, G., Di Lorenzo, G., Soldini, M., et al. (1998b). Flumazenil for hepatic coma in patients with liver cirrhosis: an Italian multicentre double-blind, placebo-controlled, crossover study. *European Journal of Emergency Medicine*, **5**, 213–8.

Bates, B. (1987). *A Guide to Physical Examination and History Taking*, 4th edn. Philadelphia: J.B. Lippincott Company.

Beck, A. T. & Steer, R. A. (1987). *Beck Depression Inventory*. New York: Harcourt Brace Jovanovich.

Beck, A. T. (1999). Cognitive aspects of personality disorders and their relation to syndromal disorders: a psychoevolutionary approach. In *Personality and Psychopathology*, ed. C. R. Cloninger, pp. 411–30. Washington, DC: American Psychiatric Press, Inc.

Benedek, D.M. & Peterson, K.A. (1995). Sertraline for treatment of pathological crying. *American Journal of Psychiatry*, **152**, 953–4.

Benson, D. F. (1981). Aphasia management: the neurologist's role. In *Seminars in Speech, Language and Hearing*, ed. R. T. Wertz, pp. 237–47. New York: Thieme-Stratton.

Benson, D. F. & Gorman, D. G. (1996). Hallucinations and delusional thinking. In *Neuropsychiatry*, ed. B. S. Fogel, R. B. Schiffer & S. M. Rao, pp. 307–24. Baltimore: Williams & Wilkins.

Benson, H. & Friedman, R. (1996). Harnessing the power of the placebo effect and renaming it "Remember Wellness". *Annual Review of Medicine*, **47**, 193–9.

Beresford, T. P. & Gomberg, E. S. L. (1995). *Alcohol and Aging*, New York: Oxford University Press.

Beresford, T., Arciniegas, D., Rojas, D., et al. (1999). Hippocampal to pituitary volume ratio: a specific measure of reciprocal neuroendocrine alterations in alcohol dependence. *Journal of Studies on Alcohol*, **60**, 586–8.

Binnie, C. D. & Prior, P. F. (1994). Electroencephalography. *Journal of Neurology, Neurosurgery, and Psychiatry*, **57**, 1308–19.

Birks, J. S. & Melzer, D. (1999) *Donepezil for Mild and Moderate Alzheimer's Disease*. Cochrane Dementia and Cognitive Impairment Groups for mild and moderate Alzheimer's disease. Cochrane Database of Systematic Reviews 3.

Book, S. W., Villarreal, G., Brawman-Mintzer, O., et al. (1997). Neuroimaging in obsessive compulsive disorder. In *Brain Imaging in Clinical Psychiatry*, ed. K. R. R. Krishnan & P. M. Doraiswamy, pp. 463–76. New York: Marcel Dekker, Inc.

Boston Collaborative Drug Surveillance. (1972). Acute adverse reactions to prednisone in relation to dosage. *Clinical Pharmacology and Therapeutics*, **13**, 694–8.

Bouchard, T .J. (1994). Genes, environment, and personality. *Science*, **264**, 1700–1.

Bridgeford, D., Arciniegas, D. B., Batkis, M., et al. (2000). Methylphenidate treatment of neuropsychiatric symptoms of central and extrapontine myelinolysis. *Journal of Studies in Alcohol*, **61**, 657–60.

Brodie, M. S., Pesold, C. & Appel, S. B. (1999). Ethanol directly excites dopaminergic ventral tegmental area reward neurons. *Alcoholism: Clinical and Experimental Research*, **23**, 1848–52.

Bronster, D. J., Boccagni, P., O'Rourke, M., et al. (1995). Loss of speech after orthotopic liver transplantation. *Transplant International*, **8**, 234–7.

Bronster, D. J., Emre, S., Boccagni, P., et al. (2000). Central nervous system complications in liver transplant recipients: incidence, timing, and long-term follow-up. *Clinical Transplantation*, **14**, 1–7.

Brooke, M. M., Patterson, D. R., Questad, K. A., et al. (1992). The treatment of agitation during initial hospitalization after traumatic brain injury. *Archives of Physical Medicine and Rehabilitation,* **73,** 917–21.

Buckely, P., Stack, J. P., Madigan, C. et al. (1993). MRI of schizophrenia-like psychoses associated with cerebral trauma: clinicopathological correlates. *American Journal of Psychiatry,* **150,** 146–8.

Busch, C. R. & Alpern, H. P. (1998). Depression after mild traumatic brain injury: a review of current research. *Neuropsychology Review,* **8,** 95–108.

Buss, A. H. (1991). The EAS theory of temperament. In *Explorations in Temperament: International Perspectives on Theory and Management. Perspectives on Individual Differences,* ed. J. Strelau & A. Angleitner, pp. 43–60. New York: Plenum.

Cadoux-Hudson, T. A., Wade, D., Taylor, D. J., et al. (1990). Persistent metabolic sequelae of severe head injury in humans *in vivo. Acta Neurochirurgica,* **104,** 1–7.

Cahn, D. A., Sullivan, E. V., Shear, P. K., et al. (1998). Neuropsychological and motor functioning after unilateral anatomically guided posterior ventral pallidotomy. Preoperative performance and three-month follow-up. *Neuropsychiatry, Neuropsychology, and Behavioral Neurology,* **11,** 136–45.

Campbell, H. E. (1969). Studies of driving and drinking. *Quarterly Journal of Studies on Alcohol,* **30,** 457–8.

Campbell, J. J., Duffy, J. D. & Salloway, S. P. (1994). Treatment strategies for patients with dysexecutive syndromes. *Journal of Neuropsychiatry and Clinical Neurosciences,* **6,** 411–18.

Campbell, J. J. & Duffy, J. D. (1997). Treatment strategies in amotivated patients. *Psychiatric Annals,* **27,** 44–9.

Cannon, W. B. (1927). The James–Lange theory of emotion: a critical examination and an alternative theory. *American Journal of Psychology,* **39,** 106–24.

Cassidy, J. W. (1994). Neuropathology. In *Neuropsychiatry of Traumatic Brain Injury,* ed. J. M. Silver, S. C. Yudofsky & R. E. Hales, pp. 43–79. Washington, DC: American Psychiatric Press, Inc.

Charles, H. C., Synderman, T. B. & Ahearn, E. (1997). Magnetic resonance spectroscopy. In *Brain Imaging in Clinical Psychiatry,* ed. K. R. R. Krishnan & P. M. Doraiswamy, pp. 13–22. New York: Marcel Dekker, Inc.

Churchland, P. S. (1986). *Neurophilosophy: Toward a Unified Science of the Mind-Brain.* Cambridge: The MIT Press.

Churchland, P. M. (1988). *Matter and Consciousness,* Revised Edition. Cambridge: The MIT Press.

Cloninger, C. R. (1986). A proposal: a unified biosocial theory of personality and its role in the development of anxiety states. *Psychiatric Developments,* **3,** 167–226.

Cloninger, C. R. (1987). A systematic method for clinical description and classification of personality variants. *Archives of General Psychiatry,* **44,** 573–88.

Cloninger, C. R., Svrakic, D. M. & Przybeck, T. R. (1993). A psychobiological model of temperament and character. *Archives of General Psychiatry,* **50,** 975–90.

Cloninger, C. R., Svrakic, D. M., Bayon, C., et al. (1999). Measurement of Psychopathology as Variants in Personality. In *Personality and Psychopathology,* ed. C.R. Cloninger, pp. 33–66. Washington, DC: American Psychiatric Press, Inc.

Cobb, S. (1952). *Foundations of Neuropsychiatry,* 5th edn. Baltimore: The Williams & Wilkins Company.

Coccaro, E. F. & Siever, L. J. (1995). The Neuropsychopharmacology of personality disorders. In *Psychopharmacology: The Fourth Generation of Progress: An Official Publication of the American College of Neuropsychopharmacology,* ed. F. E. Bloom & D. J. Kupfer, pp. 1567–79. New York: Raven Press, Ltd.

Coenen, A. M. (1998). Neuronal phenomena associated with vigilance and consciousness: from cellular mechanisms to electroencephalographic patterns. *Consciousness and Cognition, 7,* 42–53.

Costa, P. T., Williams, T. F., Somerfield, M. et al. (1996) *Recognition and initial assessment of Alzheimer's disease and related dementias. Clinical practice guideline No. 19.* U.S. Department of Health and Human Services, Public Health Service, Agency for Health Care Policy and Research. AHCPR Publication No. 97–0702.

Cottrell, S. S. & Wilson, S. A. (1926). The affective symptomatology of disseminated sclerosis. *Journal of Neurology and Psychopathology,* VII, 1–30.

Crum, R. M., Anthony, J. C., Bassett, S. S., et al. (1993). Population-based norms for the Mini-Mental State Examination by age and education level. *Journal of the American Medical Association,* **269,** 2386–91.

Cummings, J. L. & Benson, D. F. (1992). *Dementia: A Clinical Approach,* 2nd edn. Boston: Butterworth-Heinemann.

Cummings, J. L., Mega, M., Gray, K., et al. (1994). The Neuropsychiatric Inventory: comprehensive assessment of psychopathology in dementia. *Neurology,* **44,** 2308–14.

Cummings, J. L. & Masterman, D. L. (1999). Depression in patients with Parkinson's disease. *International Journal of Geriatric Psychiatry,* **14,** 711–8.

Cummings, J. L. (2000). Cholinesterase inhibitors: a new class of psychotropic compounds. *American Journal of Psychiatry,* **157,** 4–15.

Cutting, J. (1979). Differential impairment of memory in Korsakoff's syndrome. *Cortex,* **15,** 501–6.

Cutting, J. (1982). Alcoholism: neuropsychiatric complications of alcoholism. *British Journal of Hospital Medicine,* **27,** 335–42.

Dalrymple-Alford, J. C., Jamieson, C. F. & Donaldson, I. M. (1995). Effects of selegiline (deprenyl) on cognition in early Parkinson's disease. *Clinical Neuropharmacology,* **18,** 348–59.

Damasio, A. R. (1994). *Decartes' Error: Emotion, Reason, and the Human Brain.* New York: Avon Press.

Daniel, D. G., Zigun, J. R. & Weinberger, D. R. (1992). Brain imaging in neuropsychiatry. In *The Textbook of Neuropsychiatry,* 2nd edn, ed. S. C. Yudofsky & R. E. Hales, pp. 165–86. Washington, DC: American Psychiatric Press.

Danielczyk, W. (1992). Mental disorders in Parkinson's disease. *Journal of Neural Transmission,* **38**, 115–27.

Dao-Castellana, M. H., Samson, Y., Legault, F., et al. (1998). Frontal dysfunction in neurologically normal chronic alcoholic subjects: metabolic and neuropsychological findings. *Psychological Medicine,* **28**, 1039–48.

Daube, J. R. (1996). *Clinical Neurophysiology.* Philadelphia: Davis Company.

Davison, K. & Bagley, C. R. (1969). Schizophrenia-like psychoses associated with organic disorders of the central nervous system: a review of the literature. In *Current Problems in Neuropsychiatry: Schizophrenia, Epilepsy, The Temporal Lobe,* ed. R. N. Harrington, pp. 113–84. *British Journal of Psychiatry,* Special Publication No. 4.

Dawson, T. M., Steiner, J., Dawson, V. L., et al. (1993). Immunosuppressant FK506 enhances phosphorylation of nitric oxide synthase and protects against glutamate neurotoxicity. *Proceedings of the National Academy of Sciences of the United States of America,* **90**, 9808–12.

Denckla, M. B. (1985). Revised neurological examination for subtle signs. *Psychopharmacology Bulletin, 21,* 773–89.

Di Sclafani, V., Ezekiel, F., Meyerhoff, D. J., et al. (1995). Brain atrophy and cognitive function in older abstinent alcoholic men. *Alcoholism: Clinical and Experimental Research,* **19**, 1121–6.

DiMartini, A. F., Trzebacz, P. T., Pajer, K. A., et al. (1997). Neuropsychiatric side effects of FK506 vs. cyclosporine A. First-week postoperative findings. *Psychosomatics,* **38**, 565–9.

Doe, J. (1987). Alleviation of severe emotional symptoms by carbidopa-levodopa, MSD, in a Parkinson's patient: a personal report. *Journal of Nervous & Mental Disease,* **175**, 185–6.

Doezema, D., King, J. N., Tandberg, D., et al. (1991). Magnetic resonance imaging in minor head injury. *Annals of Emergency Medicine,* **20**, 1281–5.

Duffy, J. D. (1997). The neural substrates of motivation. *Psychiatric Annals,* **27**, 24–9.

Duffy, J. D. & Kant, R. (1997). Apathy secondary to neurologic disease. *Psychiatric Annals,* **27**, 39–43.

Eisenberg, L. (1986). Mindlessness and brainlessness in psychiatry. *British Journal of Psychiatry,* **148**, 497–508.

Emsley, R., Smith, R., Roberts, M., et al. (1996). Magnetic resonance imaging in alcoholic Korsakoff's syndrome: evidence for an association with alcoholic dementia. *Alcohol and Alcoholism,* **31**, 479–86.

Epstein, R. S. & Ursano, R. J. (1994). Anxiety disorders. In *Neuropsychiatry of Traumatic Brain Injury,* ed. J. M. Silver, S. C. Yudofsky & R. E. Hales, pp. 285–311. Washington, DC: American Psychiatric Press, Inc.

Evans, R. W., Gualtieri, C. T. & Patterson, D. (1987). Treatment of chronic closed head injury with psychostimulant drugs: a controlled case study and an appropriate evaluation procedure. *Journal of Nervous and Mental Disease,* **175**, 106–10.

Faber, R. & Trimble, M. R. (1991). Electroconvulsive therapy in Parkinson's disease and other movement disorders. *Movement Disorders,* **6**, 293–303.

Feinberg, T. E. & Farah, M. J. (1997). *Behavioral Neurology and Neuropsychology.* New York: McGraw-Hill.

Fields, J. A., Troster, A. I., Wilkinson, S. B., et al. (1999). Cognitive outcome following staged bilateral pallidal stimulation for the treatment of Parkinson's disease. *Clinical Neurology and Neurosurgery,* **101,** 182–8.

Fife, D. (1987). Head injury with and without hospital admission: comparison of incidence and short-term disability. *American Journal of Public Heath,* **77,** 810–12.

Filley, C. M. & Cullum, C. M. (1993). Early detection of fronto-temporal degeneration by clinical evaluation. *Archives of Clinical Neuropsychology,* **8,** 359–67.

Filley, C. M. (1995). *Neurobehavioral Anatomy,* Niwot: University Press of Colorado.

Filley, C. M. (1996). Neurobehavioral aspects of cerebral white matter disorders. In *Neuropsychiatry,* ed. B. S. Fogel, R. B. Schiffer & S. M. Rao, pp. 913–34. Baltimore: Williams & Wilkins.

Filley, C. M. (1998). The behavioral neurology of cerebral white matter. *Neurology,* **50,** 1535–40.

Fisher, H. W. & Ketonen, L. (1991). *Radiographic Neuroanatomy: A Working Atlas.* New York: McGraw Hill, Inc.

Fogel, B. S. (1996). Drug therapy in neuropsychiatry. In *Neuropsychiatry,* ed. B. S. Fogel, R. B. Schiffer & S. M. Rao, pp. 223–56. Baltimore: Williams and Wilkins.

Fogel, B. S., Schiffer, R. B. & Rao, S. M. (1996). *Neuropsychiatry.* Baltimore: Williams and Wilkins.

Folstein, M. F., Folstein, S. E. & McHugh, P. R. (1975). Mini-Mental State: a practical method for grading the cognitive state of patients for the clinician. *Journal of Psychiatry Research,* **12,** 189–98.

Forssmann-Falck, R., Christian, F. M. & O'Shanick, G. (1989). Group therapy with moderately neurologically damaged patients. *Health and Social Work,* **14,** 235–43.

Foster, G. R., Scott, D. A. & Payne, S. (1999). The use of CT scanning in dementia: a systematic review. *International Journal of Technology Assessment in HealthCare,* **15,** 406–23.

Freud, S. (1891). *On Aphasia.* New York: International Universities Press.

Freund, R. K. & Palmer, M. R. (1997). β-adrenergic sensitization of GABA receptors to ethanol involves a cyclic AMP/protein kinase A second messenger system. *Journal of Pharmacology and Experimental Therapeutics,* **280,** 1192–200.

Friberg, H., Ferrand-Drake, M., Bengtsson, F., et al. (1998). Cyclosporin A, but not FK506, protects mitochondria and neurons against hypoglycemic damage and implicates the mitochondrial permeability transition in cell death. *Journal of Neuroscience,* **18,** 5151–9.

Friedman, G., Froom, P., Sazbon, L., et al. (1999). Apolipoprotein E-ε4 genotype predicts a poor outcome in survivors of traumatic brain injury. *Neurology,* **52,** 244–8.

Fritze, J. (1993). The adrenergic–cholinergic imbalance hypothesis of depression: a review and a perspective. *Reviews in the Neurosciences,* **4,** 63–93.

Fuller, M. G., Fishman, E., Taylor, C. A., et al. (1994). Screening patients with traumatic brain injuries for substance abuse. *Journal of Neuropsychiatry and Clinical Neurosciences,* **6,** 143–6.

Gainotti, G., Caltagirone, C. & Zoccolotti, P. (1993). Left/right and cortical/subcortical dichotomies in the neuropsychological study of human emotions. *Cognitive Emotion,* **7,** 71–93.

Gainotti, G. (1997). Emotional disorders in relation to unilateral brain damage. In *Behavioral Neurology and Neuropsychology,* ed. T. E. Feinberg & M. J. Farah, pp. 691–8. New York: McGraw-Hill.

Gardner, H. (1983). *Frames of Mind: The Theory of Multiple Intelligence.* New York: Basic Books.

Gasparini, M., Fabrizio, E., Bonifati, V., et al. (1997). Cognitive improvement during tolcapone treatment in Parkinson's disease. *Journal of Neural Transmission,* **104,** 887–94.

Gold, B. G., Densmore, V., Shou, W., et al. (1999). Immunophilin FK506-binding protein 52 (not FK506-binding protein 12) mediates the neurotrophic action of FK506. *Journal of Pharmacology and Experimental Therapeutics,* **289,** 1202–10.

Goldberg, E., Gerstman, L. J., Mattis, S., et al. (1982). Effects of cholinergic treatment on post-traumatic anterograde amnesia. *Archives of Neurology,* **39,** 581–9.

Goldsmith, W. (1966). The physical processes producing head injury. In *Head Injury, Conference Proceedings,* ed.W. F. Cavaness & A. E. Walker. Philadelphia: Lippincott.

Goldstein, F. C. & Levin H. S. (1991). Question-asking strategies after severe closed head injury. *Brain and Cognition,* **17,** 23–30.

Goldstein, L. B. (1995a). Basic and clinical studies of pharmacologic effects on recovery from brain injury. *Journal of Neural Transplantation and Plasticity,* **4,** 175–92.

Goldstein, L. B. (1995b). Prescribing of potentially harmful drugs to patients admitted to hospital after head injury. *Journal of Neurology, Neurosurgery and Psychiatry,* **58,** 753–5.

Goleman, D. (1995). *Emotional Intelligence.* New York: Bantam Books, Inc.

Gorman, J. M., Kent, J. M., Sullivan, G. M., et al. (2000). Neuroanatomical hypothesis of panic disorder, revised. *American Journal of Psychiatry,* **157,** 493–505.

Grafman, J., Vance, S. C., Weingartner, H., et al. (1986). The effects of lateralized frontal lesions on mood regulation. *Brain,* **109,** 1127–48.

Grafman, J., Schwab, K., Warden, D., et al. (1996). Frontal lobe injuries, violence, and aggression: a report of the Vietnam head injury study. *Neurology,* **46,** 1231–8.

Gualtieri, C. T. & Evans, R. W. (1988). Stimulant treatment for the neurobehavioral sequelae of traumatic brain injury. *Brain Injury,* **2,** 273–90.

Gyr, K., Meier, R., Haussler, J., et al. (1996). Evaluation of the efficacy and safety of flumazenil in the treatment of portal systemic encephalopathy: a double-blind, randomised, placebo controlled multicentre study. *Gut,* **39,** 319–24.

Hagen, C., Malkmus, D. & Durham, P. (1972). *Rancho Los Amigos Scale.* Communication Disorders Service. Rancho Los Amigos Hospital.

Haines, D. E. (1991). *Neuroanatomy: An Atlas of Structures, Sections, and Systems,* 3rd edn. Baltimore: Williams and Wilkins.

Hall, R. C., Beresford, T. P., Gardner, E. R. & Popkin, M. K. (1982). The medical care of psychiatric patients. *Hospital and Community Psychiatry,* **33,** 25–34.

Halliday, A. L. (1999). Pathophysiology. In *Traumatic Brain Injury,* ed. D.W. Marion, pp. 29–38. New York: Thieme Medical Publishers, Inc.

Hansen, L. A., Natelson, B. H., Lemere, C., et al. (1991). Alcohol-induced brain changes in dogs. *Archives of Neurology,* **48,** 939–42.

Harlow, J. M. (1848). Passage of an iron rod through the head. *Boston Medical and Surgical Journal,* **39**, 389–93.

Harper, C. (1998). The neuropathology of alcohol-specific brain damage, or does alcohol damage the brain? *Journal of Neuropathology and Experimental Neurology,* **57**, 101–10.

Harris, R. A., McQuilkin, S. J., Paylor, R., et al. (1995). Mutant mice lacking the gamma isoform of protein kinase C show decreased behavioral actions of ethanol and altered function of gamma-aminobutyrate type A receptors. *Proceedings of the National Academy of Sciences,* **92**, 3658–62.

Harvey, P. D., Greenberg, B. R. & Serper, M. R. (1989). The affective lability scales: development, reliablility, and validity. *Journal of Clinical Psychology,* **45**, 786–93.

Hauser, R. A. & Zesiewicz, T. A. (1997). Sertaline for the treatment of depression in Parkinson's disease. *Movement Disorders,* **12**, 756–9.

Heilman, K. M. (1997). The neurobiology of emotional experience. In *The Neuropsychiatry of Limbic and Subcortical Disorders,* ed. S. Salloway, P. Malloy & J. L. Cummings, pp. 133–42. Washington, DC: American Psychiatric Press, Inc.

Heimer, L., Alheid, G. F., de Olmos, J. S., et al. (1997). The Accumbens. In *The Neuropsychiatry of Limbic and Subcortical Disorders,* ed. S. Salloway, P. Malloy & J. L. Cummings, pp. 43–70. Washington, DC: American Psychiatric Press, Inc.

Herpertz, S., Gretzer, A., Steinmeyer, E. M., et al. (1997). Affective instability and impulsivity in personality disorder: results of an experimental study. *Journal of Affective Disorders,* **44**, 31–7.

Herr, I., Martin-Villalba, A., Kurz, E., et al. (1999). FK506 prevents stroke-induced generation of ceramide and apoptosis signaling. *Brain Research,* **826**, 210–19.

Hinnant, D. W. (1999). Neurobehavioral consequences: assessment, treatment, and outcome. In *Traumatic Brain Injury,* ed. D.W. Marion, pp. 187–97. New York: Thieme Medical Publishers, Inc.

Hodge, C. W., Mehmert, K. K., Kelley, S. P., et al. (1999). Supersensitivity to allosteric GABA(A) receptor modulators and alcohol in mice lacking PKCε. *Nature Neuroscience,* **2**, 219–28.

Hollender, M. H. (1991). *The American Board of Psychiatry and Neurology: The First Fifty Years.* Deerfield: American Board of Psychiatry and Neurology.

Hughes, J. R. (1982). *EEG in Clinical Practice.* New York: Butterworth Publishers, Inc.

Hughes, J. R., Shanmugham, S., Wetzel, L. C., et al. (1989). The relationship between EEG changes and cognitive functions in dementia: a study in a VA population. *Clinical Electroencephalography,* **20**, 77–85.

Hughes, J. R. (1995). The EEG in psychiatry: an outline with summarized points and references. *Clinical Electroencephalography,* **26**, 92–101.

Hughes, J. R. & John, E. R. (1999). Conventional and quantitative electroencephalography in psychiatry. *Journal of Neuropsychiatry and Clinical Neurosciences,* **11**, 190–208.

Iannaccone, S. & Ferini-Strambi, L. (1996). Pharmacologic treatment of emotional lability. *Clinical Neuropharmacology,* **19**, 532–5.

Imperato, A. & Di Chiara, G. (1986). Preferential stimulation of dopamine release in the nucleus accumbens of freely moving rats by ethanol. *Journal of Pharmacology and Experimental Therapeutics,* **239**, 219–28.

Jackson, G. D. & Duncan, J. S. (1996). *MRI Neuroanatomy: A New Angle on the Brain.* New York: Churchill Livingstone.

James, W. (1884). What is an emotion? *Mind,* **9,** 188–205.

James, W. (1950). *The Principles of Psychology,* New York: Dover.

Jenike, M. A. & Brotman, A. W. (1984). The EEG in obsessive–compulsive disorder. *Journal of Clinical Psychiatry,* **45,** 122–4.

Jennett, B. & Bond, M. (1975). Assessment of outcome after severe brain damage: a practical scale. *Lancet,* **1,** 480–4.

Jennett, B. & Teasdale, G. (1981). *Management of Head Injuries.* Philadelphia: FA Davis.

Jensen, G. B. & Pakkenberg, B. (1993). Do alcoholics drink their neurons away? *Lancet,* **342,** 1201–4.

Jernigan, T. L., Butters, N., DiTraglia, G., et al. (1991). Reduced cerebral grey matter observed in alcoholics using magnetic resonance imaging. *Alcoholism: Clinical and Experimental Research,* **15,** 418–127.

Jeste, D. V., Galasko, D., Correy-Bloom, J., et al. (1996). Neuropsychiatric aspects of the schizophrenias. In *Neuropsychiatry,* ed. B. S. Fogel, R. B. Schiffer & S. M. Rao, pp. 325–44. Baltimore: Williams and Wilkins.

Johnson, K. A. & Becker, J. A. (2000). *The Whole Brain Atlas.* www.med.harvard.edu/AANLIB/home.html

Juncos, J. L. (1999). Management of psychotic aspects of Parkinson's disease. *Journal of Clinical Psychiatry,* **60,** 42–53.

Kaim, S. C. & Klett, C. J. (1972). Treatment of delirium tremens. A comparative evaluation of four drugs. *Quarterly Journal of Studies on Alcohol,* **33,** 1065–72.

Kalivas, P. W., Churchill, L. & Kliteneck, M. A. (1994). The circuitry mediating the translation of motivational stimuli into adaptive motor responses. In *Limbic Motor Circuits and Neuropsychiatry,* ed. P. W. Kalivas & C. D. Barnes. Boca Raton: CRC Press.

Kalra, S., Bergeron, C. & Lang, A. E. (1996). Lewy body disease and dementia. A review. *Archives of Internal Medicine,* **156,** 487–93.

Kant, R., Duffy, J. D. & Pivovarnik, A. (1998). Prevalence of apathy following head injury. *Brain Injury,* **12,** 87–92.

Kaplan, H. I., Saddock, B. J. & Grebb, J. A. (1994). *Synopsis of Psychiatry.* Baltimore: Williams and Wilkins.

Kaufer, D. I. & Cummings, J. L. (1997). Dementia and delirium: an overview. In *Behavioral Neurology and Neuropsychology,* ed. T. E. Feinberg & M. J. Farah, pp. 299–520. New York: McGraw-Hill Company, Inc.

Kelley, J. T. & Reilly, E. L. (1983). EEG, alcohol, and alcoholism. In *EEG and Evoked Potentials in Psychiatry and Behavioral Neurology,* ed. J. R. Hughes & W. P. Wilson, pp. 55–77. London: Butterworth.

Kelly, D. F. (1999). Emergency department management. In *Traumatic Brain Injury,* ed. D. W. Marion, pp. 67–79. New York: Thieme.

Kelly, J. P., Nichols, J. S., Filley, C. M., et al. (1991). Concussion in sports: guidelines for the prevention of catastrophic outcome. *JAMA,* **266**, 2867–9.

Kelly, J. P. & Rosenberg, J. H. (1997a). Diagnosis and management of concussion in sports. *Neurology,* **48**, 575–80.

Kelly, M. P., Johnson, C. T., Knoller, N., et al. (1997b). Substance abuse, traumatic brain injury and neuropsychological outcome. *Brain Injury,* **11**, 391–402.

Khaspekov, L., Friberg, H., Halestrap, A. P., et al. (1999). Cyclosporin A and its nonimmunosuppressive analogue N-Me-Val-4-cyclosporin A mitigate glucose/oxygen deprivation-induced damage to rat cultured hippocampal neurons. *European Journal of Neuroscience,* **11**, 3194–8.

Kido, D. K. & Sheline, Y. I. (1996). Neuroimaging for Neuropsychiatry. In *Neuropsychiatry,* ed. B. S. Fogel, R. B. Schiffer & S. M. Rao, pp. 47–64. New York: Williams and Wilkins.

Kneepkens, R. G. & Oakley, L. D. (1996). Rapid improvement in the defense style of depressed women and men. *Journal of Nervous and Mental Disease,* **184**, 358–61.

Knight, R. T. (1997). Electrophysiological Methods in Behavioral Neurology and Neuropsychology. In *Behavioral Neurology and Neuropsychology,* ed. T. E. Feinberg & M. J. Farah, pp. 101–20. New York: McGraw-Hill Companies, Inc.

Knoll, J. (1992). L-Deprenyl-medication: a strategy to modulate the age-related decline of the striatal dopaminergic system. *Journal of the American Geriatric Society,* **40**, 839–47.

Kraus, J. F. & Nourjah, P. (1988). The epidemiology of mild, uncomplicated brain injury. *Journal of Trauma-Injury, Infection and Critical Care,* **28**, 1637–43.

Kraus, J. F. & Nourjah, P. (1989). The epidemiology of mild head injury. In *Mild Head Injury,* ed. H. S. Levin, H. M. Eisenberg & A. L. Benton, pp. 8–22. New York: Oxford University Press.

Kraus, J. F. & Sorenson, S. B. (1994). Epidemiology. In *Neuropsychiatry of Traumatic Brain Injury,* 5th edn, ed. J. M. Silver, S. C. Yudofsky & R. E. Hales, pp. 3–41. Washington, DC: American Psychiatric Press, Inc.

Kraus, M. F. (2000). Neuropsychiatric sequelae: assessment and pharmacologic intervention. In *Traumatic Brain Injury,* ed. D. W. Marion, pp. 173–86. New York: Thieme Medical Publishers, Inc.

Krauss, S. W., Ghirnikar, R. B., Diamond, I., et al. (1993). Inhibition of adenosine uptake by ethanol is specific for one class of nucleoside transporters. *Molecular Pharmacology,* **44**, 1021–6.

Kril, J., Halliday, G. M., Svoboda, M. D., et al. (1997). The cerebral cortex is damaged in chronic alcoholics. *Neuroscience,* **79**, 983–98.

Krupp, B. H. (1997a). Ethical considerations in apathy syndromes. *Psychiatric Annals,* **27**, 50–4.

Krupp, B. H. & Fogel, B.S. (1997b). Motivational impairment in primary psychiatric and medical illness. *Psychiatric Annals,* **27**, 34–8.

Kunik, M. E., Snow-Turek, A.L., Iqubal, N., et al. (1999). Contribution of psychosis and depression to behavioral disturbances in geropsychiatric inpatients with dementia. *Journal of Gerontology,* **54**, M157–61.

LaBar, K. S. & LeDoux, J. E. (1997). Emotion and the brain: an overview. In *Behavioral Neurology and Neuropsychology*, ed. T. E. Feinberg & M. J. Farah, pp. 675–89. New York: McGraw-Hill Health Professions Division.

Laird, J. D. (1974). Self-attribution of emotion: the effects of expressive behavior on the quality of emotional experience. *Journal of Personality and Social Psychology*, **29**, 475–86.

Lam, R. W., Hurwitz, T. A. & Wada, J. A. (1988). The clinical use of EEG in a general psychiatric setting. *Hospital and Community Psychiatry*, **39**, 533–6.

Lambert, M. T., Trutia, C. & Petty, F. (1998). Extrapyramidal adverse effects associated with sertraline. *Progress in Neuro-Psychopharmacology and Biological Psychiatry*, **22**, 741–8.

Lange, C. G. (1887). *Uber Gemuthsbewegungen.* Leipzig: Thomas.

Lawson, I. R. & MacLeod, D. M. (1969). The use of imipramine ("Tofranil") and other psychotropic drugs in organic emotionalism. *British Journal of Psychiatry*, **115**, 281–5.

Lees, A. J. (1991). Selegiline hydrochloride and cognition. *Acta Neurologica Scandinavica*, **136** (Suppl.), 91–4.

Lerner, A. J., Strauss, M. E. & Whitehouse, P. J. (1997). Neuropsychiatric aspects of degenerative dementias associated with motor dysfunction. In *Textbook of Neuropsychiatry*, 3rd edn, ed. S. C. Yudofsky & R. B. Hales, pp. 799–822. Washington, DC: American Psychiatric Press, Inc.

Levia, D. B. (1990). The neurochemistry of mania: a hypothesis of etiology and rationale for treatment. *Progress in Neuro-Psychopharmacology and Biological Psychiatry*, **14**, 423–9.

Levin, H. S., O'Donnell, V. M. & Grossman, R. G. (1979). The Galveston Orientation and Amnesia Test: a practical scale to assess cognition after head injury. *Journal of Nervous and Mental Disease*, **167**, 675–84.

Levin, H. S., High, W. M., Goethe, K. E., et al. (1987). The neurobehavioural rating scale: assessment of the behavioural sequelae of head injury by the clinician. *Journal of Neurology, Neurosurgery and Psychiatry*, **50**, 183–93.

Levin, H. S., Eisenberg, H. M. & Benton, A. L. (1991). *Frontal Lobe Function and Dysfunction.* New York: Oxford University Press.

Levine, B., Black, S. E., Cabeza, R., et al. (1998). Episodic memory and the self in a case of isolated retrograde amnesia. *Brain*, **121**, 1951–73.

Levy, M. L. & Cummings, J. L. (1999). Parkinson's disease and parkinsonism. In *Movement Disorders in Neurology and Neuropsychiatry*, ed. A. B. Joseph & R. R. Young, pp. 171–9. Malden: Blackwell Science, Inc.

Levy, M. L. & Cummings, J. L. (2000). Parkinson's disease. In *Psychiatric Management in Neurological Disease*, ed. E. C. Lauterbach, pp. 41–70. Washington, DC: American Psychiatric Press, Inc.

Lewin, J. & Sumners, D. (1992). Successful treatment of episodic dyscontrol with carbamazepine. *British Journal of Psychiatry*, **161**, 262.

L'heureux, P. & Askenasi, R. (1991). Efficacy of flumazenil in acute alcohol intoxication: double blind placebo-controlled evaluation. *Human and Experimental Toxicology*, **10**, 235–9.

Li, C., Peoples, R. W. & Weight, F. F. (1994). Alcohol action on a neuronal membrane receptor: evidence for a direct interaction with the receptor protein. *Proceedings of the National Academy of Sciences*, **91**, 8200–4.

Lieberman, D. N. & Mody, I. (1994). Regulation of NMDA channel function by endogenous Ca^{2+}-dependent phosphatase. *Nature,* **369,** 235–9.

Lin, A.M., Bickford, P. C., Palmer, M. R., et al. (1997). Effects of ethanol and nomifensine on NE clearance in the cerebellum of young and aged Fischer 344 rats. *Brain Research,* **756,** 287–92.

Lin, M.J. & Lin-Shiau, S.Y. (1999). Enhanced spontaneous transmitter release at murine motor nerve terminals with cyclosporine. *Neuropharmacology,* **38,** 195–8.

Lishman, W.A., Jacobson, R.R. & Acker, C. (1987). Brain damage in alcoholism: current concepts. *Acta Medica Scandinavica,* **717** (Suppl.), 5–17.

Lishman, W. A. (1990). Alcohol and the brain. *British Journal of Psychiatry,* **156,** 635–44.

Litten, R. Z. & Allen, J. P. (1998). Advances in development of medications for alcoholism treatment. *Psychopharmacology,* **139,** 20–33.

Livesley, W. J., Jang, K. L., Jackson, D. N., et al. (1993). Genetic and environmental contributions to dimensions of personality disorder. *American Journal of Psychiatry,* **150,** 1826–31.

Livesley, W. J., Jang, K. L. & Vernon, P. A. (1998). Phenotypic and genetic structure of traits delineating personality disorder. *Archives of General Psychiatry,* **55,** 941–8.

Lorberboym, M., Bronster, D. J., Lidov, M., et al. (1996). Reversible cerebral perfusion abnormalities associated with cyclosporine therapy in orthotopic liver transplantation. *Journal of Nuclear Medicine,* **37,** 467–9.

Lovinger, D. M. & White, G. (1991). Ethanol potentiation of 5-hydroxytryptamine$_3$ receptor-mediated ion current in neuroblastoma cells and isolated adult mammalian neurons. *Molecular Pharmacology,* **40,** 263–70.

Lucey, M. R., Merion, R. M., Henley, K. S., et al. (1992). The selection for and outcome of liver transplant in alcoholic liver disease. *Gastroenterology,* **102,** 1736–41.

Lucey, M. R., Merion, R. M. & Beresford, T. P. (1994). *Liver Transplantation and the Alcoholic Patient.* Cambridge: Cambridge University Press.

Luria, A. R. (1966). *Higher Cortical Functions in Man,* 2nd edn. New York: Basic Books, Inc.

Lyons, W. E., Steiner, J. P., Snyder, S. H., et al. (1995). Neuronal regeneration enhances the expression of the immunophilin FKBP-12. *Journal of Neuroscience,* **15,** 2985–94.

Machu, T. K. & Harris, R. A. (1994). Alcohols and anesthetics enhance the function of 5-hydroxytryptamine$_3$ receptors expressed in Xenopus laevis oocytes. *Journal of Pharmacology and Experimental Therapeutics,* **271,** 898–905.

MacKinnon, A. J., Henderson, A. S. & Andrews, G. (1990). Genetic and environmental determinants of the lability of trait neuroticism and the symptoms of anxiety and depression. *Psychological Medicine,* **20,** 581–90.

MacLean, P. D. (1949). Psychosomatic disease and the visceral brain: recent developments bearing on the papez theory of emotion. *Psychosomatic Medicine,* **11,** 338–53.

MacLean, P. D. (1952). Some psychiatric implications of physiological studies on the frontotemporal portion of limbic systerm (visceral brain). *Electroencephalography and Clinical Neurophysiology,* **4,** 407–18.

Makatura, T. J., Lam, C. S., Leahy, B. J., et al. (1999). Standardized memory tests and the appraisal of everyday memory. *Brain Injury,* **13,** 355–67.

Mally, J. & Stone, T. W. (1999). Therapeutic and "dose-dependent" effect of repetitive micro-electroshock induced by transcranial magnetic stimulation in Parkinson's disease. *Journal of Neuroscience Research,* **57,** 935–40.

Mann, K., Batra, A., Gunthner, A., et al. (1992). Do women develop alcoholic brain damage more readily than men? *Alcoholism: Clinical and Experimental Research,* **16,** 1052–6.

Marin, R. S. (1991). Apathy: a neuropsychiatric syndrome. *Journal of Neuropsychiatry and Clinicial Neurosciences,* **3,** 243–54.

Marin, R. S., Biedrzycki, R. C. & Firinciogullari, S. (1991). Reliability and validity of the apathy evaluation scale. *Psychiatry Research,* **38,** 143–62.

Marin, R. S., Fogel, B. S., Hawkins, J., et al. (1995). Apathy: a treatable syndrome. *Journal of Neuropsychiatry and Clinical Neurosciences,* **7,** 23–30.

Marin, R. S. (1997a). Apathy – who cares? An introduction to apathy and related disorders of diminished motivation. *Psychiatric Annals,* **27,** 18–23.

Marin, R. S. (1997b). Differential diagnosis of apathy and related disorders of diminished motivation. *Psychiatric Annals,* **27,** 30–3.

Marion, D. W. (1999). Introduction. In *Traumatic Brain Injury,* ed. D. W. Marion, pp. 3–8. New York: Thieme Medical Publishers, Inc.

Martina, M., Mozrzymas, J. W., Boddeke, H. W., et al. (1996). The calcineurin inhibitor cyclosporin A-cyclophilin A complex reduces desensitization of GABA(A) mediated responses in acutely dissociated rat hippocampal neurons. *Neuroscience Letters,* **215,** 95–8.

Matsuura, K., Kabuto, H., Makino, H., et al. (1996). Cyclosporine A attenuates degeneration of dopaminergic neurons induced by 6-hydroxydopamine in the mouse brain. *Brain Research,* **733,** 101–4.

Mayberg, H. S. (1997). Limbic-cortical dysregulation. In *The Neuropsychiatry of Limbic and Subcortical Disorders,* ed. S. Salloway, P. Malloy & J. L. Cummings, pp. 167–77. Washington, DC: American Psychiatric Press.

Mayeux, R., Ottman, R., Tang, M. X., et al. (1993). Genetic susceptibility and head injury as risk factors for Alzheimer's disease among community-dwelling elderly persons and their first-degree relatives. *Annals of Neurology,* **33,** 494–501.

Mayeux, R., Ottman, R., Maestre, G., et al. (1995). Synergistic effects of traumatic head injury and apolipoprotein-E4 in patients with Alzheimer's disease. *Neurology,* **45,** 555–7.

McAllister, T. W. (1983). Overview: pseudodementia. *American Journal of Psychiatry,* **140,** 528–33.

McAllister, T. W. (1992). Neuropsychiatric sequelae of head injuries. *Psychiatric Clinics of North America,* **15,** 395–413.

McAllister, T. W. (1994). Mild traumatic brain injury and the postconcussive syndrome. In *Neuropsychiatry of Traumatic Brain Injury,* ed. J. M. Silver, S. C. Yudofsky & R. E. Hales, pp. 357–92. Washington, DC: American Psychiatric Press, Inc.

McCrea, M., Kelly, J. P., Kluge, J., et al. (1997). Standardized assessment of concussion in football players. *Neurology,* **48,** 586–8.

McIntosh, T. K., Juhler, M., Raghupathi, R., et al. (1999). Secondary brain injury: neurochemical and cellular mediators. In *Traumatic Brain Injury*, ed. D.W. Marion, pp. 39–54. New York: Thieme Medical Publishers, Inc.

Mega, M. S. & Cummings, J. L. (1994). Frontal-subcortical circuits and neuropsychiatric disorders. *Journal of Neuropsychiatry and Clinical Neurosciences*, 6, 358–70.

Mega, M. S., Cummings, J. L., Salloway, S., et al. (1997). The limbic system: an anatomic, phylogenetic, and clinical perspective. In *The Neuropsychiatry of Limbic and Subcortical Disorders*, ed. S. Salloway, P. Malloy & J. L. Cummings, pp. 3–18. Washington, DC: American Psychiatric Press, Inc.

Mega, M. S., Masterman, D. M., O'Connor, S. M., et al. (1999). The spectrum of behavioral responses to cholinesterase inhibitor therapy in Alzheimer's disease. *Archives of Neurology*, 56, 1388–93.

Mehta, K. M., Ott, A., Kalmijn, S., et al. (1999). Head trauma and risk of dementia and Alzheimer's disease: the Rotterdam study. *Neurology*, 53, 1959–62.

Mesulam, M.-M. (1985). Attention, confusional states, and neglect. In *Principles of Behavioral Neurology*, ed. M.-M. Mesulam, pp. 125–68. Philadelphia: F.A. Davis.

Mesulam, M.-M. (1998). From sensation to cognition. *Brain*, *121*, 1013–52.

Mesulam, M.-M. (2000). *Principles of Behavioral and Cognitive Neurology*. Philadelphia: F. A. Davis.

Mihic, S. J. (1999). Acute effects of ethanol on $GABA_A$ and glycine receptor function. *Neurochemistry International*, 35, 115–23.

Miller, L. (1991). Psychotherapy of the brain-injured patient: principles and practices. *Cognitive Rehabilitation*, 9, 24–30.

Miller, L. (1992). When the best help is self-help: or, everything you always wanted to know about brain injury support groups. *Journal of Cognitive Rehabilitation*, 10, 14–7.

Miller, L. (1993). *Psychotherapy of the Brain-Injured Patient: Reclaiming the Shattered Self*. New York: W. W. Norton & Company.

Miller, L. J. & Mittenberg, W. (1998). Brief cognitive behavioral interventions in mild traumatic brain injury. *Applied Neuropsychology*, 5, 172–83.

Minden, S. L. & Schiffer, R. B. (1990). Affective disorders in multiple sclerosis. *Archives of Neurology*, 47, 98–104.

Mindus, P., Rasmussen, S. A. & Lindquist, C. (1994). Neurosurgical treatment for refractory obsessive compulsive disorder: implications for understanding frontal lobe function. *Journal of Neuropsychiatry and Clinical Neurosciences*, 6, 467–77.

Mittl, R. L., Grossman, R. I., Hiele, J. F., et al. (1994). Prevalence of MR evidence of diffuse axonal injury in patients with mild head injury and normal head CT findings. *American Journal of Neuroradiology*, 15, 1583–9.

Miyakawa, T., Yagi, T., Kitazawa, H., et al. (1997). Fyn-kinase as a determinant of ethanol sensitivity: relation to NMDA-receptor function. *Science*, 278, 698–701.

Moellentine, C., Rummans, T., Ahlskog, J. E., et al. (1998). Effectiveness of ECT in patients with parkinsonism. *Journal of Neuropsychiatry and Clinical Neurosciences*, 10, 187–93.

Morioka, M., Hamada, J., Ushio, Y., et al. (1999). Potential role of calcineurin for brain ischemia and traumatic injury. *Progress in Neurobiology, 58,* 1–30.

Morrow, A. L., Janis, G. C., VanDoren, M. J., et al. (1999). Neurosteroids mediate pharmacological effects of ethanol: a new mechanism of ethanol action? *Alcoholism: Clinical and Experimental Research, 23,* 1933–40.

Mueller, J. & Fogel, B. S. (1996). Neuropsychiatric Evaluation. In *Neuropsychiatry,* ed. B. S. Fogel, R. B. Schiffer & S. M. Rao, pp. 11–28. Baltimore: Williams & Wilkins.

Mukand, J., Kaplan, M., Senno, R. G., et al. (1996). Pathological crying and laughing: treatment with sertraline. *Archives of Physical Medicine and Rehabilitation, 77,* 1309–11.

Mullen, L. S., Blanco, C., Vaughan, S. C., et al. (1999). Defense mechanisms and personality in depression. *Depression and Anxiety, 10,* 168–74.

Mutzell, S. (1991). Brain damage in alcoholics without neuropsychological impairment. A population study. *Upsala Journal of Medical Sciences, 96,* 129–40.

Mutzell, S. (1992). Computed tomography of the brain, hepatotoxic drugs and high alcohol consumption in male alcoholic patients and a random sample from the general male population. *Upsala Journal of Medical Sciences, 97,* 183–94.

Nahas, Z., Arlinghaus, K. A., Kotrla, K. J., et al. (1998). Rapid response of emotional incontinence to selective serotonin reuptake inhibitors. *Journal of Neuropsychiatry and Clinical Neurosciences, 10,* 453–5.

Naimark, D., Jackson, E., Rockwell, E., et al. (1996). Psychotic symptoms in Parkinson's disease patients with dementia. *Journal of the American Geriatrics Society, 44,* 296–9.

Nestler, E. J. & Aghajanian, G. K. (1997). Molecular and cellular basis of addiction. *Science, 278,* 58–68.

Neylan, T. C., Reynolds, C. F. & Kupfer, D. J. (1992). Electrodiagnostic techniques in neuropsychiatry. In *Textbook of Neuropsychiatry,* 3rd edn, ed. S. C. Yudofsky & R. B. Hales, pp. 165–80. Washington, DC: American Psychiatric Press, Inc.

Nicoll, J., Roberts, G. W. & Graham, D. I. (1995). Apolipoprotein E-ε4 allele is associated with deposition of amyoid β-protein following head injury. *Nature Medicine, 1,* 135–7.

Nieuwenhuys, R., Voogd, J. & van Huijzen, C. (1988). *The Human Central Nervous System: A Synopsis and Atlas,* 3rd edn. Berlin: Spinger-Verlag.

O'Shanick, G. J. (1991). Cognitive function after brain injury: pharmacologic interference and facilitation. *Neurorehabilitation, 1,* 44–9.

O'Shanick, G. J. & O'Shanick, A. M. (1994). Personality and intellectual changes. In *Neuropsychiatry of Traumatic Brain Injury,* ed. J. M. Silver, S. C. Yudofsky & R. E. Hales, pp. 163–88. Washington, DC: American Psychiatric Press, Inc.

Oishi, M., Mochizuki, Y. & Shikata, E. (1999). Corpus callosum atrophy and cerebral blood flow in chronic alcoholics. *Journal of the Neurological Sciences, 162,* 51–5.

Olafasson, K., Jørgensen, S., Jensen, H. V., et al. (1992). Fluvoxamine in the treatment of demented elderly patients: a double-blind, placebo-controlled study. *Acta Psychiatrica Scandinavica, 85,* 453–6.

Oruc, L., Verheyen, G. R., Furac, I., et al. (1997). Positive association between GABRA5 gene and unipolar recurrent major depression. *Neuropsychobiology*, **36**, 62–4.

Oslin, D., Atkinson, R. M., Smith, D. M., et al. (1998). Alcohol related dementia: proposed clinical criteria. *International Journal of Geriatric Psychiatry*, **13**, 203–12.

Ovsiew, F. (1992). Bedside neuropsychiatry: eliciting the clinical phenomena of neuropsychiatric illness. In *Textbook of Neuropsychiatry*, 2nd edn, ed. S. C. Yudofsky & R. E. Hales, pp. 89–126. Washington, DC: American Psychiatric Press, Inc.

Palmer, A. M., Marion, D. W., Botscheller, M. L., et al. (1994). Increased transmitter amino acid concentration in human ventricular CSF after brain trauma. *Neuroreport*, **6**, 153–6.

Papez, J. W. (1937). A proposed mechanism of emotion. *Archives of Neurological Psychiatry*, **79**, 217–24.

Paulus, W. & Jellinger, K. (1991). The neuropathologic basis of different clinical subgroups of Parkinson's disease. *Journal of Neuropathology and Experimental Neurology*, **50**, 743–55.

Perros, P., Young, E. S., Ritson, J. J., et al. (1992). Power spectral EEG analysis and EEG variability in obsessive–compulsive disorder. *Brain Topography*, **4**, 187–92.

Perry, J. C. & Ianni, F. F. (1998). Observer-rated measures of defense mechanisms. *Journal of Personality*, **66**, 993–1024.

Petty, F. (1995). GABA and mood disorders: a brief review and hypothesis. *Journal of Affective Disorders*, **34**, 275–81.

Pfefferbaum, A., Sullivan, E. V., Mathalon, D. H., et al. (1993). Increase in brain cerebrospinal fluid volume is greater in older than in younger alcoholic patients: a replication study and CT/MRI comparison. *Psychiatric Research*, **50**, 257–74.

Pfefferbaum, A., Sullivan, E. V., Mathalon, D. H., et al. (1997). Frontal lobe volume loss observed with magnetic resonance imaging in older chronic alcoholics. *Alcoholism: Clinical and Experimental Research*, **21**, 521–9.

Pfefferbaum, A., Sullivan, E. V., Rosenbloom, M. J., et al. (1998). A controlled study of cortical gray matter and ventricular changes in alcoholic men over a 5-year interval. *Archives of General Psychiatry*, **55**, 905–12.

Piccini, C., Bracco, L. & Amaducci, L. (1998). Treatable and reversible dementias: an update. *Journal of the Neurological Sciences*, **153**, 172–81.

Pincus, J. H. & Tucker, G. J. (1974). *Behavioral Neurology*. London: Oxford University Press.

Plomin, R., Chuiper, H. M. & Lehlin, J. C. (1990). Behavioral Genetics and Personality. In *Handbook of Personality Theory and Research*, ed. L. A. Pervin. New York: Guilford Press.

Poeck, K. (1969). Pathophysiology of emotional disorders associated with brain damage. *Handbook of Clinical Neurology*, **3**, 343–67.

Poeck, K. & Fredericks, J. A. M. (1985). Pathological laughter and crying. *Handbook of Clinical Neurology*, **45**, 219–25.

Portin, R. & Rinne, U. K. (1983). The effect of deprenyl (selegiline) on cognition and emotion in parkinsonian patients undergoing long-term levodopa treatment. *Acta Neurologica Scandinavica*, **95** (Suppl), 135–44.

Price, B. H., Adams, R. D. & Coyle, J. T. (2000). Neurology and psychiatry: closing the great divide. *Neurology,* **54,** 8–14.

Prichep, L. S., Mas, F., Hollander, E., et al. (1993). Quantitative electroencephalographic (QEEG) subtyping of obsessive-compulsive disorder. *Psychiatry Research,* **50,** 25–32.

Rabins, P. V. (1989). Developing treatment guidelines for Alzheimer's disease and other dementias. *Journal of Clinical Psychiatry,* **59,** S17–S19.

Rabins, P. V., Lyketsos, C. G. & Steele, C. D. (1999). *Practical Dementia Care.* New York: Oxford University Press.

Reeve, A. (1996). Clinical neurophysiology in neuropsychiatry. In *Neuropsychiatry,* ed. B. S. Fogel, R. B. Schiffer & S. M. Rao, pp. 65–92. Baltimore: Williams & Wilkins.

Rich, S. S. & Friedman, J. H. (1995). Treatment of psychosis in Parkinson's disease. In *Medical Psychiatric Practice,* vol. 3, ed. A. Stoudemire & B. S. Fogel, pp. 151–82. Washington, DC: American Psychiatric Press, Inc.

Richard, I. H. & Kurlan, R. (1997). A survey of antidepressant drug use in Parkinson's disease. Parkinson Study Group. *Neurology,* **49,** 1168–70.

Ritter, J. L. & Alexander, B. (1997). Retrospective study of selegiline-antidepressant drug interactions and a review of the literature. *Annals of Clinical Psychiatry,* **9,** 7–13.

Rizzo, M. & Tranel, D. (1996). Head Injury and Postconcussive Syndrome. New York: Churchill Livingstone.

Robbins, T. W. (1997). Arousal systems and attentional processes. *Biological Psychology,* **45,** 57–71.

Robertson, M. M. & Yakeley, J. (1996). Gilles de la Tourette Syndrome and Obsessive-Compulsive Disorder. In *Neuropsychiatry,* ed. B. S. Fogel, R. B. Schiffer & S. M. Rao, pp. 827–70. Baltimore: Williams and Wilkins.

Robinson, R. G., Kubos, K. L., Starr, L. B., et al. (1983). Mood changes in stroke patients: relationship to lesion location. *Comprehensive Psychiatry,* **24,** 555–66.

Robinson, R. G., Kubos, K. L., Starr, L. B., et al. (1984). Mood disorders in stroke patients: importance in locaton of lesion. *Brain,* **107,** 81–93.

Robinson, R. G., Parikh, R. M., Lipsey, J. R., et al. (1993). Pathological laughing and crying following stroke: validation of a measurement scale and a double-blind treatment study. *American Journal of Psychiatry,* **150,** 286–93.

Robinson, R. G. & Jorge, R. (1994). Mood disorders. In *Neuropsychiatry of Traumatic Brain Injury,* ed. J. M. Silver, S. C. Yudofsky & R. E. Hales, pp. 219–50. Washington, DC: American Psychiatric Press, Inc.

Rodd-Henricks, Z. A., McKinzie, D. L., Shaikh, S. R., et al. (2000). Alcohol deprivation effect is prolonged in the alcohol preferring (P) rat after repeated deprivations. *Alcoholism: Clinical and Experimental Research,* **24,** 8–16.

Rojas, D. C., Arciniegas, D. B., Teale, P. D., et al. (1999). Magnetoencephalography and magnetic source imaging: technology overview and applications in psychiatric neuroimaging. *CNS Spectrums,* **4,** 37–43.

Ronty, H., Ahonen, A., Tolonen, U., et al. (1997). Cerebral trauma and alcohol abuse. *European Journal of Clinical Investigation,* **23,** 182–7.

Ross, B. & Michaelis, T. (1994). Clinical applications of magnetic resonance spectroscopy. *Magnetic Resonance Quarterly,* **10**, 191–247.

Ross, E. D. & Mesulam, M. M. (1979). Dominant language functions of the right hemisphere: prosody and emotional gesturing. *Archives of Neurology,* **36**, 144–8.

Ross, E. D. (1981). The aprosodias: functional-anatomic organization of the affective components of language in the right hemisphere. *Archives of Neurology,* **38**, 645–748.

Ross, E. D. (1997). The aprosodias. In *Behavioral Neurology and Neuropsychology,* ed. T. E. Feinberg & M. J. Farah, pp. 699–709. New York: McGraw-Hill Health Professions Division.

Rothbart, M. (1991). Temperament: a developmental framework. In *Explorations in Temperament,* ed. J. Strelau & A. Angleitner, pp. 61–74. New York: Plenum.

Ruff, R. M., Levin, H. S., Mather, S., et al. (1989). Recovery of memory after mild head injury: a three-center study. In *Mild Head Injury,* ed. H. S. Levin, H. M. Eisenberg & A. L. Benton, pp. 176–88. New York: Oxford University Press.

Ruff, R., Camenzuli, L. & Mueller, J. (1999). Miserable minority: emotional risk factors that influence the outcome of mild traumatic brain injury. *Brain Injury,* **10**, 551–65.

Ruff, R. M. & Jurica, P. (1999). In search of a unified definition for mild traumatic brain injury. *Brain Injury,* **13**, 943–52.

Russell, W. R. & Smith, A. (1961). Post-traumatic amnesia in closed head injury. *Archives of Neurology,* **5**, 16–29.

Rutter, M. (1987). Temperament, personality, and personality disorder. *British Journal of Psychiatry,* **150**, 443–58.

Sackeim, H. A., Greenberg, M. S., Weiman, A. L., et al. (1982). Hemispheric asymmetry in the expression of positive and negative emotions. *Archives of Neurology,* **39**, 210–8.

Samson, H. H., Hodge, C. W., Erickson, H. L., et al. (1997). The effects of local application of ethanol in the nucleus accumbens on dopamine overflow and clearance. *Alcohol,* **14**, 485–92.

Satz, P., Forney, D. L., Zaucha, K., et al. (1998). Depression, cognition, and functional correlates of recovery outcome after traumatic brain injury. *Brain Injury,* **12**, 537–53.

Schiffer, R. B., Herndon, R. M. & Rudick, R. A. (1985). Treatment of pathological laughing and weeping with amitriptyline. *New England Journal of Medicine,* **312**, 1480–2.

Schomerus, H. & Hamster, W. (1998). Neuropsychological aspects of portal-systemic encephalopathy. *Metabolic Brain Disease,* **13**, 361–77.

Selby, R., Ramirez, C. B., Singh, R., et al. (1997). Brain abscess in solid organ transplant recipients receiving cyclosporine-based immunosuppression. *Archives of Surgery,* **132**, 304–10.

Selden, N. R., Gitelman, D. R., Salamon-Murayama, N., et al. (1998). Trajectories of cholinergic pathways within the cerebral hemispheres of the human brain. *Brain,* **121**, 2249–57.

Serkova, N., Brand, A., Christians, U., et al. (1996). Evaluation of the effects of immunosuppressants on neuronal and glial cells in vitro by multinuclear magnetic resonance spectroscopy. *Biochimica et Biophysica Acta,* **8**, 93–104.

Shear, P. K., Sullivan, E. V., Lane, B., et al. (1996). Mammillary body and cerebellar shrinkage in chronic alcoholics with and without amnesia. *Alcoholism: Clinical and Experimental Research,* **20**, 1489–95.

Shuto, H., Kataoka, Y., Kanaya, A., et al. (1998). Enhancement of serotonergic neural activity contributes to cyclosporine-induced tremors in mice. *European Journal of Pharmacology*, **341**, 33–7.

Shuto, H., Kataoka, Y., Fujisaki, K., et al. (1999). Inhibition of GABA system involved in cyclosporine-induced convulsions. *Life Sciences*, **65**, 879–87.

Silva, S. G. & Marin, R. S. (1999). Apathy in neuropsychiatric disorders. *CNS Spectrum*, **4**, 31–50.

Silver, J. M. & Yudofsky, S. C. (1994a). Aggressive disorders. In *Neuropsychiatry of Traumatic Brain Injury*, ed. J. M. Silver, S. C. Yudofsky & R. E. Hales, pp. 313–53. Washington, DC: American Psychiatric Press, Inc.

Silver, J. M. & Yudofsky, S. C. (1994b). Psychopharmacology. In *Neuropsychiatry of Traumatic Brain Injury*, ed. J. M. Silver, S. C. Yudofsky & R. E. Hales, pp. 631–70. Washington, DC: American Psychiatric Press, Inc.

Silver, J. M. Yudofsky, S. C. & Hales, R. E. (eds). (1994). *Neuropsychiatry of Traumatic Brain Injury*. Washington, DC: American Psychiatric Press, Inc.

Silver, J. M., Yudofsky, S. C., Slater, J. A., et al. (1999). Propranolol treatment of chronically hospitalized aggressive inpatients. *Journal of Neuropsychiatry and Clinical Neurosciences*, **11**, 328–35.

Silverman, J. S. & Loychik, S. G. (1990). Brain-mapping abnormalities in a family with three obsessive-compulsive children. *Journal of Neuropsychiatry and Clinical Neurosciences*, **2**, 319–22.

Singh, N., Bonham, A. & Fukui, M. (2000). Immunosuppressive-associated leukoencephalopathy in organ transplant recipients. *Transplantation*, **69**, 467–72.

Sloan, R. L., Brown, K. W. & Pentland, B. (1992). Fluoxetine as a treatment for emotional lability after brain injury. *Brain Injury*, **6**, 315–9.

Smith, D. M. & Atkinson, R. M. (1995). Alcoholism and dementia. *International Journal of the Addictions*, **30**, 1843–69.

Spreen, O. & Strauss, E. (1998). *A Compendium of Neuropsychological Tests: Administration, Norms, and Commentary*, 2nd edn. New York: Oxford University Press.

Starkstein, S. E., Federoff, J. P., Price, T. R., Leiguardo, R. C. & Robinson, R. G. (1994). Neuropsychological and neurodiologic correlates of emotional prosody comprehension. *Neurology*, **44**, 515–22.

Starkstein, S. E., Mayberg, H. S., Berthier, M. L., et al. (1990). Mania after brain injury: neuroradiological and metabolic findings. *Annals of Neurology*, **27**, 652–9.

Starkstein, S. E., Migliorelli, R., Teson, A., et al. (1995). Prevalence and clinical correlates of pathological affective display in Alzheimer's disease. *Journal of Neurology, Neurosurgery and Psychiatry*, **59**, 55–60.

Starkstein, S. E. & Robinson, R. G. (1989a). Affective disorders and cerebrovascular disease. *British Journal of Psychiatry*, **154**, 170–82.

Starkstein, S. E., Robinson, R. G. & Price, T. R. (1988). Comparison of patients with and without poststroke major depression matched for size and location of lesion. *Archives of General Psychiatry*, **45**, 247–52.

Starkstein, S. E., Robinson, R. G., Honig, M. A., et al. (1989b). Mood changes after right-hemisphere lesions. *British Journal of Psychiatry*, **155**, 70–85.

Stein, S. C., O'Malley, K. F. & Ross, S. E. (1991). Is routine computed tomography scanning too expensive for mild head injury? *Annals of Emergency Medicine, 20*, 1286–9.

Steiner, J. P., Hamilton, G. S., Ross, D. T., et al. (1997). Neurotrophic immunophilin ligands stimulate structural and functional recovery in neurodegenerative animal models. *Proceedings of the National Academy of Sciences of the United States of America, 94*, 2019–24.

Strub, R. L. & Black, W. B. (1985). *The Mental Status Examination in Neurology,* 2nd edn. Philadelphia: F.A. Davis Company.

Strub, R. L. & Black, F. W. (1988). *Neurobehavioral Disorders: A Clinical Approach.* Philadelphia: F. A. Davis Company.

Strub, R. L. & Black, F. W. (1997). The mental status exam. In *Behavioral Neurology and Neuropsychology,* ed. T. E. Feinberg & M. J. Farah. New York: McGraw-Hill.

Stuss, D. T., Gow, C. A. & Hetherington, C. R. (1992). "No longer Gage": frontal lobe - dysfunction and emotional changes. *Journal of Consulting and Clinical Psychology, 60*, 349–59.

Sullivan, E. V., Marsh, L., Mathalon, D. H., et al. (1995). Anterior hippocampal volume deficits in nonamnesic, aging chronic alcoholics. *Alcoholism: Clinical and Experimental Research, 19*, 110–22.

Sullivan, E. V., Marsh, L., Mathalon, D. H., et al. (1996). Relationship between alcohol withdrawal seizures and temporal lobe white matter deficits. *Alcoholism: Clinical and Experimental Research, 20*, 348–54.

Sullivan, E. V., Mathalon, D. H., Lim, K. O., et al. (1998). Patterns of regional cortical dysmorphology distinguishing schizophrenia and chronic alcoholism. *Biological Psychiatry, 43*, 118–31.

Tarczy, M. & Szirmai, I. (1995). Failure of dopamine metabolism: borderlines of parkinsonism and dementia. *Acta Bio-Medica de Ateneo Parmense, 66*, 93–7.

Taylor, A. E., Cox, C. A. & Mailis, A. (1996). Persistent neuropsychological deficits following whiplash: evidence for chronic mild traumatic brain injury? *Archives of Physical Medicine and Rehabilitation, 77*, 529–35.

Taylor, M. A. (1999). *The Fundamentals of Clinical Neuropsychiatry.* New York: Oxford University Press.

Teasdale, G. & Jennett, B. (1974). Assessment of coma and impaired consciousness. A practical scale. *Lancet, 2*, 81–4.

Teasdale, G. & Mendelow, D. (1984). Pathophysiology of head injuries. In *Closed Head Injury: Psychological, Social, and Family Consequences,* ed. N. Brooks, pp. 4–36. New York: Oxford University Press.

Teasdale, G. M., Nicoll, J. A. R., Murray, G., et al. (1997). Association of apolipoprotein E polymorphism with outcome after head injury. *Lancet, 350*, 1069–71.

Thatcher, R. W., Walker, R. A., Gerson, I., et al. (1989). EEG discriminant analyses of mild head trauma. *Electroencephalography and Clinical Neurophysiology, 73*, 93–106.

Thatcher, R. W., Cantor, D. S., McAlaster, R., et al. (1991). Comprehensive predictions of outcome in closed head-injured patients: the development of prognostic equations. *Annals of New York Academy of Sciences,* **620**, 82–101.

Thatcher, R. W., Camacho, M., Salazar, A., et al. (1997). Quantitative MRI of the gray-white matter distribution in traumatic brain injury. *Journal of Neurotrauma,* **14**, 1–14.

Thatcher, R. W., Biver, C., McAlaster, R., et al. (1998a). Biophysical linkage between MRI and EEG amplitude in closed head injury. *Neuroimage,* **7**, 352–67.

Thatcher, R. W., Biver, C., McAlaster, R., et al. (1998b). Biophysical linkage between MRI and EEG coherence in traumatic brain injury. *Neuroimage,* **8**, 307–26.

Thatcher, R. W., Moore, N., John, E. R., et al. (1999). QEEG and traumatic brain injury: rebuttal of the American Academy of Neurology 1997 report by the EEG and Clinical Neuroscience Society. *Clinical Electroencephalography,* **30**, 94–8.

Tomkins, S. S. (1962). *Affect, Imagery, and Consciousness,* vol. 2, *The Positive Affects.* New York: Springer.

Tomkins, S. S. (1963). *Affect, Imagery, and Consciousness,* vol. 2, *The Negative Affects.* New York: Springer.

Torner, J. C., Choi, S. & Barnes, T. Y. (1999). Epidemiology. In *Traumatic Brain Injury,* ed. D.W. Marion, pp. 9–28. New York: Thieme Medical Publishers, Inc.

Trimble, M. R. (1981). *Neuropsychiatry.* Chichester: John Wiley and Sons.

Troster, A. I., Fields, J. A., Wilkinson, S. B., et al. (1997). Unilateral pallidal stimulation for Parkinson's disease: neurobehavioral functioning before and 3 months after electrode implantation. *Neurology,* **49**, 1078–83.

Trzepacz, P. T., Brenner, R. & Van Thiel, D. H. (1989). A psychiatric study of 247 liver transplantation candidates. *Psychosomatics,* **30**, 147–53.

Trzepacz, P. T. & Baker, R. W. (1993). *The Psychiatric Mental Status Examination.* New York: Oxford University Press.

Trzepacz, P. T. (1994). Delirium. In *Neuropsychiatry of Traumatic Brain Injury,* ed. J. M. Silver, S. C. Yudofsky & R. E. Hales, pp. 189–218. Washington, DC: American Psychiatric Press, Inc.

Udaka, F., Yamao, S., Nagata, H., et al. (1984). Pathologic laughing and crying treated with Levodopa. *Neurology,* **41**, 1095–6.

Vaillant, G. E. (1977). *Adaptation to Life.* Boston: Little, Brown.

Vaillant, G. E. (1979). Natural history of male psychologic health: effects of mental health on physical health. *New England Journal of Medicine,* **301**, 1249–54.

Vaillant, G. E. (1993). *The Wisdom of the Ego.* Boston: Harvard University Press.

Vaillant, G. E. (1995). *The Natural History of Alcoholism, Revisited.* Cambridge: Harvard University Press.

Vaillant, G. E., Bond, M. & Vaillant, C. O. (1986). An empirically validated hierarchy of defense mechanisms. *Archives of General Psychiatry,* **43**, 786–94.

Vaillant, G. E. & Koury, S. H. (1993). Late midlife development. In *The Course of Life,* vol. 6, Late Childhood, ed. G. H. Pollock, S. I. Greenspan et al., pp. 1–22. Madison: International Universities Press, Inc.

VanDoren, M. J., Matthews, D. B., Janis, G. C., et al. (2000). Neuroactive steroid 3alpha-hydroxy-5alpha-pregnan-20-one modulates electrophysiological and behavioral actions of ethanol. *Journal of Neuroscience*, **20**, 1982–9.

Victor, M., Adams, R. D. & Collins, G. H. (1971). *The Wernicke-Korsakoff Syndrome*. Philadelphia: F.A. Davis.

Vingerhoets, G., Van der Linden, C., Lannoo, E., et al. (2000). Cognitive outcome after unilateral pallidal stimulation in Parkinson's disease. *Journal of Neurology, Neurosurgery & Psychiatry*, **66**, 297–304.

Vlaardingerbroek, M. T. & den Boer, J. A. (1999). *Magnetic Resonance Imaging*, 2nd edn. Berlin: Springer.

Walker, Z., Grace, J., Overshot, R., et al. (1999). Olanzapine in dementia with Lewy bodies: a clinical study. *International Journal of Geriatric Psychiatry*, **14**, 459–66.

Wang, Y., Palmer, M. R., Cline, E. J., et al. (1997). Effects of ethanol on striatal dopamine overflow and clearance: an *in vivo* electrochemical study. *Alcohol*, **14**, 593–601.

Weiner, J. L., Valenzuela, C. F., Watson, P. L., et al. (1997). Elevation of basal protein kinase C activity increases ethanol sensitivity of GABA$_A$ receptors in rat hippocampal CA1 pyramidal neurons. *Journal of Neurochemistry*, **68**, 1949–59.

Weiner, J. L., Dunwiddie, T. V. & Valenzuela, C. F. (1999). Ethanol inhibition of synaptically evoked kainate responses in rat hippocampal CA3 pyramidal neurons. *Molecular Pharmacology*, **56**, 85–90.

Wester, K. & Hugdahl, K. (1997). Thalamotomy and thalamic stimulation: effects on cognition. *Stereotactic and Functional Neurosurgery*, **69**, 80–5.

White, K. E. & Cummings, J. L. (1997). Neuropsychiatric Aspects of Alzheimer's Disease and Other Dementing Illnesses. In *Textbook of Neuropsychiatry*, 3rd edn, ed. S. C. Yudofsky & R. E. Hales, pp. 823–54. Washington, DC: American Psychiatric Press, Inc.

Whitehouse, P. J., Price, D. L., Struble, R. G., et al. (1982). Alzheimer's disease and senile dementia: loss of neurons in the basal forebrain. *Science*, **215**, 1237–9.

Whitehouse, P. J., Martino, A. M., Antuono, P. G., et al. (1986). Nicotinic acetylcholine binding sites in Alzheimer's disease. *Brain Research*, **371**, 146–51.

Wijdicks, E. F., Wiesner, R. H. & Krom, R. A. (1995). Neurotoxicity in liver transplant recipients with cyclosporine immunosuppression. *Neurology*, **45**, 1962–4.

Wijdicks, E. F., Plevak, D. J., Wiesner, R. H., et al. (1996). Causes and outcome of seizures in liver transplant recipients. *Neurology*, **47**, 1523–5.

Williams, K. H. & Goldstein, G. (1979). Cognitive and affective responses to lithium in patients with organic brain syndrome. *American Journal of Psychiatry*, **136**, 800–3.

Wilson, S. A. K. (1924). Some problems in neurology. II. Pathological laughing and crying. *Journal of Neurology and Psychopathology*, **16**, 299–333.

Wolf, J. K., Santana, H. B. & Thorpy, M. (1979). Treatment of "emotional incontinence" with levodopa. *Neurology*, **29**, 1435–6.

Wolters, E. C. (1999). Dopaminomimetic psychosis in Parkinson's disease patients: diagnosis and treatment. *Neurology*, **52**, S10–3.

Wong, M. & Yamada, K. A. (2000). Cyclosporine induces epileptiform activity in an *in vitro* seizure model. *Epilepsia,* **41**, 271–6.

Wood, A. M. & Bristow, D. R. (1998). N-methyl-D-aspartate receptor desensitization is neuro-protective by inhibiting glutamate-induced apoptotic-like death. *Journal of Neurochemistry,* **70**, 677–87.

Workman, R. H., Orengo, C. A., Bakey, A. A., et al. (1997). The use of risperdone for psychosis and agitation in demented patients with Parkinson's disease. *Journal of Neuropsychiatry and Clinical Neurosciences,* **9**, 594–7.

Woyshville, M. J., Lackamp, J. M., Eisengart, J. A., et al. (1999). On the meaning and measure-ment of affective instability: clues from chaos theory. *Biological Psychiatry,* **45**, 261–9.

Wroblewski, B. A., McColgan, K., Smith, K., et al. (1990). The incidence of seizures during tri-cyclic antidepressant drug treatment in a brain-injured population. *Journal of Clinical Psychopharmacology,* **10**, 124–8.

Wroblewski, B. A., Leary, J. M., Phelan, A. M., et al. (1992). Methylphenidate and seizure fre-quency in brain injured patients with seizure disorders. *Journal of Clinical Psychiatry,* **53**, 86–9.

Wroblewski, B., Glenn, M. B., Cornblatt, R., et al. (1993). Protriptyline as an alternative stimu-lant medication in patients with brain injury: a series of case reports. *Brain Injury,* **7**, 353–62.

Wroblewski, B. A., Joseph, A. B. & Cornblatt, R. R. (1996). Antidepressant pharmacotherapy and the treatment of depression in patients with severe traumatic brain injury: a controlled, pros-pective study. *Journal of Clinical Psychiatry,* **57**, 582–7.

Wroblewski, B. A., Joseph, A. B., Kupfer, J., et al. (1997). Effectiveness of valproic acid on destruc-tive and aggressive behaviours in patients with acquired brain injury. *Brain Injury,* **11**, 37–47.

Yoshimura, M. & Tabakoff, B. (1999). Ethanol's actions on cAMP-mediated signaling in cells transfected with type VII adenylyl cyclase. *Alcoholism: Clinical and Experimental Research,* **23**, 1457–61.

Yudofsky, S. C. & Hales, R. E. (1992). *Textbook of Neuropsychiatry.* Washington, DC: American Psychiatric Press.

Yudofsky, S. C. & Hales, R. E. (1997). *Textbook of Neuropsychiatry,* 2nd edn. Washington, DC: American Psychiatric Press.

Yuh, W. T., Simonson, T. M., D'Alessandro, M. P., et al. (1995). Temporal changes of MR findings in central pontine myelinolysis. *American Journal of Neuroradiology,* **16**, 975–7.

Zhou, Q., Verdoorn, T. A. & Lovinger, D. M. (1998). Alcohols potentiate the function of 5-HT$_3$ receptor channels on NCB-20 neuroblastoma cells by favouring and stabilizing the open channel state. *Journal of Physiology,* **507**, 335–52.

Zimatkin, S. M. & Deitrich, R. A. (1995). Aldehyde dehydrogenase activities in the brains of rats and mice genetically selected for different sensitivity to alcohol. *Alcoholism: Clinical & Experimental Research,* **19**, 1300–6.

Appendix

Neuropsychiatry evaluation and consultation form

Date(s): _____

Time(s): _____

Patient: _____

Evaluator: _____

Location: _____

Chief Complaint:

History of Present Illness (onset and duration, quality, intensity, relationship to precipitating and palliating factors, context in which symptoms occur, treatments to-date; include report of symptoms by others and collateral information, where available; if other medical/neurological/psychiatric disorders are present, note temporal and contextual relationship of the presenting problems to these other conditions):

_____

_____

_____

_____

_____

_____

_____

_____

_____

_____

_____

_____

_____

_____

_____

_____

_____

_____

_____

_____

_____

_____

_____

Neuropsychiatry evaluation and consultation form

Past Medical and Surgical History (include diagnoses, past treatments/outcomes, and hospitalizations; ask specifically about seizures or "spells," and also about concussions or other head trauma):

_____
_____
_____
_____
_____
_____
_____
_____

Past Psychiatric History (include diagnoses, treatments/outcomes, suicide attempts, violence toward property and persons, and hospitalizations, if any):

_____
_____
_____
_____
_____
_____
_____
_____
_____

Current Medications:

_____
_____
_____
_____
_____
_____

Allergies:

_____
_____

Neuropsychiatry evaluation and consultation form

Substance History (include past and current use of alcohol, drugs, tobacco, and caffeine; note any tolerance, withdrawal, loss of control, or use despite adverse consequences with each; ask CAGE questions):

_____

_____

_____

_____

_____

_____

_____

Social History (include development, academic performance/problems, employment, military history, legal history, relationships and present marital status, financial status/medical coverage):

_____

_____

_____

_____

_____

_____

_____

_____

_____

_____

Family History (include medical, neurological, and psychiatric conditions):

_____

_____

_____

_____

_____

_____

_____

Neuropsychiatry evaluation and consultation form

Review of Systems and Symptoms:

(1) Cognition (attention, language, memory, praxis, recognition, complex cognition):

_____
_____
_____
_____
_____
_____
_____

(2) Emotion (distinguish between mood and affect, subjective and objective components of each, and specify the duration, variability, intensity, appropriateness, and degree of voluntary control over problems reported):

_____
_____
_____
_____
_____
_____
_____

(3) Behavior (include motivation/apathy, impulsivity, violence/aggression, and any other functionally significant or distressing behavioral problem):

_____
_____
_____
_____
_____
_____

(4) Physical (include HEENT, cor/pulm, hepatic/renal, GI/GU, heme/onc, endocrine, musculoskeletal, neurological, etc.):

_____
_____
_____
_____
_____

Neuropsychiatry evaluation and consultation form

(1) General Physical Examination (include at least vital signs, weight, general appearance; others as clinically indicated):

(2) Elemental Neurological Examination:

Cranial Nerves

I (olfactory):

II (optic) – Pupils:

      Fundi:

      visual fields:

III, IV, VI (EOM):

V (trigeminal):

VII (facial):

VIII (auditory/vestibular)

IX, X, XII (tongue, palate, gag):

XI (accessory):

Motor Examination (*tone/resistance to passive manipulation, bulk, strength, abnormal involuntary movements, pronator drift*)

Sensory Examination (*pin-prick, light touch, vibration, proprioception*)

Coordination (*finger-to-nose, fine finger movements, rapid alternating movements, heel-to-shin*)

Gait (*base/station, toe walking, heel walking, tandem gait, turning; assess for Romberg sign*)

Reflexes (*including primitive reflexes*)

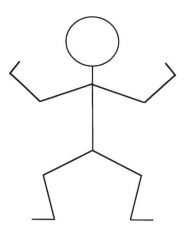

Glabellar   _____

Snout   _____

Palmomental (R)___(L)___

Grasp   _____

Rooting   _____

Suck   _____

Hoffman's   _____

Neuropsychiatry evaluation and consultation form

Mental Status Examination

General Examination (appearance and behavior, speech, thought process, thought content including illusions and hallucinations, delusions, obsessions, recurrent or dominant themes, suicidality, homicidality, current mood and affect)

Cognitive Examination (arousal, attention, language, memory, praxis, recognition, complex cognition; perform at least the Mini-Mental State Examination and record score)

Level of Arousal (circle one):   coma   hypoaroused   alert   hyperaroused

Stimulus level needed to
arouse patient: N/A   conversational verbal   loud verbal   light physical   noxious physical

Patient's response to stimulus:

Attention (general observations during examination):

	Forward	Reverse			Time	Errors
Digit Span	*(check if done correctly)*					
2-9	_____	_____	**Verbal Trials A** (count from 1 to 15)		_____	_____
1-6-3	_____	_____				
9-4-7-2	_____	_____	**Verbal Trials B** (1-a, 2-b, 3-c, etc.)		_____	_____
3-7-9-4-1	_____	_____				
2-5-3-6-9-2	_____	_____				
7-3-8-2-6-5-1	_____	_____	**Registration of Items**		**# Correct**	**Trials**
5-2-9-3-1-4-6-2	_____	_____	(e.g., apple pie, red Cadillac, honesty)			
6-1-9-4-2-8-1-5-3	_____	_____				

_____ _____ _____ _____ _____

Language:
Fluency
Spontaneous:
Writing a sentence:

Word finding problems?	**Y**	**N**
Agrammatisms?	**Y**	**N**
Circumlocutions?	**Y**	**N**
Substitutions?	**Y**	**N**
Other paraphasic errors?	**Y**	**N**

Naming
Objects:
Parts of objects:

Comprehension
General conversation:
Reading a sentence:
Yes/No statements:
True/False statements:
Brief story:

Repetition
Simple statement:
Long statement:
Agrammatic statement ('no ifs, ands, or buts')

Neuropsychiatry evaluation and consultation form

Memory:

	Number Recalled	Verbatim Responses
Spontaneous recall of three objects used in Registration (above):	_____	_____
		_____
		_____
If missing any items, then facilitate recall with semantic cues:	_____	_____
		_____
		_____
If still missing items, then facilitate recall via recognition cues:	_____	_____
		_____
		_____

Orientation (enter responses given):

Time: Day _____ Date _____ Month _____ Year _____ Season _____

Place: Name _____ Floor _____ City _____ County _____ State _____

Situation (reason for coming to clinic): _____

_____

Remote Memory (including historical events, famous dates and people; personal history if verifiable with collateral information):

Praxis:

Limb-kinetic (e.g., pantomime buttoning a shirt; if unable to pantomime, have the patient try to execute this task on a real shirt)

Ideomotor (e.g., pantomime brushing teeth, brushing hair, throwing a ball, hammering wood; if unable to pantomime, give patient real objects with which to try such tasks)

Ideational

Three-step task ("take this piece of paper, fold it in half, and place it on the table"):
Cross-midline task ("cover your left eye with your right hand"):
Three-step cross-midline task with a temporal qualifier ("touch your right hand to your left ear after you point to the ceiling")

Recognition:

	Right	Left
Stereognosis:	_____	_____
Graphesthesia:	_____	_____

Neuropsychiatry evaluation and consultation form

Visuospatial Skills:

Figure Copy:

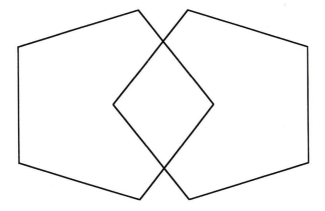

Clock Drawing Task *(use space below):*

Neuropsychiatry evaluation and consultation form

Executive Function: (Note also performance on Trails B and Reverse Digit Span in this section)

	Task	Number	Repeats	Intrusions (non-target)
Word Fluency	Letter 1: _____	_____	_____	_____
	Letter 2: _____	_____	_____	_____
	Letter 3: _____	_____	_____	_____
	Category 1: _____	_____	_____	_____
	Category 2: _____	_____	_____	_____

Alternating Sequences: (use a separate sheet of paper, record results here):

Abstraction:

Similarities

Apple/Orange:
Table/Chair:
Father/Niece:
Sun/Moon
Painting/Poem:
Fly/Tree:

Proverbs

"The grass is always greener on the other side"

"People who live in glass houses shouldn't throw stones"

"Even monkeys fall from trees:

"The tongue is the enemy of the neck"

Fund of Information (current events, historical and geographical information; public figures such as politicians, actors, musicians, and the situations or eras with which they are most closely associated):

Problem Solving:
Mathematical Problems

Real-Life Situations

Judgment:

Insight:

(attach additional sheets used for sentence writing, alternating sequences, serial math problems, etc.)

Neuropsychiatry evaluation and consultation form

Laboratory Evaluation:

Blood Work

Electroencephalography

Neuroimaging

Neuropsychological Testing

Other Pertinent Results

Impression:

_____

_____

_____

_____

_____

_____

_____

_____

_____

_____

_____

_____

_____

_____

Neuropsychiatry evaluation and consultation form

Plan:

_____

_____

_____

_____

_____

_____

_____

_____

_____

_____

_____

_____

_____

_____

Resident Name/Signature Date	Attending Name/Signature Date

Index